Lecture Notes in Statistics-Proceedings 1205

Edited by
P. Bickel
P.J. Diggle
S.E. Fienberg
U. Gather
I. Olkin
S. Zeger

For further volumes:
http://www.springer.com/series/8440

Thomas R. Fleming • Bruce S. Weir

Editors

Proceedings of the Fourth Seattle Symposium in Biostatistics: Clinical Trials

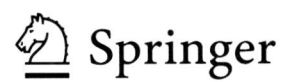 Springer

Editors
Thomas R. Fleming
Department of Biostatistics
University of Washington
Seattle, WA 98195-7232, USA

Bruce S. Weir
Department of Biostatistics
University of Washington
Seattle, WA 98195-7232, USA

ISSN 1869-7240
ISBN 978-1-4614-5244-7   ISBN 978-1-4614-5245-4 (eBook)
DOI 10.1007/978-1-4614-5245-4
Springer New York Heidelberg Dordrecht London

Library of Congress Control Number: 2012952276

Printed on acid-free paper

Springer is part of Springer Science+Business Media (www.springer.com)

Preface

Continuing the tradition, once every half decade, of hosting a major biostatistical meeting, where thought leaders can gather to address scientific issues of current and compelling importance, the organizing committee and sponsors held the Fourth Seattle Symposium on Biostatistics on November 22 and 23, 2010. The topic area for this successful meeting was clinical trials, with focus on the use of biomarkers, issues in multi-regional clinical trials, and identifying and addressing safety signals. The event was sponsored by Axio Research, Bristol-Myers Squibb, Genentech, Novartis and Onyx and was co-sponsored by the UW School of Public Health and the Division of Public Health Sciences at the Fred Hutchinson Cancer Research Center (FHCRC). The symposium featured keynote lectures by Robert O'Neill, Ross Prentice and Robert Temple, as well as invited talks by Jesse Berlin, Christy Chuang-Stein, David DeMets, Bill DuMouchel, Susan Ellenberg, Thomas Fleming, Laurence Freedman, Margaret Pepe, Steve Self, Richard Simon, Bruce Weir, John Whittaker and Janet Wittes. Invited panelists included Jesse Berlin, Bruce Binkowitz, Christy Chuang-Stein, Bill DuMouchel, Susan Ellenberg, Thomas Fleming, Henry Fuchs, Dominic Labriola, Robert O'Neill, Robert Temple and Janet Wittes. There were 200 attendees at the symposium. In addition, more than 100 people attended short courses delivered on November 20 and 21, 2010. At these short courses, "Statistical Design of Sequential Clinical Trials in R" was taught by Scott Emerson and Dan Gillen, "The Use of Genetic Marker Data in Clinical Trials" was taught by Bruce Weir and Patrick Heagerty, "Data Monitoring Committees: A Practical Approach" was taught by Susan Ellenberg, Thomas Fleming and David DeMets, "Statistical Evaluation of Markers for Classification and Prediction" was taught by Margaret Pepe and "Practice Issues in the Conduct and Reporting of Large-Scale Clinical Trials: The Women's Health Initiative Experience" was taught by Garnet Anderson and Andrea LeCroix.

When the UW School of Public Health was formed in 1970, biostatistics as a discipline was very young. In the subsequent 40 years, both the field and the UW Department of Biostatistics have evolved in many exciting ways. The department had only seven faculty when it moved from the School of Medicine to the new School of Public Health and Community Medicine in 1970. The faculty roster currently lists 49 regular and research faculty and 34 adjunct and affiliate faculty. Ed Perrin was the Department Chair in 1970, succeeded by Donovan Thompson, Norman Breslow, Thomas Fleming and presently Bruce Weir. The faculty have been actively involved in methodological and collaborative research in addition to graduate teaching. The choice of *Clinical Trials* as the theme for the *Fourth Seattle Symposium in Biostatistics* was a tribute to the significant contributions made by the UW and FHCRC faculty to this important area of statistical science.

The Symposium Organizing Committee consisted of Susan Ellenberg, Scott Emerson, Nathalie Ezzet, Thomas Fleming (Chair), Henry Fuchs, Lee Hooks, Dominic Labriola, Michael Ostland, Ross Prentice and Bruce Weir. The staff of the Department of Biostatistics, especially Sandra Coke, provided great administrative support to the symposium. The UW School of Public Health Dean Howard Frumkin, the Department Chair Bruce Weir and the Organizing Committee Chair Thomas Fleming delivered the opening remarks. The scientific sessions were chaired by Bruce Weir, Scott Emerson, Thomas Fleming, Lee Hooks, Henry Fuchs, Michael Ostland, Susan Ellenberg, Nathalie Ezzet and Dominic Labriola. We are grateful to the aforementioned people as well as all the speakers and participants for making the symposium a great success.

This volume contains most of the papers presented at the symposium, as well as some of the science presented at the short courses. These papers encompass recent methodological advances on several important topics, summaries of the state of the art of methodology in key areas of clinical trials, as well as innovative applications of the existing theory and methods. This collection serves as a reference for those working in several key areas of clinical trials.

Each of the 12 papers in this volume was referred by two or three peer reviewers, and their comments were incorporated by the authors into the final versions of the papers. The referees are listed at the end of this book. We are indebted to them for their time and efforts. We also appreciate the guidance and assistance by Marc Springer of Springer-Verlag.

Contents

Part IV Safety

Part V Special Topics

Part I
Biomarkers: Role in the Design and Interpretation of Clinical Trials

The Role and Potential of Surrogate Outcomes in Clinical Trials: Have We Made Any Progress in the Past Decade?

David L. DeMets

Abstract Randomized clinical trials are the standard method for evaluating new interventions or comparing existing ones. Trials which use clinical outcomes as the primary outcome can be large, require lengthy follow-up, and can be expensive. For these reasons, researchers have sought to use intermediate outcomes such as biomarkers as a substitute or surrogate for the clinical outcome. Over a decade ago, this practice had become common. Fleming and DeMets (Ann Intern Med 125:605–613, 1996) reported many cases where the use of a biomarker as a surrogate outcome failed to reliably assess the effect of the intervention, in some cases missing harmful effects including mortality. Recently, the Institute of Medicine (IOM) reviewed the state of the art and came to similar conclusions that biomarkers have often proved to be unreliable as a surrogate [Committee on Qualifications of Biomarkers and Surrogate Endpoints in Chronic Disease, Michael C, Ball J (eds) (2010) Evaluation of biomarkers and surrogate endpoints in chronic disease. National Academies Press, Washington]. They proposed that biomarkers must meet certain criteria including analytic validity, strong correlation with the clinical outcome and the ability to capture the full effects of the intervention. The use of a biomarker as a surrogate must be done so in the context of its intended use, and done so with great caution. While the IOM report further clarifies the necessary requirements of a potential biomarker as a surrogate, the report still recommends caution in using surrogate outcomes in final phases of intervention evaluation as did Fleming and DeMets (Ann Intern Med 125:605–613, 2004).

D.L. DeMets (✉)
Department of Biostatistics & Medical Informatics, University of Wisconsin-Madison,
610 Walnut Street, Madison, WI, 53726 USA
e-mail: demets@biostat.wisc.edu

T.R. Fleming and B.S. Weir (eds.), *Proceedings of the Fourth Seattle Symposium in Biostatistics: Clinical Trials*, Lecture Notes in Statistics 1205, DOI 10.1007/978-1-4614-5245-4_1, © Springer Science+Business Media New York 2013

1 Introduction

Clinical trials have been the primary method for evaluating new interventions or strategies for disease diagnosis, prevention, and treatment over the past four decades. These interventions may be drugs, biologics, devices, procedures, and dietary or behavioral modifications. While the ultimate test of a new intervention would be the modification of a clinically important outcome, trials with such a design can be large, lengthy, and costly. Attempts to improve trial efficiency have included a substitute outcome for the clinically important outcome that may be easier, cheaper, or quicker to measure and may also result in a smaller trial. The intermediate outcomes or biomarkers used for this purpose are often referred to as surrogate outcomes, defined as a biomarker that is intended to be used as a substitute for a clinical outcome in evaluating a new intervention [1].

Examples of such intermediate markers that have been used previously in the evaluation of new interventions are blood pressure and cholesterol levels as a substitute for cardiovascular events such as death or nonfatal myocardial infarction. While the use of surrogate outcomes has become common in recent years, in 1996 Fleming and DeMets reviewed the experience at that point as to whether or not the use of biomarkers as surrogates in clinical trials had proven to be reliable [1]. Their conclusion was that there were many examples in several disciplines where the use of biomarkers as surrogate outcomes had been misleading with regard to benefit and risk for new interventions. Recently, the Institute of Medicine (IOM) reviewed the same subject in the context of use of biomarkers as surrogates for nutritional intervention claims and came to similar conclusions [2]. In addition, the IOM report presents a structure for the evaluation of a biomarker for potential use as a surrogate outcome. This paper will provide a brief overview of the requirements for a biomarker to be a valid surrogate with some early and more recent examples of biomarkers not being reliable as surrogates.

2 Basic Requirements for a Potential Surrogate

In 2010, the Institute of Medicine (IOM) of the National Academies issued a report "Evaluation of Biomarkers and Surrogate Endpoints in Chronic Disease" which reviewed the requirements for a potential biomarker to be used as a surrogate end point [2]. While the initial stimulus for this evaluation was for nutritional biomarkers as a surrogate for health claims, the IOM report provided a general structure for evaluation of any biomarker for such use. Biomarkers measure some biological process and include, for example, not only physiological and blood measurements but also genetic or genomic signatures. Biomarkers can be used to describe risk, risk exposure, or intermediate response to an intervention or as surrogates or substitutes for clinical outcomes in evaluating a new intervention. The report argues that the Food and Drug Administration (FDA) and other regulatory agencies should use the same degree of scientific rigor across all categories of products including drugs,

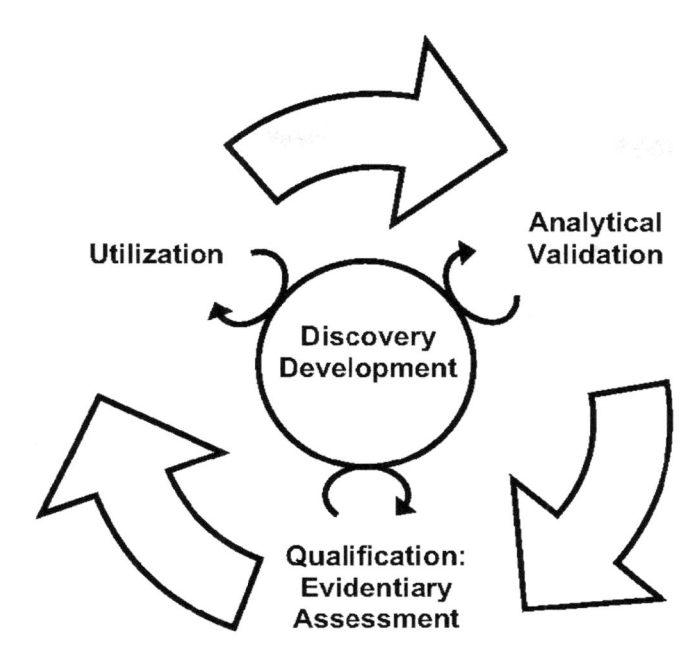

Fig. 1 The steps of the evaluation framework are interdependent. While a validated test is required before qualification and utilization can be completed, biomarker uses inform test development, and the evidence suggests possible biomarker uses. In addition, the circle in the center signifies ongoing processes that should continually inform each step in the biomarker evaluation process

biologics, devices, foods, and supplements. The evaluation process for a biomarker to be a surrogate should have three steps (1) analytical validation, (2) qualification, and (3) utilization (Fig. 1).

For analytic validation, the IOM report defined this as an assessment of the measurement assay and performance [2]. They recommended that a biomarker must be evaluated for its limit of detection, limit of quantification, reliability, and reproducibility across different laboratories. In addition, to be a surrogate outcome, a biomarker must have adequate sensitivity and specificity. Sources of variability in the biomarker measurement must be understood and controlled to the extent possible through good clinical laboratory and quality control practices. While similar to routine laboratory validation, according to the IOM report, there is still no uniform set of criterion for biomarker assay validation [2].

The second step of qualification of a biomarker as a surrogate has two parts (1) demonstrating a correlation between the biomarker and the true clinical outcome and (2) demonstrating that the total clinical impact of the intervention is captured by the biomarker. Prentice [3] described in detail these statistical criteria. The first requirement is easy to understand but a common misconception is that if a biomarker is highly correlated with a true clinical outcome, it can be used as a surrogate. However, as stated by Fleming and DeMets, "a correlate does not make a surrogate" [1]. The second criterion is a necessary and much stronger condition than just correlation. Figure 2 illustrates the simple conception of a biomarker as a surrogate. The disease process can be measured by a biomarker which is in the causal pathway to the true clinical outcome. Correlation between the biomarker and the clinical outcome would be very high in this scenario. If this were the case, then any intervention on the disease process which modified the biomarker would capture the clinical effect. However, biology is almost surely more complicated than this simple pathway. Figure 3 depicts three alternative and more complicated pathways. These are only a sample of potential pathways. In Fig. 3, the biomarker would be correlated to some degree with the clinical outcome in all cases. However, there is not a single or direct pathway between the biomarker and the clinical outcome. For example, in case A, the biomarker is not at all in the causal pathway but affected simultaneously with the clinical outcome by the disease process, thus producing a high correlation that has no associated causation. Any intervention could have a profound effect on the biomarker but have absolutely no impact on the clinical outcome. In case B, the biomarker is in the causal pathway but there is at least one other pathway where the biomarker plays no role. An intervention might affect the biomarker and have some degree of impact on the clinical outcome, but it could be overwhelmed by the other pathway. For example, the intervention might have the desired effect on the biomarker but have a negative or harmful effect through the other pathway that would not be identified if only the biomarker was measured. In case C, an intervention might have no effect on the biomarker but still have a direct effect through another pathway on the clinical outcome. In this case, a partially effective intervention might be totally missed. A great deal of statistical research has been focused on this issue of what criteria is adequate for a biomarker to be a clinical surrogate but the criteria set forth by Prentice captures the essence of the challenge [4–17]. That is, the biomarker must be highly correlated with the clinically relevant outcome and must capture all, or nearly all, of the effect of the intervention on the clinical outcome. While these criteria are challenging to meet, failure to meet those requirements can lead to interventions becoming part of clinical practice and yet have no or even harmful effects as illustrated by examples described below.

Even if Fig. 2 were the correct pathway, the effect of the intervention seen in the biomarker could be misleading. The effect could be underestimated if there is considerable noise or measurement error in the biomarker. Alternatively, the effect could be overestimated if the effect on the biomarker is of sufficient size to produce a meaningful clinical effect.

The third step in the IOM recommendation is to take into consideration the intended use of the biomarker as a surrogate. For example, a biomarker might be suitable for identifying disease risk without any reference to intervention effect. That is, the correlation of the biomarker with the clinical outcome might be sufficiently high to have utility in describing risk. A biomarker might also be a useful intermediate or surrogate in the drug or device development process. For example, in developing a new drug, device, or intervention to reduce cardiovascular risk, assessing the impact on reducing blood pressure might be useful to rule out interventions which do not have this intended effect. However, as indicated above, other non-intended affects might not be captured by total reliance on this biomarker.

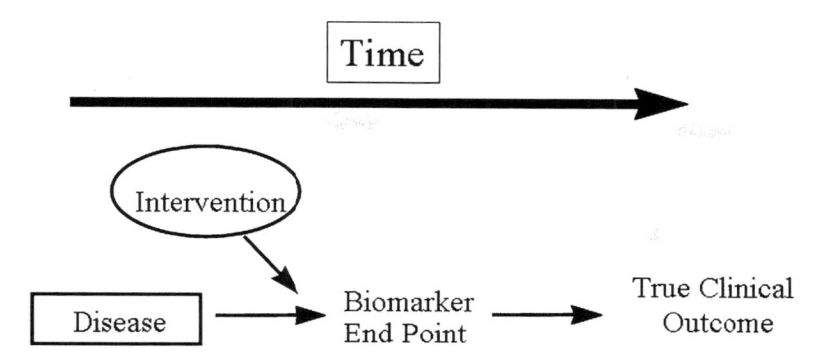

Fig. 2 Common misconception of a causal pathway and a biomarker. The setting that provides the greatest potential for the surrogate endpoint to be valid. Reprinted from Ann Intern Med 1996; 125:605–613

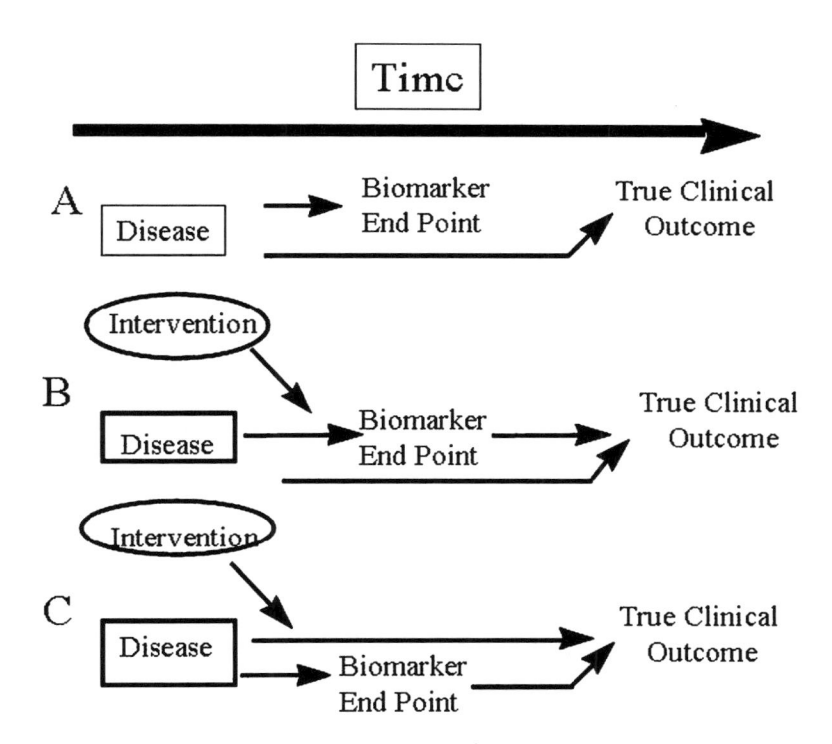

Fig. 3 Possible causal pathways relative to a biomarker. Reasons for failure of biomarker end points: (A) The biomarker is not in the causal pathway of the disease process; (B) Of several causal pathways of disease, the intervention affects only the pathway mediated through the biomarker; (C) The biomarker is not the pathway of the intervention's effect or is insensitive to its effect

3 Some Earlier Examples

While there are examples of a biomarker being successful in risk assessment or intervention development, there are many examples of failures when a biomarker was relied on as a valid surrogate. Unfortunately, we may not always have the complete clinical outcome data to assess whether the biomarker was indeed a valid surrogate. In addition, an example where the biomarker captures the effect for one specific intervention does not guarantee that it will be reliable for the next intervention of a different class or type, or even a variation within the same class. We shall briefly summarize a few of the examples described by Fleming and DeMets [1] and by the IOM report [2]. What is so remarkable is that these cases of biomarker failure can be found across a wide variety of disease areas, across a wide variety of interventions and even within a class of interventions where one biomarker success did not translate into other interventions even of the same class.

Perhaps one of the most dramatic and important examples of a biomarker failure as a surrogate outcome comes from the field of cardiology and the use of arrhythmia suppressing drugs to reduce death from cardiovascular complications. Observational data had shown that ventricular arrhythmias were shown to have as much as a four-fold increase in cardiovascular death [18, 19]. This observation led to the arrhythmia suppression hypothesis that reducing cardiac arrhythmias would reduce sudden death. Drugs were developed to suppress these arrhythmias and approved by the FDA for use in high-risk patients. The assumption was that, in general, suppressing these arrhythmias would result in a reduction of cardiovascular death and in fact some drugs with this arrhythmia suppressing effect began to be used beyond just the highest risk patients. That is, many clinicians practiced as if biomarker arrhythmia suppression would be an adequate surrogate for survival. The Cardiac Arrhythmia Suppression Trial (CAST) was a double-blind placebo-controlled trial of three such drugs (encainide, flecainide, and moricizine) to test the hypothesis that these drugs would reduce the risk of cardiovascular death in patients with a recent myocardial infarction and at least 10 premature ventricular beats per minute [18]. Each drug had a matching placebo. In order to be eligible, a patient had to have a suppressible arrhythmia as determined in a run-in phase. Initially, the data monitoring committee was blinded to drug assignment. The moricizine arm got a late start so the data for the other two arms were monitored initially by a data monitoring committee blinded to treatment assignment. Early trends in mortality were assumed to be beneficial, as expected, based on clinical practice and a belief that arrhythmia suppression was a valid surrogate. When these early trends became stronger, the data monitoring committee was unblinded and startled to learn that the trends were contrary to expectation. At the time the data monitoring committee recommended trial termination, as 56 deaths were observed on the two drug arms compared to 22 in the matching placebo arm. When the follow-up data for these randomized patients was completed, there were 63 deaths on the two drug arms compared to 26 in the placebo arm [19]. Similarly, there were 43 sudden deaths on drugs and 16 on placebo. Later, when the results for the moricizine arm became available, this arm was terminated as well with an increased risk [20]. In this third arm, the brief run-in period was modified after the results of the other two drugs arms became available to be randomized to either moricizine or placebo. If patient's arrhythmias were suppressed during the short run-in period, they were randomized to drug or placebo as before. Even exposure to moricizine during the run-in period demonstrated a strong trend for increased risk compared to the placebo. This case has several important lessons. First, the observational data was convincing about arrhythmia suppression as a surrogate and the biology seemed plausible. Assumptions were made about the clinical effect. A large number of patients were exposed to these very harmful drugs. Furthermore, the second half of CAST demonstrated that even a short exposure to moricizine was risky. This suggests that clinicians in their normal practice could not detect this increased risk in a group of patients who were already at risk due to a prior heart attack. Before these drugs were used routinely in clinical practice, the definitive test using clinical outcomes, in retrospect, should have been done.

While the lessons from CAST are dramatic, this is not a unique example in cardiology for this particular patient diagnosis. Other drugs such as quinidine and lidocaine with known arrhythmia controlling activity were shown to have increased mortality risk [21–23].

4   Lipid-Lowering Interventions

The Framingham Heart Study identified that high cholesterol levels including low density lipids (LDL) were associated with increased cardiovascular mortality [24]. Strategies to lower lipid values were identified including drug interventions such as niacin and clofibrate. The Coronary Drug Project (CDP) was a multi-armed randomized placebo-controlled trial of these two drugs as well as high and low doses of estrogen, also known to reduce cholesterol levels, to test the lipid lowering hypothesis [25]. The CDP was a trial with a planned 7 years of follow-up with death and death from coronary heart disease as the primary outcomes. The two estrogen arms were terminated early with increased cardiovascular risk probably due to increased clotting risk. Neither the niacin or clofibrate arm reduced total mortality although there was a favorable trend for niacin [25]. Several other lipid-lowering trials combined in a meta-analysis did not show a reduction in total mortality but actually had an increase in noncardiovascular death which offset a reduction in cardiovascular death [26]. Despite the consistent correlation between high cholesterol levels and increased risk, this reduction of serum lipid values was not an adequate biomarker to be used as a valid surrogate.

While several interventions existed which reduce cholesterol, the clinical benefit was not demonstrated until the Scandinavian Simvastatin Survival Study (4S) was done [27]. The multicenter randomized double-blind placebo-controlled trial evaluated one of the statins and observed a 25% reduction in cholesterol with a 30% reduction in total mortality. This trial has had a major impact on clinical practice. However, just because one statin had a beneficial effect does not mean that cholesterol lowering with a statin qualifies that as a surrogate. One statin trial (Baycol) was terminated early with an increase in mortality [28]. In another study, the trial ILLUMINATE evaluated a member of a new class of drugs, torcetrapib, that decreased LDL cholesterol (the bad cholesterol) and increased HDL cholesterol (the good cholesterol) but was terminated early because of an increase in death and cardiac events [29].

Several large epidemiological studies demonstrated a strong correlation between hormone replacement treatment (HRT) usage, either estrogen or estrogen-progestin supplementation, and a decreased risk in cardiovascular risk [30, 31]. HRT is known to reduce cholesterol levels and reduce bone density loss in post-menopausal women. Estrogen alone is used for women with a hysterectomy and an estrogen–progestin combination for women with an intact uterus. HRT supplementation became one of the most widely prescribed medicines, assuming that cholesterol reduction was a surrogate for cardiovascular risk. The Women's Health Initiative (WHI) was a factorial trial evaluating the impact of low-fat diets, hormone replacement therapy (HRT), and calcium supplementation [32, 33]. The HRT component was actually two trials, one comparing estrogen and placebo in women without a uterus and the other comparing estrogen–progestin with placebo in women with an intact uterus, with clinical outcomes of cardiovascular death or cardiovascular events such as nonfatal heart attack or nonfatal stroke. As expected, HRT lowered LDL cholesterol and reduced bone density loss with an accompanying reduction in major fractures. However, both trials were terminated early with increased cardiovascular risk, with clotting problems being the major issue. For the estrogen–progestin arms, there was also an increase in cases of uterine cancer. These results clearly refuted the assumption that cholesterol reduction with HRT was an adequate surrogate for cardiovascular risk. Unfortunately, millions of women were treated with HRT under the false assumption of cardiovascular benefit. Interestingly, three decades earlier, men given low and high doses of estrogen also experienced increased risk due to clotting problems even though LDL was lowered [34]. This early CDP lesson on the failure of cholesterol reduction as a surrogate was missed in later research such as in design of the WHI. While the intervention effect of lowering LDL was observed, the clotting problem was not anticipated for women taking HRT (Fig. 4).

As described by Fleming and DeMets [1], there are many other examples in cardiology involving biomarkers which failed to be reliable surrogates for cardiovascular risk. These include blood pressure lowering [35–39] for cardiovascular morbidity and exercise tolerance for congestive heart failure [40–42]. Cardiology has several classic examples of biomarker failure to be a surrogate but other disciplines have such examples as well.

Cancer is the second leading cause of mortality with an associate morbidity. Cancer treatment trials have often used the biomarker tumor shrinkage as a surrogate for clinical response in drug development, for example, in breast cancer, colon cancer, and lung cancer [43]. Responses are often categorized as a complete response (no remaining tumor visible), partial response (a 50% reduction in tumor volume), no change or progression. Tumor volume has an initial challenge of

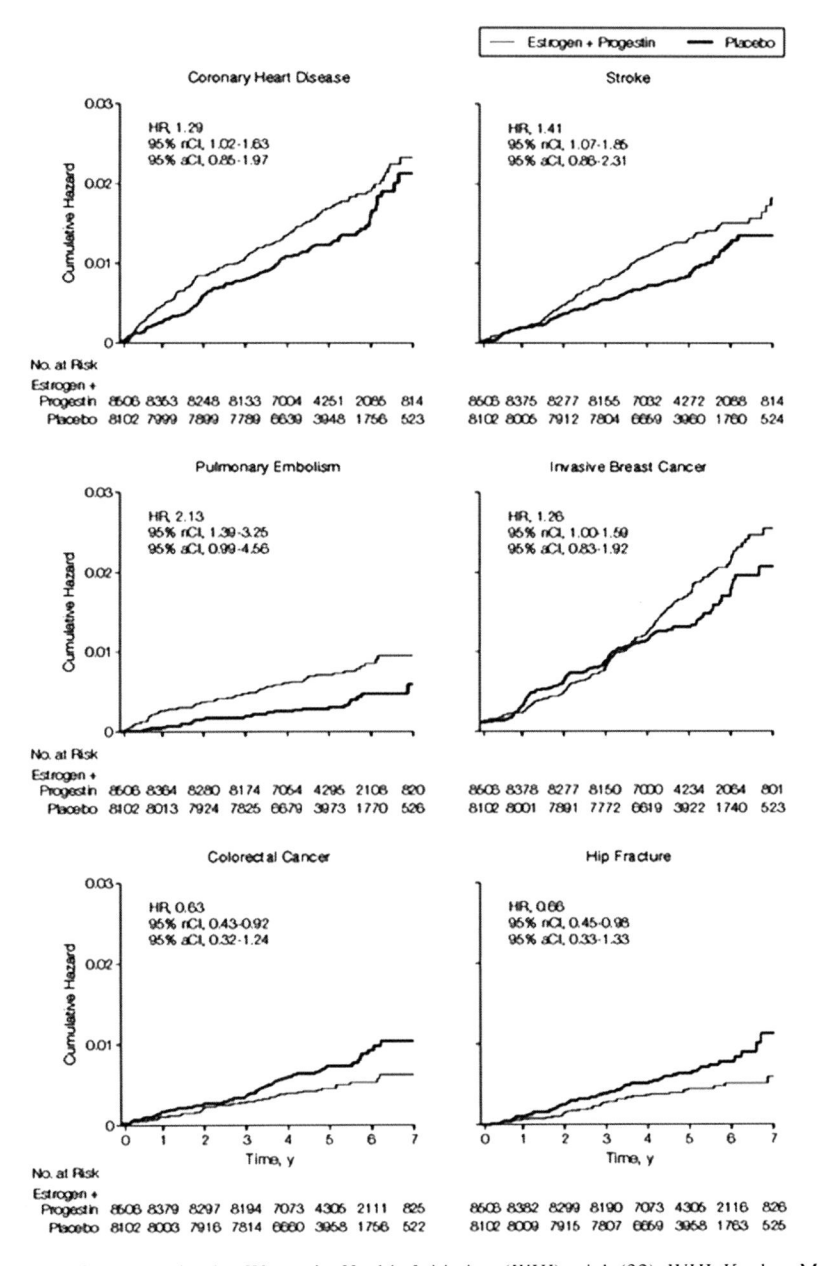

Fig. 4 (a) Outcomes in the Women's Health Initiative (*WHI*) trial (32) WHI Kaplan–Meier estimates of cumulative hazards for selected clinical outcomes

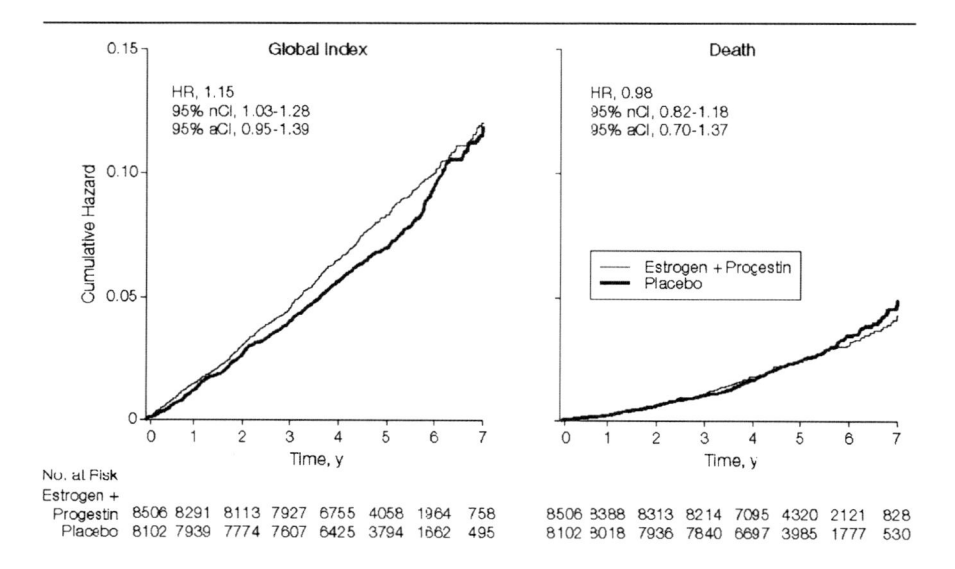

Fig. 4 (b) WHI Kaplan–Meier estimates of cumulative hazards for Global Index and Death. HR = hazard ratio; nCI = nominal confidence interval; aCI = adjusted confidence interval. JAMA 2002; 288(3):321–333

validation since measurement of tumor volume is highly variable depending on methodology. Tumor response has been widely used for drug development and early phase trials in cancer [44]. In addition, tumor volume reduction has not always been a reliable biomarker for survival [6, 45, 46]. Tumor response was also used as a surrogate for approval of cancer therapy drugs in the 1970s but later the FDA requested that a clinical survival benefit or quality of life benefit be demonstrated as well. However, with the urgency of new and effective cancer treatments, in 1996 the FDA utilized the accelerated approval process using surrogate outcomes such as progression-free survival, meaning survival with no tumor recurrence or progression [46, 47]. The assumption was that post-approval trials demonstrating a survival benefit would follow but this has not happened consistently.

A specific cancer example is the use of 5-fluorouracil plus leucovorin compared to 5-fluorouracil alone in colon cancer. The combination showed a complete plus partial response rate of 23% compared to 5-fluorouracil alone of 11%. Yet, this difference in tumor response biomarker provided no improvement in survival. These results came from a meta-analysis of over 1400 patients [48]. These disappointing results could be due to the poor effect of the combination or that the combination has other unintended adverse effects.

Other important diseases such as AIDS, osteoporosis, and infectious diseases also provide excellent examples of the failure of biomarkers [1]. Given that Fleming and DeMets discussed these problems in 1996, it is natural to ask if any progress in successful use of biomarkers as valid surrogates has been observed since. The IOM report [2] is a more recent review of this question.

5 Other Recent Examples

As discussed above, cancer is the second leading cause of mortality. Nutritional researchers observed that individuals with low levels of beta-carotene intake had a higher risk for lung cancer [49]. Beta-carotene is a plant carotenoid which is partially converted into vitamin A which is an important nutrient for many functions, including vision, gene expression, growth, and immune function. These observations were based on measures of dietary intake but were confirmed by blood level measurements. On the basis of the epidemiologic observations, the notion of increasing intake levels of beta-carotene emerged. Qualification of the biomarker, serum beta-carotene, as a surrogate outcome is itself a challenge and not given much attention[2]. Three large prevention trials were launched to test the hypothesis that increasing levels of serum beta-carotene would result in reduced risk of cancer, lung cancer in particular. [50–52].

The Alpha Tocopherol Beta-Carotene (ATBC) trial began in 1985, randomized over 29,000 Finnish smokers in a factorial trial, alpha tocopherol vs. placebo and bet-carotene vs. placebo [50]. Subjects were followed for 5–8 years using the Finnish cancer registry. Results for the beta-carotene vs. placebo component demonstrated a statistically significant increase in lung cancer incidence and lung cancer mortality for those patients receiving a beta-carotene containing study drug. While this result was unexpected, it was essentially replicated by a trial conducted in the USA, referred to as CARET [51]. CARET was a randomized placebo controlled trial of over 18,000 smokers or workers exposed to asbestos. Lung cancer mortality and coronary heart disease mortality were significantly higher for those participants on beta-carotene compared to the control arm. The relative risk for developing lung cancer was 1.28 (1.04–1.57) and 1.46 (1.07–2.0) for lung cancer death. Given that these results paralleled the ATBC results, CARET was terminated early. A third trial, the Physicians Health Study-I (PHS-I) was a randomized double-blind factorial trial of beta-carotene and aspirin compared to a matching placebo [52]. Participants were US male physicians who were largely nonsmokers. Contrary to the two other trials of smokers or workers exposed to asbestos, the PHS-I trial showed neither a benefit nor a harm with a relative risk of 0.98. In addition, there were no trends for benefit or harm in total mortality or cardiovascular events. More recently, a Women's Antioxidant Cardiovascular Study (WACS) also used a randomized factorial trial to evaluate beta-carotene, vitamin C, or vitamin E compared to a placebo [53]. The results indicated no benefit or harm for beta-carotene with a relative risk of 1.02. Another trial in women, the Women's Health Study (WHS) found no beneficial or harmful effects of beta-carotene supplementation for cancer or cardiovascular disease [54]. The first two trials involve participants who were at higher risk for lung cancer while the latter three trials involved participants at lower risk. For three of the trials [50–52], the placebo arm confirmed the observation that low serum beta-carotene was associated with higher risk of lung cancer, despite either harmful or no effects from increasing those levels when compared to a placebo arm. Clearly, serum beta-carotene as a useful biomarker for risk failed as a surrogate for clinically meaningful outcomes.

Cardiology provides two more recent examples of biomarkers, C-reactive protein (CRP) and troponin, neither of which qualified as a surrogate [2] for cardiovascular outcomes. Although mortality from heart disease has fallen, it remains the leading cause of death in the USA so research for more prevention and intervention continues. Beyond the known risk factors of lipids, blood pressure, diabetes and obesity, inflammation is now considered to have an impact on the progression of cardiovascular disease [55]. One inflammation biomarker is CRP which is low in normal individuals but increases with acute episodes such as a heart attack. CRP has some predictive ability for future coronary events. There are now standardized low-cost assays for CRP that meet criteria for analytical validation.

While CRP is correlated with cardiovascular events and thus can be used as a predictor of risk, it is not known whether it is in the causal pathway. That is, even if CRP is just tracking along with other unknown biomarkers that are on the causal pathway, it will still correlate with the clinical outcome and thus be useful for risk assessment. However, it will not be useful to monitor change in CRP since it is not on the causal pathway. Thus this biomarker of inflammation does not qualify as a surrogate outcome without further studies. One major randomized placebo-controlled trial, JUPITER, evaluated the effect of a statin, rosuvastatin, in preventing cardiovascular events in individuals with high CRP but lower or moderate values of LDL cholesterol. JUPITER showed a reduction in new cardiovascular events using this particular statin [56]. However, further analyses showed that LDL reductions and CRP reductions were weakly correlated. Thus, JUPITER was not able to demonstrate that CRP is in the causal pathway and thus not a validated surrogate. However, it may have utility as a predictor of cardiovascular risk and be used in that manner [2].

Troponin is another biomarker of interest. In fact, troponin is used as a biomarker in the current definition of a myocardial infarction or heart attack but in combination with other factors such as changes in electrocardiograms and myocardial enzyme measurements [57–59]. It is a protein that is involved with the function of both cardiac and skeletal muscle function. Subunits of troponin can be defined which are cardiac muscle specific. High levels of troponin do not automatically suggest an acute myocardial event, so it is not in the primary causal pathway. However, it is the preferred biomarker included in the definition of a heart attack and has met accepted standards of good clinical laboratory measurement. Still, the analytic validation is not complete [2]. Clinical data indicate that high levels of troponin indicate a higher risk of mortality. Thus, it passes the first requirement for surrogate qualification. However, to date there is limited evidence that suggests reducing troponin levels would improve mortality risk.

Finally, we examine the use of epogen in kidney failure patients to maintain hematocrit levels. Clinicians believe that it is important to treat anemia to maintain an adequate hematocrit level. A class of erythropoietin-stimulating agents was developed to increase hematocrit levels. One such drug, epogen, was evaluated in a randomized placebo clinical trial called TREAT (Trial to Reduce cardiovascular Events with Aranesp Therapy), which was a randomized placebo-controlled clinical trial, epogen vs. placebo plus standard of care, in type 2 diabetes patients with kidney failure [60]. This drug was known to significantly improve hematocrit levels, considered to be a biomarker for type 2 diabetes risk and a surrogate for clinical outcome. Many investigators believed that TREAT was even unethical to start since the evidence that epogen increased hematocrit was established, and thus presumed to produce a resulting clinical benefit, breaking their equipoise between epogen and placebo[60]. Slightly over two thousand patients were randomized to each intervention. Compliance to the study medication was excellent and the resulting hemoglobin levels were statistically and clinically higher on the epogen-treated patients compared to placebo treated. Nevertheless, the composite endpoint of death, nonfatal heart attack, nonfatal stroke, heart failure, and myocardial ischemia had a hazard ratio of 1.05 (0.94–1.17), in favor of placebo. The outcome of end-stage renal disease or death had a hazard ratio of 1.06 (0.95–1.19), similar to the composite outcome. There was a significant difference in fatal and nonfatal stroke frequency, with a hazard ratio of 1.92 (1.38–2.68, $P < 0.001$) in favor of placebo. Thus, the biomarker of hemoglobin levels would not qualify as a surrogate since this trial demonstrated a dramatic effect on hemoglobin level increase with no effect on clinical outcomes, but with a significant adverse effect in fatal and nonfatal stroke. Obviously, not all of the clinical effect of epogen was captured by simply measuring hematocrit.

In early AIDS research, measures of immune response such as CD4 cell counts were used as biomarkers with the hope of being a valid surrogate. AIDS is a disease that compromises the body's immune system. One therapeutic strategy is to help the immune system recover as measured by CD4 cell counts. Low CD4 cell count was considered a predictor of mortality and morbidity in AIDS patients. Fleming and DeMets [1] report several examples where improved or positive changes in CD4 cell count did not convey clinical benefit in either mortality or morbidity. Recently, another study group has reported similar results [61]. Two separate trials evaluating two cohorts defined by their baseline CD4 counts compared interleukin-2 plus antiretroviral therapy with antiretroviral therapy alone. Despite substantial and sustained elevations of CD4 count over several years, there was no significant clinical benefit in either study.

6 Summary

The need for randomized clinical trials to evaluate new interventions will continue to be the best and primary methodology. As a result, interest in efficient trial designs will include the potential use of biomarkers as a surrogate for clinical outcomes. As described, besides being able to measure the biomarker adequately, there are two critical requirements before it can be relied on completely. Those requirements are that a reasonably strong correlation exists between the biomarker and the clinical outcome, and reasonable certainty that the biomarker is capturing all of the effects of the intervention including harmful effects. Ideally, there should be perfect correlation and 100% certainty. These stringent conditions are rarely met.

How strong the correlation must be and how certain we are about capturing all of the effects will depend on the context of the intended use. That is the point of the IOM's third criterion [2]. Thus, no specific correlation and level of certainty can be specified without considering the context of intended use. With alarming frequency, reliance on a biomarker as a surrogate for clinical outcomes has resulted in numerous interventions being utilized without appreciation of other effects, especially harmful effects. Only later, when subsequent trials were conducted were the harmful effects discovered. Biomarkers will, however, continue to play a critical role in the development of new drugs, devices, and other interventions. Some biomarkers may also be useful in identifying patient risk. However, for now the recent IOM report [2] is consistent with the recommendations of Fleming and DeMets [1] made a decade earlier that biomarkers should not be relied upon as a surrogate for clinically relevant outcomes in Phase III clinical trials.

References

1. Fleming TR, DeMets DL (1996) Surrogate endpoints in clinical trials: are we being mislead? Ann Intern Med 125:605–613
2. Committee on Qualifications of Biomarkers and Surrogate Endpoints in Chronic Disease, Michael C, Ball J (eds) (2010) Evaluation of biomarkers and surrogate endpoints in chronic disease. National Academies Press, Washington
3. Prentice RL (1989) Surrogate endpoints in clinical trials: definition and operational criteria. Stat Med 8:431–440
4. Fleming TR (1992) Evaluating therapeutic interventions: some issues and experiences (with discussion and rejoinder). Stat Sci 7:428–456
5. Fleming TR (1990) Evaluation of active control trials in AIDS. J Acquir Immun Defic Syndr 3(Suppl 2):S82–S87
6. Johnson JR, Temple R (1985) Food and Drug Administration requirements for approval of new anticancer drugs. Cancer Treat Rep 69:1155–1159
7. Ellenberg SS, Hamilton JM (1989) Surrogate endpoints in clinical trials: cancer. Stat Med 8:405–413
8. Fleming TR, Prentice RL, Pepe MS, Glidden D (1994) Surrogate and auxiliary endpoints in clinical trials, with potential applications in cancer and AIDS research. Stat Med 3:955–968
9. Herson J (1989) The use of surrogate endpoints in clinical trials. Stat Med 8:403–404
10. Kosorok MR, Fleming TR (1993) Using surrogate failure time data to increase cost effectiveness in clinical trials. Biometrika 80:823–833
11. Machado SG, Gail MH, Ellengerg SS (1990) On the use of laboratory markers as surrogates for clinical endpoints in the evaluation of treatment for HIV infection. J Acquir Immune Defic Syndr 3:1065–1073
12. Pepe MS, Reilly M, Fleming TR (1994) Auxiliary outcome data and the mean score method. J Stat Plan Inference 42:137–160
13. Wittes J, Lakatos E, Probstfield J (1989) Surrogate endpoints in clinical trials: cardiovascular diseases. Stat Med 8:415–425
14. Ellenberg SS (1991) Surrogate end points in clinical trials [Editorial]. BMJ 302:63–64
15. Fleming TR (1994) Surrogate markers in AIDS and cancer trials. Stat Med 13:1423–1435
16. Lagakos SW, Hoth DF (1992) Surrogate markers in AIDS: where are we? Ann Intern Med 116:599–601
17. Boissel JP, Collet JP, Moleur P, Haugh M (1992) Surrogate endpoints: a basis for a rationale approach. Eur J Clin Pharmacol 43:235–244

18. The Cardiac Arrhythmia Suppression Trial (CAST) Investigators (1989) Preliminary report: effect of encainide and flecainide on mortality in a randomized trial of arrhythmia suppression after myocardial infarction. N Engl J Med 321:406–412
19. Echt DS, Liebson PR, Mitchell LB, Peters RW, Obias-Manno D, Barker AH et al (1991) Mortality and morbidity in patients receiving encainide, flecainide, or placebo. The Cardiac Arrhythmia Suppression Trial. N Engl J Med 324:781–788
20. The Cardiac Arrhythmia Suppression Trial Investigators (1992) Effect of the antiarrhythmic agent moricizine on survival after myocardial infarction. N Engl J Med 327:227–233
21. Coplen SE, Antman EM, Berlin JA, Hewitt P, Chalmers TC (1990) Efficacy and safety of quinidine therapy for maintenance of sinus rhythm after cardioversion. A meta-analysis of randomized control trials. Circulation 82:1106–1116
22. Hine LK, Laird N, Hewitt P, Chalmers TC (1989) Meta-analytic evidence against prophylactic use of lidocaine in acute myocardial infarction. Arch Intern Med 149:2694–2698
23. MacMahon S, Collins R, Peto R, Koster RW, Yusuf S (1988) Effects of prophylactic lidocaine in suspected acute myocardial infarction. An overview of results from the randomized, controlled trials. JAMA 260:1910–1916
24. Rossouw JE, Lewis B, Rifkind BM (1990) The value of lowering cholesterol after myocardial infarction. N Engl J Med 323:1112–1119
25. The Coronary Drug Project Research Group (1975) Clofibrate and niacin in coronary heart disease. JAMA 231:360–381
26. Gordon DJ (1994) Cholesterol lowering and total mortality. In: Rifkind BM (ed) Contemporary issues in cholesterol lowering: clinical and population aspects. Marcel Dekker, New York
27. (1994) Randomised trial of cholesterol lower in 4444 patients with coronary heart disease: the Scandinavian Simvastatin Survival Study (4S). Lancet 344:1383–1389
28. Fogoros RN (2001) The Baycol recall, what it means, Heart Health Center, About.com, Aug 13, 2001
29. Barter PJ, Caulfield M, Eriksson M, Grundy SM, Kastelein JJ, Komajda M, Lopez-Sendon J, Mosca L, Tardiff JC, Waters DD, Shear CL, Revkin JH, Buhr KA, Fisher MR, Tall AR, Brewer B, ILLUMINATE Investigators (2007) Effects of torcetrapib in patients at high risk for coronary events. N Engl J Med 357:2109–2122
30. Stampfer M, Colditz G (1991) Estrogen replacement therapy and coronary heart disease, a quantitative assessment of the epidemiological evidence. Prev Med 20:47–63
31. Grady D, Rueben SB, Pettiti DB et al (1992) Hormone therapy to prevent heart disease and prolong life in postmenopausal women. Ann Int Med 117:1102–1109
32. Writing Group for the Women's Health Initiative Investigators (2002) Risks and benefits of estrogen plus progestin in healthy postmenopausal women. Principal results from the Women's Health Initiative randomized controlled trial. JAMA 288(3):321–333
33. Women's Health Initiative Investigators Steering Committee (2004) Effects of conjugated equine estrogen in postmenopausal women with a hysterectomy: the Women's Health Initiative randomized clinical trial. JAMA 291:1701–1712
34. Coronary Drug Project Research Group (1973) The Coronary Drug Project: Findings leading to discontinuation of the 2.5-mg/day estrogen group. JAMA 226:652–657
35. Collins R, Peto R, MacMahon S, Hebert P, Fiebach NH, Eberlein KA et al (1990) Blood pressure, stroke and coronary heart disease. Part 2, short-term reduction in blood pressure: overview of randomized drug trials in their epidemiological context. Lancet 335:827–838
36. Hypertension Detection and Follow-up Program Cooperative Group (1979) Five-year finding of the hypertension detection and follow-up program. 1. Reduction in mortality of persons with high blood pressure: including mild hypertension. JAMA 242:2562–2571
37. Furberg CD, Berglund G, Manolio TA, Psaty BM (1994) Overtreatment and undertreatment of hypertension. J Intern Med 235:387–397
38. Psaty BM, Heckbert SR, Koepsell TD, Siscovick DS, Lemaitre R, Smith NL et al (1996) The risk of incident myocardial infarction associated with anti-hypertensive drug therapies [Abstract]. Circulation 91:925

39. Held PH, Yusuf S, Furberg CD (1989) Calcium channel blockers in acute myocardial infarction and unstable angina: an overview. BMJ 299:1187–1192
40. Feldman AM, Bristow MR, Parmley WW, Carson PE, Pepine CJ, Gilbert EM et al (1993) Effects of vesnarinone on morbidity and mortality in patients with heart failure. Vesnarinone Study Group. N Engl J Med 329:149–155
41. Packer M, Carver JR, Rodehoffer JR, Ivanhoe RJ, DiBianco R, Zeldis SM et al (1991) Effect of oral milrinone on mortality in severe chronic heart failure. The PROMISE Study Research Group. N Engl J Med 325:1468–1475
42. Packer M, Rouleau J, Swedberg K, Pitt B, Fisher L, Klepper M et al (1993) Effect of flosequinan on survival in chronic heart failure: preliminary results of the PROFILE study [Abstract]. Circulation 88(Suppl I):I–301
43. Moertel CG (1984) Improving the efficiency of clinical trials: a medical perspective. Stat Med 3:455–468
44. Sargent DJ, Rubinstein L, Schwarz L, Dancey JE, Gastonis C, Dodd E, Shankar LK (2009) Validation of novel imaging methodologies for use as cancer clinical trial end-points. Eur J Cancer 45:290–299
45. IOM (2007) Cancer-biomarkers: The promises and challenges of improving detection and treatment. The National Academies Press, Washington
46. IOM (2009) Accelerating the development of biomarkers for drug safety. The National Academies Press, Washington
47. Sargent DJ, Wieand HS, Haller DG, Gray R et al (2005) Disease-free survival vs overall survival as primary end point for adjuvant colon cancer cancer studies: individual patient data from 20,898 patients on 18 randomized trials. J Clin Oncol 23:8664–8670
48. (1992) Modulation of fluorouracil by leucovorin in patients with advanced colorectal cancer: evidence in terms of response rate. Advanced Colorectal Cancer Meta-Analysis Project. J Clin Oncol 10:896–903
49. Peto R, Doll R, Buckley JD, Sporn MB (1981) Can dietary beta-carotene materially reduce cancer rates? Nature 290:201–208
50. The ATBC Study Group (2003) Incidence of cancer and mortality following α-tocopherol and β-carotene supplementation. A postintervention follow-up. JAMA 290(4):476–485
51. Omenn GS, Goodman GE, Thornquist MD, Balmes J, Cullen MR, Glass A, Keogh JP, Meyskens FL, Valanis B, Williams JH, Barnhart S, Hammar S (1996) Effects of a combination of beta carotene and vitamin A on lung cancer and cardiovascular disease. N Engl J Med 334:1150–1155
52. Hennekens CH, Buring JE, Manson JE, Stampfer M, Rosner B, Cook N, Belanger C, LaMotte F, Gaziano JM, Ridker PM, Willett W, Peto R (1996) Lack of effect of long term supplementation with beta carotene on the incidence of malignant neoplasms and cardiovascular disease. N Engl J Med 334(18):1145–1149
53. Kang JH, Cook NR, Manson JE, Buring JE, Albert CM, Grodstein F (2009) Vitamin E, vitamin C, beta carotene, and cognitive function among women with or at risk of cardiovascular disease: The Women's Antioxidant and Cardiovascular Study. Circulation 119:2772–2780
54. Lee IM, Cook IR, Manson JE, Buring JE, Hennekens CH (1999) Beta-carotene supplementation and incidence of cancer and cardiovascular disease: the Women's Health Study. J Natl Cancer Inst 91:2102–2106
55. Ridker PM, Cushman M, Stampfer MJ, Tracy RP, Hennekens CH (1997) Inflammation, aspirin, and the risk of cardiovascular disease in apparently healthy men. N Engl J Med 336:973–979
56. Hlatky M (2011) The cost-effectiveness of rosuvastatin therapy JUPITER (justification for the use of statins in prevention: an intervention trial evaluating rosuvastatin). J Am Coll Cardiol 57:792–793
57. Heidenreich PA, Alloggiamento T, Melsop K, McDonald KM, Go AS, Hlatky MA (2001) The prognostic value of troponin in patients with non-ST elevation acute coronary syndromes. J Am Coll Cardiol 38:478–485
58. Wallace TW, Abdullah SM, Drazner MH et al (2006) Prevalence and determinants of troponin T elevation in the general population. Circulation 113:1958–1965

59. Thygesen K, Alpert J, White H et al (2007) Joint Task Force for the redefinition of myocardial infarction, Universal definition of myocardial infarction. Eur Heart J 28:2525–2538
60. Solomon SD, Uno H, Lewis EF, Eckardt KU, Lin J, Burdmann EA, de Zeeuw D, Ivanovich P, Levey AS, Parfrey P, Remuzzi G, Singh AK, Toto R, Huang F, Rossert J, McMurray JJ, Pfeffer MA (2010) Trial to Reduce Cardiovascular Events with Aranesp Therapy (TREAT) Investigators. N Engl J Med 363(12):1146–1155
61. INSIGHT-ESPIRIT Study Group and SILCAAT Steering Committee (2009) Interleukin-2 therapy in patients with HIV infection. N Engl J Med 361:1548–1559

On the Use of Biomarkers to Elucidate Clinical Trial Results: Examples from the Women's Health Initiative

Ross L. Prentice and Shanshan Zhao

Abstract Biomarkers provide opportunities to maximize the knowledge gained from randomized controlled trials. Applications may include the identification of subpopulations that experience differential treatment effects; the assessment of adherence to treatment or intervention goals; and the elucidation of key biological pathways through which the treatments affect clinical outcomes. This last biomarker role also has implications for the development and initial testing of potential treatments. These types of applications are illustrated using biomarker studies in the Women's Health Initiative postmenopausal hormone therapy and low-fat dietary pattern trials. Related topics are also described where further methodology developments would be helpful.

1 Introduction

The Women's Health Initiative (WHI) is a large-scale epidemiologic research program focused on the prevention of chronic disease among postmenopausal women. A total of 161,808 postmenopausal women, in the age range 50–79, were enrolled at 40 U.S. Clinical Centers during 1993–1998. The centerpiece of the WHI is a multifaceted clinical trial of four preventive interventions, in a partial factorial design [1]. A total of 10,739 post-hysterectomy women were randomized to the E-alone trial of 0.625 mg/day of conjugated equine estrogens (Premarin) or placebo; 16,608 women with uterus were randomized to the E + P trial of this same estrogen

R.L. Prentice (✉)
Public Health Sciences, Fred Hutchinson Cancer Center, 1100 Fairview Ave. N.,
Seattle, WA, 98109 USA
e-mail: rprentic@WHI.org

S. Zhao
University of Washington, Seattle, WA, USA
e-mail: zhaoss41@gmail.com

T.R. Fleming and B.S. Weir (eds.), *Proceedings of the Fourth Seattle Symposium in Biostatistics: Clinical Trials*, Lecture Notes in Statistics 1205, DOI 10.1007/978-1-4614-5245-4_2, © Springer Science+Business Media New York 2013

Table 1 Clinical outcomes in the WHI postmenopausal hormone therapy trials

Outcomes	E + P trial		E-alone trial	
	Hazard ratio	95% CI [a]	Hazard ratio	95% CI [a]
Coronary heart disease	**1.29**	**1.02–1.63**	**0.91**	**0.75–1.12**
Stroke	1.41	1.07–1.85	1.39	1.10–1.77
Venous thromboembolism	2.11	1.58–2.82	1.33	0.99–1.79
Invasive breast cancer	**1.26**	**1.00–1.59**	**0.77**	**0.59–1.01**
Colorectal cancer	0.63	0.43–0.92	1.08	0.75–1.55
Endometrial cancer	0.83	0.47–1.47		
Hip fracture	0.66	0.45–0.98	0.61	0.41–0.91
Death due to other causes	0.92	0.74–1.14	1.08	0.88–1.32
Global index	1.15	1.03–1.28	1.01	0.91–1.12
Number of women	8,506	8,102	5,310	5,429
Follow-up time, mean (SD), mo	62.2 (16.1)	61.2 (15.0)	81.6 (19.3)	81.9 (19.7)

[a] *CI* confidence interval, from a proportional hazards model stratified by age (5-year categories), and randomization status in the DM trial

preparation plus 2.5 mg/day medroxyprogesterone acetate (Prempro) or placebo; and 48,835 women were randomized to a low-fat dietary pattern (40%) or usual diet (60%). At their one-year anniversary following randomization into either or both of the hormone therapy (HT) or dietary modification (DM) components, participating women were given the opportunity for further randomization to a dietary supplementation trial of 1,000 mg/day calcium carbonate plus 400 international units of vitamin D3 or placebo, and 36,282 women did so. The WHI program is strengthened by the inclusion of a companion cohort study among 93,676 postmenopausal women in the same age range, recruited from essentially the same catchment populations, with much commonality with the clinical trial in methodology, and in data and biospecimen collection.

Table 1 shows key findings from the hormone therapy trials [2, 3] with findings for the designated primary CHD outcome, and the designated primary adverse outcome highlighted. The E + P trial was stopped early in 2002 when health risks were judged to exceed benefits over a 5.6-year average intervention period. The risks included an early elevation in coronary heart disease incidence, the primary trial outcome for which an important risk reduction had been hypothesized, and elevations in stroke and venous thromboembolism incidence. An elevation in breast cancer incidence and a reduction in fracture incidence were also observed, as was hypothesized in trial design [1]. A global index, defined as the time to the earliest of the outcomes listed above it in Table 1 was in the unfavorable direction, and contributed to early stopping considerations. The E-alone trial also stopped early, in 2004, after an intervention period that averaged 7.1 years, substantially because of a stroke elevation of similar magnitude as that observed for E + P, though health risks and benefits and the global index were rather balanced in this trial.

Analyses beyond the summary hazard ratios (HRs) shown in Table 1 took place for each clinical outcome, as well as for some additional important outcomes (e.g., cognition and dementia). These included analyses of HR form as a function of time,

Table 2 Comparison of cancer incidence rates between intervention and comparison groups in the Women's Health Initiative (WHI) dietary modification trial

Incidence per 1,000 person-years (number of cases)				
Cancer site	Intervention	Comparison	p [a]	HR (95% CI) [b]
Breast	4.15(655)	4.52(1, 072)	0.09	0.91 (0.83–1.01)
Colorectal	1.27(201)	1.18(279)	0.29	1.08 (0.90–1.29)
Ovary	0.36(57)	0.43(103)	0.03	0.83 (0.60–1.14)
Endometrium	0.79(125)	0.71(170)	0.18	1.11 (0.88–1.40)
All other sites	4.56(720)	4.81(1, 140)	0.30	0.95 (0.86–1.04)
Total cancer	10.69(1, 687)	11.22(2, 661)	0.10	0.95 (0.89–1.01)

Trial includes 19,541 women in the intervention group and 29,294 women in the comparison group
[a] Weighted log-rank test (two-sided) stratified by age (5-year categories) and randomization status in the WHI hormone therapy trial. Weights increase linearly from zero at random assignment to a maximum of 1.0 at 10 years
[b] *HR* hazard ratio, *CI* confidence interval, from a proportional hazards model stratified by age (5-year categories), and randomization status in the WHI hormone therapy trial

analyses of HRs among women adherent to their assigned intervention, and various subgroup analyses (with appropriate caveats). Participating women were actively followed beyond the cessation of intervention, giving rise to a range of additional analyses of public health importance [4, 5].

To cite but one example, the more detailed studies of breast cancer incidence in the E + P trial showed an HR that increased unfavorably and approximately linearly to about 1.6 following 5 years of use, and dropped back to basal levels by 2–3 years following trial stoppage. When analyses focused on adherent women, a more dramatic increase to an HR of about 2.5 after 5 years of use was estimated, again with dissipation by 2–3 years following cessation of use [6]. These patterns, in conjunction with the approximately six million women using this estrogen plus progestin preparation in the USA, about 70% of whom stopped shortly after initial trial results [1] were announced, projected a national reduction in breast cancer incidence of about 15,000 women per year as a result of this change in usage patterns, as agrees with subsequent U.S. breast cancer incidence rates [7].

The WHI low-fat dietary pattern trial had dietary intervention goals of equal or less than 20% of energy from fat; five or more fruit and vegetable servings/day, and six or more grain servings/day, with breast and colorectal cancer as primary outcomes, and with ovary and endometrial cancer as additional diet-related cancers that may benefit from this intervention. Table 2 shows principal cancer incidence results from this trial, which proceeded to its planned termination with an 8.1-year average intervention period. The trial design projected a reduction in breast cancer risk with an overall HR of 0.87. The principal targeted dietary change was a reduction in percent of energy from fat, but only about 70% of the hypothesized change was achieved. In correspondence the estimated breast cancer HR of 0.91 [8] differed from unity by about 70% of that projected, but was not significantly different from one (weighted logrank p = 0.09). The corresponding contrast for ovarian cancer incidence [9] was nominally significant (p = 0.03), providing an important lead for a disease having few known modifiable risk factors. For both breast [8] and ovarian cancer [9], there was a significant interaction between baseline percent of energy from fat and HR, with stronger evidence for an intervention effect among women having a high fat content in their customary diet. These women made a comparatively larger reduction in percent of energy from fat, if assigned to the dietary intervention group.

The calcium and vitamin trial did not provide significant evidence of a treatment effect, either for its primary hip fracture outcome [10], or secondary outcomes (colorectal cancer, other fractures).

2 Biomarkers and Variations in Clinical Trial Intervention Effects

Even though it is good clinical trial practice to focus primarily on overall treatment effects as opposed to those in subsets of a study population, it needs to be recognized that hazard ratios may, and often do, vary according to specific characteristics of the study population. Notably, HRs provide but one way of summarizing a treatment effect over time, and lack of variation on an HR scale may differ from corresponding lack of variation on other assessment scales. That said, however, HR or other ratio measures (e.g., odds ratios) seem particularly useful in leading to simple models, wherein the joint association of treatment and study subject characteristics or exposures on clinical outcomes often seems to depart little from a multiplicative model.

For example, for breast cancer incidence, no interacting demographic or clinical variables were found for E + P [11], whereas for E-alone a suggested reduction in risk seemed to be largely confined to lower risk women, specifically those without benign breast disease or a family history of breast cancer [12].

Several nested case–control studies within the HT trial cohorts were conducted in an attempt to identify biomarkers that may interact with hormone therapy HRs, or that may mediate the observed intervention effects on clinical outcomes. These studies primarily focused on biochemical and genetic markers that were recognized risk indicators for the clinical outcomes under study. For example, a Cardiovascular Disease Biomarker Study focused on markers of inflammation, coagulation/thrombosis, lipids and lipoproteins, and related genetic variants, for each of coronary heart disease, stroke, and venous thromboembolism. These studies [13, 14] generally confirmed associations with disease risk, but there were few interacting factors identified and none of the observed biomarker changes following intervention activities appeared to meaningfully mediate the observed treatment effects, a topic that will be discussed further below. As an example of an interacting variable, women having a relatively high baseline low-density lipoprotein (LDL) cholesterol who were assigned to active hormone therapy evidently experienced a comparatively larger early elevation in coronary heart disease risk [13].

Some high-dimensional genotype biomarker studies were also conducted, in an attempt to understand more of the biology related to observed clinical effects in the WHI trials. For example, a breast cancer nested case–control study involved the genotyping of 9,039 single nucleotide polymorphisms (SNPs) for 2,166 women who developed breast cancer during the trial intervention period. A randomized trial context is well suited to genotype by treatment interaction testing in that "case-only" analyses, which require genotype data only on study subjects developing disease, have efficiency about the same as if genotyping had been conducted on the full cohort.

More specifically, let $V = 1$ and $V = 0$ denote active and control randomization assignments, and $z = 0$, 1, or 2 denote the number of minor alleles of an SNP. A simple Cox model that stratifies on SNP genotype, and allows a separate HR parameter for treatment at each value of z, can be written

$$\lambda (t;\ V,\ z) = \lambda_{0z} (t) \exp\{\beta_0 I (z = 0) + \beta_1 I (z = 1) + \beta_2 I (z = 2)\},$$

where $I(\cdot)$ denotes an indicator variable, and $e^{\beta z}$ is the HR for women having SNP genotype z, for $z = 0$, 1, or 2. From this expression,

$$\text{logit} (V|X = t,\ z) = \text{logit} (V|X \geq t, z) + \sum_{i=0}^{2} \beta_i I (z = z_i) ,$$

where $X = t$ denotes disease occurrence at time t following randomization. The important feature here is that V is orthogonal to z by virtue of randomization so that if the disease is rare one has, to a good approximation

$$\text{logit} (V|T \geq t,\ z) = \log \{q/ (1 - q)\} ,$$

where $q = \text{pr}(V = 1)$ is the randomization fraction for the active treatment group. It follows that one can estimate intervention HRs at each SNP genotype by ordinary logistic regression of the randomization indicator V on indicator variables for the number of minor SNP alleles, with $\log \{q/(1 - q)\}$ as an "offset." Breast cancer analyses of this type yielded nominally significant variations in the intervention HR with a SNP (rs3750817) in intron 2 of the fibroblast growth factor receptor gene on chromosome 10 for both E + P and E-alone [15] and for the dietary modification intervention in the subset of women (denoted DMQ) who were in the upper quartile of percent of energy from fat in their baseline diet [16]. These analyses also drew attention (nominal $p < 0.05$) to a SNP (rs7705343) in the mitochondrial ribosomal protein S30 region of chromosome five [17] for each of E-alone, DMQ, and for the calcium and vitamin D intervention (for which there was no breast cancer "main" effect). For either SNP the more favorable intervention effects were evidently localized among women who were homozygous for the SNP minor allele (TT genotype for rs3750817; AA for rs7705343). A challenge with these types of suggestive findings is the identification of a research strategy for replication. Observational studies pertinent to these intervention topics may be limited in their assessment of related exposures (e.g., hormonal or dietary exposures), and may be subject to important confounding or measurement biases. In general, the methods for identification of genotype by environmental factor interaction evaluation are at an early stage of development, and large-scale clinical trial settings have much to offer in this arena.

3   Biomarkers of Intervention Adherence and Exposure

As mentioned above, the Dietary Modification trial evidently achieved only about 70% of its projected intervention versus control group difference for the principal dietary intervention target, percent of energy from fat. Even this 70% assessment relies on self-reported dietary information from participating women. Specifically, based on food frequency questionnaire (FFQ) assessments, intervention group women reported a 10.7% average lower percent of energy from fat compared to the control group at 1-year following randomization; 9.5% at 3 years after randomization; and 8.1% at 6 years after randomization. However, the FFQ data also indicate a differential total energy consumption by about 100 kilocalories/day, which is not consistent with the weight changes experienced by trial participants (2–3 kg greater weight loss in intervention group compared to usual diet control group at 1-year, which mostly dissipated over the subsequent 5 years). If the greater underreporting of energy by intervention group women pertained disproportionately to fat calories, then percent of energy from fat would also be differentially reported and the power of the DM trial accordingly affected.

In fact, the dietary assessment measurement issue is even more acute in observational nutritional epidemiology studies, where systematic and random assessment errors could well distort the very associations under study, rather than simply reducing study power as in the intervention trial setting. In either context, however, biomarkers provide important avenues for strengthening the research agenda.

Two nutritional biomarker substudies have been conducted in WHI cohorts, and a controlled human feeding study that aims to develop biomarkers for additional nutrients and foods is currently underway. The first, the Nutrient Biomarker Study (NBS) included energy [18] and protein [19] biomarkers and a concurrent FFQ, among a representative 544 weight-stable women in the DM trial. The second, the Nutrition and Physical Activity Assessment Study included these biomarkers and self-reports of dietary frequencies, records and recalls, along with a biomarker of activity-related energy expenditure and three types of physical activity self-report, among 450 representative women from the WHI Observational (cohort) Study. By simple linear regression of log-biomarker assessments on corresponding log self-reports and on readily available study subject characteristic data (body mass index, age, and ethnicity), calibrated consumption estimates were developed for energy, protein, and percent of energy from protein. For example, for energy, even though the log self-report data explained only a few percent (e.g., 3–4% for the FFQ) of the variation in log-biomarker values, the inclusion of these other factors in the regression equation raised this percentage to the 40–45% range. Upon extracting the temporal variation in the biomarker, this increased to about 70% of the average daily energy consumption variation over a 1-year study period [20]. The NBS equations were used to develop calibrated-energy, protein, and percent of energy from protein estimates throughout the WHI cohorts, and positive associations between energy and several major cancers [21] as well as coronary disease [22] and diabetes [23] were found that were not apparent without calibration. The role of body mass index in these analyses is complex [24], and the associations just mentioned seemed substantially, if not entirely, explained by body fat accumulation over time.

This nutritional epidemiology research area and the similarly important physical activity epidemiology area are ripe for further development, with a substantial use of biomarkers providing a logical next step in the overall research agenda.

The energy biomarker data indicates severe underreporting using the FFQ, by about 30% overall, and with much greater underreporting among overweight and obese women, along with greater underreporting by younger compared to older postmenopausal women. These analyses also suggest some energy underreporting by intervention compared to control group women also, by about 100 kcal/day, allowing the weight change data mentioned above to align with corresponding calibrated energy consumption in the DM trial.

4 Biomarkers as Mediators of Clinical Trial Intervention Effects

Again let $V = 1$ or 0 denote active and control randomization assignments in a clinical trial, but now let z denote a biomarker change following some period of intervention activities. Analyses may aim to understand the extent to which intervention effects on the clinical outcome are mediated by z. A traditional mediation analysis would compare the coefficient of V in a regression analysis that doesn't include z with a corresponding analysis including z, with evidence for mediation if the coefficient for V moves substantially toward the null when z is added to the regression model.

A key statistical difference is evident between the type of interaction analysis discussed in Sect. 2, where V and z are independent by study design, and mediation analyses where V and z may be highly correlated. This is a critical point. In the extreme, for example, if the biomarker doesn't change in the control group ($z = 0$) and changes by exactly the same amount ($z = c$, for some $c \neq 0$) among all study subjects in the intervention group, then z and V will be perfectly correlated, and it will not be possible to carry out an analysis that simultaneously models V and z. As a plausible departure from this scenario, suppose that z is constant in both groups, but that z is assessed with some technical measurement error. As amplified below, the regression analyses will then be possible, but z may then appear not to mediate, even though the biomarker change in question may be central to explaining the intervention effects on clinical outcomes.

To elaborate just a little, consider baseline, x_0, and post-intervention, x_1, biomarker values, and suppose that the biomarker fully mediates an intervention effect in a linear model for a quantitative response Y. Hence, $E(Y; x_0, x_1, V) = a + a_0 x_0 + a_1 x_1$, with $a_1 \neq 0$. Under a bivariate normal model for (x_0, x_1) with mean $(\mu_0, \mu_1 + dV)$, common variance σ^2 and correlation ρ, one can derive

$$E(Y; x_0, V) = a' + a'_0 x_0 + (a_1 d) V,$$

where a' and a'_0 are simple functions of the response and biomarker parameters, so that a mediation analysis would compare an estimate of $a_1 d$ to an estimate of the coefficient of V (zero) when x_1 is added to the regression model.

Now suppose that x_0 and x_1 incorporate classical normal measurement error, so that one measures $w_0 = x_0 + e_0$ and $w_1 = x_1 + e_1$ where e_0 and e_1 are independent mean zero normal variates having variance σ_e^2. It is straightforward to show that the coefficient of V in $E(Y; w_0, V)$ is again $a_1 d$, unaffected by measurement error owing to the independence between x_0 and V, but that for V in $E(Y \mid w_0, w_1, V)$ is a complicated function of model parameters that approaches $(a_0 + a_1)d/(2 + \delta^2)$ as $\rho \to 1$, where $\delta^2 = \sigma_e^2/\sigma^2$. This limiting coefficient can be very far from zero even if δ^2 is small! This rather counter-intuitive result arises because of the diminishing ability to distinguish the biomarker effect from the overall treatment effect on Y, as $\rho \to 1$. It follows that careful modeling of the biomarker and its measurement process may be needed to reliably assess mediation, or more generally, to assess treatment effects after allowing for certain biomarker changes.

As noted above, none of the candidate biomarkers studied appeared to mediate HT effects on cardiovascular diseases in the WHI hormone therapy trials. We undertook additional "discovery" research to identify blood biomarkers that are risk markers for these diseases, and that are affected by hormone therapy. This work focused on protein expression, using an Intact Protein Analysis System [25] having the capability of quantitatively comparing concentrations between pairs of specimens for about 350–400 proteins across a substantial dynamic range. Specifically, concentrations based on blood collected 1-year after randomization were compared to corresponding baseline concentrations for 50 women adherent to active E-alone, and 50 women adherent to active E + P, over the first year of HT trial participation. For throughput reasons IPAS analyses were based on pools formed from equal volumes of serum from 10 women. A total of 378 proteins were quantified for change. Of these, a remarkable 44.7% (169/378) had evidence of change (p < 0.05) following intervention with E-alone or E + P [26, 27]. The protein changes were mostly quite similar for E-alone and E + P, and included proteins in multiple biological pathways relevant to observed clinical effects, including inflammation, coagulation, immune function, cell adhesion, growth factors, and osteogenesis, among others.

Corresponding analyses were then conducted, using the same proteomic platform, to compare baseline blood protein concentrations between women who went on to develop CHD or stroke and corresponding matched controls, with cases and controls drawn from the WHI Observational Study. This time larger pools of size

100 were employed. There were eight such pool pairs for each of these diseases, as well as for breast cancer. From the resulting data [28] there were 37 proteins having nominal p < 0.05 for a CHD case versus control difference compared to 17.3 expected by chance; and 47 for stroke compared to 18.3 expected by chance. Several of these had estimated false discovery rates <0.05 and most of these were among the proteins evidently affected by E-alone and/or E + P. These provide novel candidates for mechanistic effects of HT on these cardiovascular diseases.

We are still at an early stage of evaluating these candidates for mediation in the HT trials. An initial evaluation involving beta-2 microglobulin, a highly ranked protein for CHD association, and insulin-like growth factor binding protein 4 (IGFBP4), a highly ranked protein for stroke association, confirmed the association of these proteins with disease incidence in the WHI trials but, once again, change in protein concentration following hormone therapy treatment did not seem to mediate intervention effects on these diseases, at least not without explicit account of the biomarker measurement error process. Further, analyses with these analytes revealed that HT hazard ratios, in the presence of baseline and 1-year biomarker measurements were quite sensitive to the ratio (δ^2) of the measurement error variance to the underlying biomarker variance for both E-alone and E + P, with larger δ^2 values consistent with full mediation.

These preliminary analyses reinforce the need for enhanced statistical methods for identifying the important biological intermediaries of intervention effects in clinical trials. Adequate modeling of the underlying biomarker process, and of the departure of such models from corresponding measured biomarker values, may typically require biomarker assessments at more than two time points in conjunction with large case and control sample sizes. This topic, and methods for correcting treatment hazard ratio estimates for the biomarker measurement process, will be discussed in more detail elsewhere.

5   Biomarkers for Intervention Development

In recent years biomarkers have come to play a rather central role in treatment development, particularly in the therapeutics area. For example, the molecular characteristics of patient tumors may identify key therapeutic targets for disruption by potential treatments. High-dimensional data, including gene expression profiles, may help to focus developmental efforts toward therapeutic benefit or toward the avoidance of certain adverse effects.

The development and initial testing of preventive interventions is a rather under-developed aspect of the chronic disease prevention research agenda. Sometimes it is attractive to move interventions from therapeutics to primary prevention. Examples include statins for heart disease prevention; tamoxifen, SERMS, or aromatase inhibitors for breast cancer prevention; or biphosphonates for fracture prevention. However, this approach seems unlikely to lead to the behavioral changes, for example, in the diet and physical activity area, that arguably provide the ultimate preventive approaches needed. Observational epidemiology has much to offer for identifying preventive approaches, but findings may lack the needed specificity and force to fuel needed behavioral, regulatory, or policy changes. For example, one can contrast the influence of the rather extensive body of observational research on postmenopausal hormones, with that of the comparatively few clinical trials that eventually were able to be conducted.

Intermediate outcome trials, which have outcomes on putative pathways between treatments and clinical outcomes of interest, have considerable potential to add to these other data sources for preventive intervention development. For example, a trial of moderate size, called the Postmenopausal Estrogen Progestin Intervention (PEPI) trial was initiated in advance of the WHI trials to compare various hormone regimens in respect to cardiovascular disease risk factors, uterine hyperplasia, and other intermediate outcomes [29, 30]. This trial had an influence on the choice of regimens studied in the WHI trials, but it did not warn, for example, concerning the observed early elevation in CHD, or the sustained elevation in stroke that emerged in the WHI hormone therapy trials.

Intermediate outcome trials that combine changes in major risk factors for clinical outcomes of interest with more agnostic, possibly high-dimensional, changes in blood or other biospecimens, may offer a more comprehensive approach to the selection and initial evaluation of preventive interventions. For example, the agnostic aspect could entail study of potential intervention effects on the plasma proteome and metabolome. These data, whether for a few emergent candidates or for a high-dimensional set of changes, could then be merged with observational analyses relating the entire set of intermediate variables to clinical outcomes of interest, to develop projections of intervention effects on each such outcome. This approach could be considered for behavioral as well as chemopreventive interventions. The two data sources to be combined would each involve studies having a small fraction of the cost of a full-scale prevention trial. While not sufficient in itself, such an approach could augment the value of intermediate outcome trials and, in particular, may help to filter intervention options arising from the traditional data sources mentioned above, thereby permitting a focus on the more strongly justified concepts for full-scale trial consideration with clinical outcomes.

6 Discussion and Summary

Biomarkers have potential to play several important roles in the development, conduct, analysis, and reporting of clinical trials. Specifically, biomarkers may permit stratification of study subjects according to the magnitude of beneficial or adverse treatment effects, possibly leading to the identification of persons for whom the treatment can be particularly recommended or should be avoided.

Though not much emphasized here, biomarkers typically play a key role in the assessment of adherence to intervention goals, and in the assessment of adherence-adjusted treatment effects. Biomarkers also provide the principal approach to identifying the important biological pathways whereby a treatment may influence a clinical outcome of interest. The utility of biomarkers for each of these purposes, but especially for the elucidation of disease mechanisms can be expected to depend strongly on the properties of the biomarker measurement process, and on the ability to adequately model and correct for measurement error in data analyses.

The adherence-adjustment and mediation applications of biomarkers are sometimes posed using a potential outcomes, and a principal stratification formulation [31]. The principal stratification "framework," however, seems too restrictive to be very useful in this type of biomedical research context [32, 33], and the important measurement error issue discussed here does not seem to have been addressed in the potential outcomes context.

Finally, high-dimensional biomarkers from discovery platforms evidently have an important role to play in intervention development, though this concept has yet to be much explored to date for preventive intervention development.

Acknowledgements This work was supported by NIH/NCI grants P01-CA53996, R01-CA119171, R21HL109527, R01CA149135 U01-CA86368-06, and U19-CA148065-01; and the National Heart, Lung, and Blood Institute, National Institutes of Health, U.S. Department of Health and Human Services through contract N01WH22110.

References

1. The Women's Health Initiative Study Group (1998) Design of the Women's Health Initiative clinical trial and observational study. Control Clin Trials 19(1):61–109
2. Rossouw JE, Anderson GL, Prentice RL, LaCroix AZ, Kooperberg C, Stefanick ML, Jackson RD, Beresford SA, Howard BV, Johnson KC, Kotchen JM, Ockene J, Writing Group for the Women's Health Initiative Investigators (2002) Risks and benefits of estrogen plus progestin in healthy postmenopausal women: principal results from the Women's Health Initiative randomized controlled trial. JAMA 288(3):321–333
3. Anderson GL, Limacher M, Assaf AR, Bassford T, Beresford SA, Black H, Bonds D, Brunner R, Brzyski R, Caan B, Chlebowski R, Curb D, Gass M, Hays J, Heiss G, Hendrix S, Howard BV, Hsia J, Hubbell A, Jackson R, Johnson KC, Judd H, Kotchen JM, Kuller L, LaCroix AZ, Lane D, Langer RD, Lasser N, Lewis CE, Manson J, Margolis K, Ockene J, O'Sullivan MJ, Phillips L, Prentice RL, Ritenbaugh C, Robbins J, Rossouw JE, Sarto G, Stefanick ML, Van Horn L, Wactawski-Wende J, Wallace R, Wassertheil-Smoller S, Women's Health Initiative Steering Committee (2004) Effects of conjugated equine estrogen in postmenopausal women with hysterectomy: The Women's Health Initiative randomized controlled trial. JAMA 291(14):1701–1712
4. Heiss G, Wallace R, Anderson GL, Aragaki A, Beresford SA, Brzyski R, Chlebowski RT, Gass M, LaCroix A, Manson JE, Prentice RL, Rossouw J, Stefanick ML, WHI Investigators (2008) Health risks and benefits 3 years after stopping randomized treatment with estrogen and progestin. JAMA 299(9):1036–1045
5. LaCroix AZ, Chlebowski RT, Manson JE, Aragaki AK, Johnson KC, Martin L, Margolis KL, Stefanick ML, Brzyski R, Curb JD, Howard BV, Lewis CE, Wactawski-Wende J, WHI Investigators (2011) Health outcomes after stopping conjugated equine estrogens among postmenopausal women with prior hysterectomy: a randomized controlled trial. JAMA 305(13):1305–1314

6. Chlebowski RT, Kuller LH, Prentice RL, Stefanick ML, Manson JE, Gass M, Aragaki AK, Ockene JK, Lane DS, Sarto GE, Rajkovic A, Schenken R, Hendrix SL, Ravdin PM, Rohan TE, Yasmeen S, Anderson G, WHI Investigators (2009) Breast cancer after use of estrogen plus progestin in postmenopausal women. N Engl J Med 360(6):573–587

7. Ravdin PM, Cronin KA, Howlader N, Berg CD, Chlebowski RT, Feuer EJ, Edwards BK, Berry DA (2007) The decrease in breast-cancer incidence in 2003 in the United States. N Engl J Med 356(16):1670–1674

8. Prentice RL, Caan B, Chlebowski RT, Patterson R, Kuller LH, Ockene JK, Margolis KL, Limacher MC, Manson JE, Parker LM, Paskett E, Phillips L, Robbins J, Rossouw JE, Sarto GE, Shikany JM, Stefanick ML, Thomson CA, Van Horn L, Vitolins MZ, Wactawski-Wende J, Wallace RB, Wassertheil-Smoller S, Whitlock E, Yano K, Adams-Campbell L, Anderson GL, Assaf AR, Beresford SA, Black HR, Brunner RL, Brzyski RG, Ford L, Gass M, Hays J, Heber D, Heiss G, Hendrix SL, Hsia J, Hubbell FA, Jackson RD, Johnson KC, Kotchen JM, LaCroix AZ, Lane DS, Langer RD, Lasser NL, Henderson MM (2006) Low-fat dietary pattern and risk of invasive breast cancer: The Women's Health Initiative Randomized Controlled Dietary Modification Trial. JAMA 295(6):629–642

9. Prentice RL, Thomson CA, Caan B, Hubbell FA, Anderson GL, Beresford SAA, Pettinger M, Lane DS, Lessin L, Yasmeen S, Singh B, Khandekar J, Shikany JM, Satterfield S, Chlebowski RT (2007) Low-fat dietary pattern and cancer incidence in the Women's Health Initiative Dietary Modification Randomized Controlled Trial. J Natl Cancer Inst 99(20):1534–1543

10. Jackson RD, LaCroix AZ, Gass M, Wallace RB, Robbins J, Lewis CE, Bassford T, Beresford SA, Black HR, Blanchette P, Bonds DE, Brunner RL, Brzyski RG, Caan B, Cauley JA, Chlebowski RT, Cummings SR, Granek I, Hays J, Heiss G, Hendrix SL, Howard BV, Hsia J, Hubbell FA, Johnson KC, Judd H, Kotchen JM, Kuller LH, Langer RD, Lasser NL, Limacher MC, Ludlam S, Manson JE, Margolis KL, McGowan J, Ockene JK, O'Sullivan MJ, Phillips L, Prentice RL, Sarto GE, Stefanick ML, Van Horn L, Wactawski-Wende J, Whitlock E, Anderson GL, Assaf AR, Barad D, Women's Health Initiative Investigators (2006) Calcium plus vitamin D supplementation and the risk of fractures. N Engl J Med 354(7):669–683

11. Chlebowski RT, Hendrix SL, Langer RD, Stefanick ML, Gass M, Lane D, Rodabough RJ, Gilligan MA, Cyr MG, Thomson CA, Khandekar J, Petrovitch H, McTiernan A, WHI Investigators (2003) Influence of estrogen plus progestin on breast cancer and mammography in healthy postmenopausal women: the Women's Health Initiative Randomized Trial. JAMA 289(24):3243–3253

12. Stefanick ML, Anderson GL, Margolis KL, Hendrix SL, Rodabough RJ, Paskett ED, Lane DS, Hubbell FA, Assaf AR, Sarto GE, Schenken RS, Yasmeen S, Lessin L, Chlebowski RT, WHI Investigators (2006) Effects of conjugated equine estrogens on breast cancer and mammography screening in postmenopausal women with hysterectomy. JAMA 295(14):1647–1657

13. Rossouw JE, Cushman M, Greenland P, Lloyd-Jones DM, Bray P, Kooperberg C, Pettinger M, Robinson J, Hendrix S, Hsia J (2008) Inflammatory, lipid, thrombotic, and genetic markers of coronary heart disease risk in the Women's Health Initiative trials of hormone therapy. Arch Intern Med 168(20):2245–2253

14. Kooperberg C, Cushman M, Hsia J, Robinson J, Aragaki A, Lynch J, Baird A, Johnson K, Kuller L, Beresford S, Rodriguez B (2007) Can biomarkers identify women at increased stroke risk? The Women's Health Initiative hormone trials. PLoS Clin Trials 2(6):e28

15. Prentice RL, Huang Y, Hinds DA, Peters U, Pettinger M, Cox DR, Beilharz E, Chlebowski RT, Rossouw JE, Caan B, Ballinger DG (2009) Variation in the FGFR2 gene and the effects of postmenopausal hormone therapy on invasive breast cancer. Cancer Epidemiol Biomarker Prev 18(11):3079–3085

16. Prentice RL, Huang Y, Hinds DA, Peters U, Cox DR, Beilharz E, Chlebowski RT, Rossouw JE, Caan B, Ballinger DG (2010) Variation in the FGFR2 gene and the effect of a low-fat dietary pattern on invasive breast cancer. Cancer Epidemiol Biomarker Prev 19:74–79

17. Huang Y, Ballinger DG, Dai J, Peters U, Hinds DA, Cox DR, Beilharz E, Chlebowski RT, Rossouw JE, McTiernan A, Rohan T, Prentice RL (2011) Genetic variants in the MRPS30 region and postmenopausal breast cancer risk. Genome Med 3:42

18. Schoeller DA (1999) Recent advances from application of doubly labeled water to measurement of human energy expenditure. J Nutr 129(10):1765–1768
19. Bingham S (1994) The use of 24-h urine samples and energy expenditure to validate dietary assessments. Am J Clin Nutr 59(1):2275–2315
20. Prentice RL, Mossavar-Rahmani Y, Huang Y, Van Horn L, Beresford SAA, Caan B, Tinker LF, Schoeller D, Bingham S, Eaton CB, Thomson C, Johnson KC, Ockene J, Sarto G, Heiss G, Neuhouser ML (2011) Evaluation and comparison of food records, recalls and frequencies for energy and protein assessment using recovery biomarkers. Am J Epidemiol 174(5):591–603
21. Prentice RL, Shaw PA, Bingham SA, Beresford SA, Caan B, Neuhouser ML, Patterson RE, Stefanick ML, Satterfield S, Thomson CA, Snetselaar L, Thomas A, Tinker LF (2009) Biomarker-calibrated energy and protein consumption and increased cancer risk among postmenopausal women. Am J Epidemiol 169(8):977–989
22. Prentice RL, Huang Y, Kuller LH, Tinker LF, Van Horn L, Stefanick ML, Sarto G, Ockene J, Johnson KJ (2011) Biomarker-calibrated energy and protein consumption and cardiovascular disease risk among postmenopausal women. Epidemiology 22(2):170–179
23. Tinker LF, Sarto GE, Howard BV, Huang Y, Neuhouser ML, Mossavar-Rahmani Y, Beasley JM, Margolis KL, Eaton CB, Phillips LS, Prentice RL (2011) Biomarker-calibrated dietary energy and protein intake association with diabetes risk among postmenopausal women from the WHI. Am J Clin Nutr 94(6):1600–1606, Epub 2011 Nov 9
24. Prentice RL, Huang Y (2011) Measurement error modeling and nutritional epidemiology association analyses. Can J Statistics 39:498–509. doi:10.1002/cjs
25. Faca V, Coram M, Phanstiel D, Glukhova V, Zhang Q, Fitzgibbon M, McIntosh M, Hanash S (2006) Quantitative analysis of acrylamide labeled serum proteins by LC-MS/MS. J Proteome Res 5(8):2009–2018
26. Katayama H, Pacznesny S, Prentice RL, Aragaki A, Faca VM, Pitteri SJ, Zhang Q, Wang H, Silva M, Kennedy J, Rossouw J, Jackson R, Hsia J, Chlebowski R, Manson J, Hanash S (2009) Application of serum proteomics to the Women's Health Initiative conjugated equine estrogens trial reveals a multitude of effects relevant to clinical findings. Genome Med 1(4):47.1–47.16
27. Pitteri SJ, Hanash SM, Aragaki A, Amon L, Chen L, Busald Buson T, Paczesny S, Katayama H, Wang H, Johnson MM, Zhang Q, McIntosh M, Wang P, Kooperberg C, Rossouw JE, Jackson R, Manson JE, Hsia J, Liu S, Martin L, Prentice RL (2009) Postmenopausal estrogen and progestin effects on the serum proteome. Genome Med 1(12):121.1–121.14
28. Prentice RL, Paczesny SJ, Aragaki A, Amon LM, Chen L, Pitteri SJ, McIntosh M, Wang P, Busald Buson T, Hsia J, Jackson RD, Rossouw JE, Manson JE, Johnson K, Eaton C, Hanash SM (2010) Novel proteins associated with risk for coronary heart disease or stroke among postmenopausal women identified by in-depth plasma proteome profiling. Genome Med 2(7):48–60
29. PEPI Trial Writing Group (1995) Effects of estrogen or estrogen/progestin regimes on heart disease risk factors in postmenopausal women: the Postmenopausal Estrogen/Progestin Interventions (PEPI) Trial. JAMA 273(3):199–208
30. PEPI Trial Writing Group (1996) Effects of hormone replacement therapy on endometrial histology in postmenopausal women: the Postmenopausal Estrogen/Progestin Interventions (PEPI) Trial. JAMA 275(5):370–375
31. Frangakis CE, Rubin DB (2002) Principal stratification in causal inference. Biometrics 58:21–29
32. Pearl J (2011) Principal stratification – a goal or a tool? Int J Biostat 7(1). pii: Article 20
33. Prentice RL (2011) Invited commentary on pearl and principal stratification. Int J Biostat 7(1):Article 30

On the Use of Biomarkers in Vaccine Research and Development

Steven G. Self

Abstract Biomarkers are characteristics that are objectively measured and evaluated as indicators of normal or pathogenic biologic processes. There are a multitude of ways that biomarkers are used including diagnosis of disease, prognosis of clinical outcomes, patient staging and treatment selection, indication of response to a prior natural exposure, and characterization of response to a biomedical intervention. In the general setting of vaccine trials for infectious diseases, the identification of biomarkers ultimately depends on the specifics of the vaccine and the pathogen and typically focuses on aspects of the immune response to vaccine and/or detection and typing of the pathogen. A central use of immune response biomarkers in vaccine research is as primary endpoints for early phase vaccine trials. At one end of the spectrum, these biomarkers define the extent to which the vaccine is biologically active while at the other end they characterize the nature of the response with sufficient detail to provide some sense of the plausibility that the responses would be clinically protective.

This general theme of identification and validation of immune response biomarkers as surrogate endpoints is a specific area of interest in vaccine trials. In contrast, pathogen-based biomarkers are often used as components of clinical endpoints in situations where clinical outcomes may be attributed to causes other than the pathogen targeted by vaccination. Such biomarkers can lend specificity to trial endpoints that increases sensitivity to detect meaningful vaccine effects. A final important use of both immune response and pathogen-based biomarkers in vaccine trials is the identification of clues that can help to guide the iterative development of vaccines.

S.G. Self (✉)
Vaccine and Infectious Disease Division, Fred Hutchinson Cancer Research Center, 1100 Fairview Ave. N., Seattle, WA 98109, USA
e-mail: sself@fhcrc.org

T.R. Fleming and B.S. Weir (eds.), *Proceedings of the Fourth Seattle Symposium in Biostatistics: Clinical Trials*, Lecture Notes in Statistics 1205, DOI 10.1007/978-1-4614-5245-4_3, © Springer Science+Business Media New York 2013

1 Introduction

Biomarkers are characteristics that are objectively measured and evaluated as indicators of normal or pathogenic biologic processes. There are a multitude of ways that biomarkers are used including diagnosis of disease, prognosis of clinical outcomes, patient staging and treatment selection, indication of response to a prior natural exposure, and characterization of response to a biomedical intervention.

The use of biomarkers is ubiquitous in the clinical evaluation of biomedical interventions. In this application, biomarkers are typically used as endpoints in early phase clinical trials as a means for quickly and efficiently assessing the plausibility for clinical efficacy. Biomarkers are also sometimes used in later phase clinical trials as either a component of primary clinical endpoints to increase the sensitivity to detect intervention effects or as replacements for primary clinical endpoints to increase the efficiency with which efficacy evaluations are performed. Finally, in some circumstances, biomarkers are used in pivotal efficacy trials as secondary endpoints for analyses aimed at elucidating a deeper understanding of the biological basis for efficacy that can then be used to guide development of improved intervention strategies.

In the general setting of vaccine trials for infectious diseases, the identification of biomarkers ultimately depends on the specifics of the vaccine and the pathogen. However, there are a couple elements of commonality that make it possible to discuss biomarkers quite generally for vaccine trials and each of these elements maps directly to a specific class of biomarkers.

The first element of commonality is simply the collection of interventions defined as vaccines and the associated class of biomarkers is comprised of the measured immune responses to vaccines. Prophylactic vaccines for infectious pathogens all exploit the concept of immunologic memory in that they use some part of the pathogen (or something produced by the pathogen such as a toxin) as a design prototype, delivered to the immune system to prime it in a way to produce a protective response upon subsequent exposure to the pathogen. Although complex and not completely understood, the immune response to natural infection can provide a blueprint for protection and parts of the pathogen itself provide a blueprint for vaccine design. There is an impressive catalog of protective immune responses against a variety of pathogens that are induced by natural exposure (and recovery) to the pathogen or by receipt of an FDA-approved efficacious vaccine. A systematic characterization of these protective immune responses has not been performed. Even though there are undoubtedly pathogen-specific aspects to these vaccines, it is reasonable to believe there are common aspects as well and the latter provides the potential for a knowledge base that will help solve current vaccine development problems.

The second element of commonality is the target infectious pathogen, which in this work could refer to a virus, a bacterium or a parasite, and the associated class of biomarkers is comprised of measures of the invading pathogen with respect to its presence, abundance, locality, and specificity. For our purposes, the pathogen can be characterized without reference to a human host. This makes infectious diseases conceptually distinct compared to cancer, for example. With cancer, the "pathogen" is a transformed cell but it is not a foreign invader of our body per se. It is a cell that was originally part of "us" and through a series of subtle genetic changes, joined the other team. It is quite difficult to pin down the precise event or set of events that make a cell a cancerous turncoat. Even when this is possible, the events are usually in reference to a specific individual host because of the unique genetic background within which these events occur. It is even more difficult to define the triggering causal event for metabolic diseases such as diabetes. Compare that to an infectious pathogen which is clearly "the other" from the start and engages the host in a relatively well-defined event called infection that then initiates the pathogenic process leading to disease. There is also the clear causal role that the pathogen plays. This easy grasp of causality is something that is hard to come by in other areas of biomedicine. But having said this, it is also true that the infection event is very early on in pathogenesis and any grasp on causal pathways easily slips away in getting from infection to the disease outcome.

A central use of immune response biomarkers in vaccine research is as primary endpoints for early phase vaccine trials. At one end of the spectrum, these biomarkers define the extent to which the vaccine is biologically active while at the other end they characterize the nature of the response with sufficient detail to provide some sense of the plausibility that the responses would be clinically protective.

This general theme of identification and validation of immune response biomarkers as surrogate endpoints is a specific area of interest in vaccine trials. The prospect for use of such biomarkers as surrogate endpoints in vaccine trials is particularly intriguing because the causal pathway to an infectious disease goes through a well-defined pathogen and that measurements of specific immune effector mechanisms can be made that are responsible at least in part for protection. However, there is a limit to the specificity with which pathogenesis and mechanisms of vaccine-induced protective immune responses are understood which rightfully tempers the enthusiasm for the use of surrogate endpoints in vaccine trials.

Pathogen-based biomarkers are often used as components of clinical endpoints in situations where clinical outcomes may be attributed to causes other than the pathogen targeted by vaccination. Such biomarkers can lend specificity to trial endpoints that increases sensitivity to detect meaningful vaccine effects.

A final important use of immune response and pathogen-based biomarkers in vaccine trials is the identification of clues that can help to guide the iterative development of vaccines. Modern vaccines are constructed as molecular machines that can potentially be reengineered to tailor the immune response in a way that can improve upon immune responses and increase protective efficacy. Analyses of immune response biomarkers to identify the quality and/or quantity of specific immune responses that are predictive of vaccine-induced protection and pathogen-based biomarkers to identify differential vaccine efficacy across a landscape of antigenic variation can provide exactly such guidance for improved vaccine design.

2   Immune Response to Vaccines

Measurements of immune response, together with safety, are the standard primary endpoints for early phase vaccine trials. There is a basic logic that connects these measurements of immune response to vaccine to subsequent vaccine-induced protection, which is simply that immune responses to the vaccine will be generally recapitulated upon subsequent exposure to a pathogen. The technical aspects of these assays may vary but they generally expose a biological specimen to an antigen preparation and then measure a response relative to that without such exposure. For example, antibody responses in serum may be measured for their ability to bind to antigen or to functionally interfere with the pathogen life-cycle (neutralization) in vitro; cellular responses in peripheral blood may be measured for the ability of CD4+ and/or CD8+ T-lymphocytes to produce cytokine and chemokine molecules involved in their protective responses to infection in response to exposure to peptide or protein antigens. The collection of these assays has the potential to ascertain basic reactivity ("take"), type of response (e.g., humoral, cellular, innate), specificity of response (e.g., to level of pathogen, strain, protein, epitope), and magnitude of response. They can provide a remarkably detailed (albeit biologically quite incomplete) profile of immune response.

A primary use of these immune response measurements is to assess the plausibility for efficacy of a vaccine candidate either in absolute terms or relative to that for another candidate in a setting where clinical efficacy has not yet been directly established. The reliability and interpretability of these immunogenicity studies is critical as important decisions are based on them. Decisions to drop a candidate vaccine from continued development might be made if immune responses to the vaccine do not meet criteria to make clinically significant efficacy plausible; decisions to drop one of two candidate vaccines and advance the other in clinical development might be made based on comparison of their immune response profiles. Although the immediate clinical consequences of such decisions are not high, the long-term consequences of making erroneous choices can be significant.

A specific cautionary tale in this regard is the direct comparison of immune responses and clinical efficacy of a 2-component and a 5-component acellular pertussis vaccines [1], which found a clear ordering of the vaccines in binding antibody responses to two key antigens (pertussis toxin, filamentous hemagglutinin) and a clear but opposite ordering of the vaccines in directly measured clinical efficacy. A somewhat extreme example of the use of immune responses to assess plausibility of clinical efficacy is the accelerated approval process for vaccines used by the US FDA. In this case, plausibility for clinical efficacy may be deemed so high based on demonstrated immune responses as to grant a provisional license for the vaccine subject to completion of a future trial to directly characterize clinical efficacy.

A second important use of these measurements occurs when vaccine efficacy has been established in one setting and prediction of vaccine efficacy in another setting is needed. This "bridging" function of immune responses to vaccines is used in support of a variety of different types of decisions. For example, comparability of immune responses across different production lots of vaccine or from a current to a new method of vaccine production is used to predict comparability of clinical efficacy across lots [2] or from old to new production methods [3]. Another example of bridging is the use of demonstrated non-inferiority in immune responses and safety to a currently licensed vaccine as the basis for licensure under the US accelerated approval regulations. Comparability of antibody responses in the serum hemagglutination-inhibition assay (HA) to the licensed influenza vaccine for seasonal flu was the basis for the recent licensure of Fluarix [4].

Immune responses are also used to bridge vaccine efficacy across populations. For example, clinical efficacy of the two currently licensed HPV vaccines was established in randomized controlled trials performed in young adult women (age 15–25 for Cervarix, age 16–26 for Guardasil). Equivalence in immune responses to vaccines specific for each of the serotypes in the vaccine formulations was the basis for bridging efficacy observed in young women to adolescent girls [5, 6]. An important cautionary tale for bridging across populations may be found in the development of vaccines for genital herpes where comparable immune responses to a glycoprotein-D-adjuvant vaccine were found for men and women while clinical outcomes differed with substantial vaccine efficacy observed in women (estimated to be 73%) but no efficacy observed among men.

Probably the most extreme example of using immune responses to bridge clinical efficacy is the "animal rule" developed by the US FDA for licensure of vaccines for highly lethal pathogens for which human efficacy trials are impossible. Under this regulation, vaccines may be licensed based on clinical efficacy and immunogenicity data obtained in animal models combined with human safety and immunogenicity data (as described in the US FDA Code of Federal Regulations CFR 21 314.600). A strong and quite interesting case has been made for licensure of a vaccine for Ebola virus under the animal rule [7], but no vaccine has been licensed as yet due to lack of market incentives. Efforts to develop of a new generation anthrax vaccine via the animal rule are in a similar state.

A third important use of immune response biomarkers is for guiding new vaccine designs that will improve upon designs that are only partly efficacious. In this iterative model of vaccine development, specific immune responses to a partly efficacious vaccine are empirically related to vaccine-induced protection. These associations generate hypotheses that higher levels of clinical efficacy would obtain for a new vaccine design that amplifies those specific responses. The new recombinant genomic and other molecular techniques that can be used to design and construct novel immunogens provide the ability to deliver new vaccine constructs targeting different immune response profiles in a way that was impossible for previous generation vaccine developers [8]. Thus, vaccinologists are increasingly able to execute this program when suitable leads are provided from analyses relating immune responses to vaccine efficacy. Even though this use of immune response biomarkers is quite different than their use as surrogate endpoints for bridging vaccine efficacy, the analytic program to evaluate immune responses as surrogates is essentially the same as would be used for this hypothesis generation.

A framework for the empirical assessment of immune responses as surrogates or predictors of vaccine efficacy [9] distinguished correlates of risk (CoR) from surrogates of protection (SoP). In this framework, a CoR is defined as an immune response to vaccine that is related to the rate or level of a study endpoint used to measure efficacy in a defined population (established using statistical regression modeling). An SoP is defined as an immune response that is a CoR within a defined population of vaccinees that is also predictive of vaccine efficacy in specific analyses that contrast patterns of risk and its relationship to immune response between vaccines and placebo recipients. Two general approaches for evaluating an SoP in the setting of a single efficacy trial have been described. First is the direct application of the Prentice Criterion for surrogacy [10]. A second more recent approach is based on the causal inference framework of principal stratification [11].

Specific statistical designs and analytic methods for the causal inference approach involve collection of additional information to augment the basic data obtained in the efficacy trial [12]. This additional information includes baseline measurements from the entire study cohort that is predictive of immune responses to vaccine and immune responses to vaccine delivered to the control group subjects at the end of the trial follow-up period. The causal estimand in these methods is the vaccine efficacy conditional on the (counterfactual) immune response if a subject were to be vaccinated. Conceptually, this is the degree of protection conferred by the vaccine to an individual with a given measured immune response to vaccination.

Neither the Prentice Criterion nor the causal inference approach formally addresses the problem of bridging efficacy to a different setting. For this problem, a meta-analytic approach is proposed [9] based on earlier more general work [13–15] that requires data from multiple vaccine efficacy trials selected to reflect the variation over which efficacy is to be bridged.

Example: Herpes zoster (shingles) is characterized by a vesicular rash and associated pain caused by reactivation of latent varicella-zoster virus (VZV) within sensory ganglia. The original VZV infection typically occurs during childhood and causes the well-known condition called "chicken pox." The incidence and severity of shingles, along with the rate of debilitating long-term complications (postherpetic neuralgia), increase with advancing age. The pain and discomfort associated with shingles can be prolonged and disabling with impact on quality of life and ability to function to a degree comparable to that of congestive heart failure, myocardial infarction, type 2 diabetes, and major depression. The age-related increase in incidence and severity of disease was observed to be correlated with the corresponding age-related decline in VZV-specific T-cell responses while VZV-specific antibody responses, which do not decline with age, appeared to not play a significant role. Moreover, shingles was observed to more frequently occur in circumstances with VZV-specific cellular responses were depressed such as cancer patients undergoing bone marrow transplantation. These observations led to the hypothesis that a vaccine which induced a strong VZV-specific cellular immune response could prevent the occurrence and severity of shingles.

A live, attenuated VZV vaccine was developed that induced a strong cellular and antibody responses to VZV as measured by interferon-γ enzyme-linked immunospot (ELISPOT) assay and enzyme-linked immunosorbent assay against VZV glycoproteins (gpELISA), respectively. In an evaluation of immune responses to VZV conducted as a substudy of a shingles vaccine efficacy trial, the age-dependence of VZV-specific cellular responses but not VZV-specific antibody responses was confirmed using pre-vaccination samples and the vaccine induced both cellular and antibody responses measured 6 weeks post-vaccination that were significantly greater in magnitude than those observed among placebo recipients [16]. These observations strongly supported the plausibility for efficacy of the vaccine. However, the absolute magnitude of cellular responses to vaccine was seen to decline with increasing age of the vaccinee raising the prospect that vaccine efficacy may itself be age-dependent. The estimated vaccine efficacy from the parent efficacy trial [17] was 61% for a burden-of-illness endpoint, 66% for postherpetic neuralgia endpoint and 51% for shingles endpoint. Interestingly, the vaccine efficacy for shingles among subjects 70 years or older was only 38% compared to 64% among subjects younger than 70 years. Thus, the prospect for age-dependent vaccine efficacy suggested from trends in VZV-specific cellular immune responses was realized in this direct evaluation of efficacy.

Cellular and antibody immune responses to vaccine measured 6 weeks post-vaccination were assessed as correlates of risk using a case–control study design nested within the vaccine efficacy trial. Both types VZV-specific immune responses to vaccination were found to be significantly associated with subsequent risk for shingles [16]. Although statistically significant, the strength of association was not strong enough to provide a good predictor of the potential protective effect of vaccination. A similar analysis was performed using samples obtained at the last study visit before the diagnosis of shingles and at comparable times for controls matched to each shingles case [18]. In this analysis, the status of VZV-specific cellular immune response was associated with risk for shingles while VZV-specific antibody responses were not.

Subsequent to demonstration of vaccine efficacy, VZV-specific immune responses were used in a bridging study to demonstrate comparable immunogenicity of a frozen formulation and a refrigerator-stable formulation of the vaccine [19] Interestingly, VZV-specific antibody responses were used as the basis for this bridging study even though VZV-specific cellular responses are thought to be the key to protective efficacy of the vaccine.

3 Presence and Specificity of the Target Pathogen

The link between the clinical outcome of interest in a vaccine trial and a pathogen that is targeted by a vaccine is not always one to one. Multiple pathogens may cause the same clinical syndrome while only a single pathogen may be targeted by the vaccine; a single pathogen may exhibit antigenic variability and only a subset of antigenic types may be targeted by the vaccine; the pathogen may exhibit genetic variability that is not obviously reflected in a discrete set of antigenic types so that it is unclear what pathogen types might be "covered" by the vaccine. In these cases, a clinical efficacy endpoint is typically augmented with a biomarker-based assessment of whether the endpoint is associated with (or attributable to) a specific variant (genetic, antigenic) of the pathogen. The pathogen identity associated with a clinical endpoint may be called a "mark."

The mark that annotates a clinical endpoint might be binary, simply encoding whether the pathogen is of the "vaccine type" (VT) or "non-vaccine-type" (NVT), and vaccine efficacy is reported in primary analyses of vaccine trials as the degree of protection against VT pathogens. The mark may also be complex including multiple antigenic and/or genetic types of the pathogen; in the extreme, the mark might include the entire genomic sequence of the pathogen. The addition of a biomarker-based mark to the clinical endpoint provides specificity of vaccine effects on the pathogens explicitly targeted by the vaccine. However if multiple pathogens or non-vaccine types of the target pathogen are also associated with clinical outcomes, then the true clinical impact the vaccine at the population level can be obfuscated by primary reporting of type-specific outcomes. Variable vaccine efficacy across types, shifts in the prevalence of types over time and interference amongst types can all contribute to complexity that may be the subject of secondary explanatory analyses of type-specific outcomes.

Biomarkers specifying pathogen type associated with clinical endpoints can form the basis for exploratory analyses to generate specific hypotheses for improving the design of vaccines with partial efficacy just as the aforementioned analyses of immune responses as surrogates of protection. In this approach, the antigenic and/or genetic variation of pathogens that is captured in the endpoint marks is explored for gradients in mark-specific vaccine efficacy. Generally, pathogen types that are more likely to be immunologically cross-reactive with the vaccine antigens are expected to have high mark-specific vaccine efficacy; those pathogen types less likely to be cross-reactive with vaccine antigens are expected to have lower mark-specific vaccine efficacy. This notion gives rise to the concept of immunologically relevant distance and the methods of sieve analysis [20–24], which aim to characterize gradients in vaccine efficacy along distances computed from pathogen-specific marks and vaccine antigens using data from vaccine efficacy trials.

Although the basic statistical framework for sieve analysis has changed little from its inception, there have been considerable increases in the sophistication of immunologically relevant distances used. Advances in the informatics of immunology [25] have delivered predictors of vaccine-responsive CD4+ and CD8+ T-cell epitopes conditional on the HLA genotype of the vaccine that are being used to construct distances for exploring vaccine targets of protective cellular immune responses. Advances in structural biology and associated computational modeling have provided predictions for loci of interactions between vaccine-induced antibodies and the surface of target pathogen proteins and structures (scaffolds) that can be used to test these predictions [26]. These advances are being used to focus sieve analyses on highly specific regions of a pathogen's proteome to explore vaccine targets of protective antibody responses. These and other methods such as the peptide microarray [27] have also been used to add specificity to immune response assays so that sieve analyses can be further focused on specific regions of the pathogen proteome to which specific vaccine responses are directed. Suppose an immune response to vaccine directed at a specific locus in the pathogen proteome is shown to be a correlate of risk. Then additional evidence that the immune response may also be a surrogate of protection can be provided by a sieve analyses focused on the same site that show gradients in vaccine efficacy are associated with variation at that site.

The following examples serve to illustrate some of the aforementioned ideas.

Example 1: Rotavirus-associated acute gastroenteritis (rAGE) is a significant burden of mortality in children worldwide accounting for nearly two million deaths annually. Nearly all of these deaths occur in developing countries where life-saving rehydration therapy for severe diarrhea is not readily available. There are multiple causes of acute gastroenteritis (AGE) and, in the course of regular annual epidemics, rotavirus accounts for about 1/3 of all such deaths. There are two rotavirus vaccines, each containing multiple antigens that cover the major rotavirus serotypes that are highly efficacious in preventing severe rAGE in the developed world. However these vaccines are only 30–40% efficacious in the developing world where the disease burden is so high. Thus, even though there are two licensed vaccines, rotavirus vaccine research is still an important and active field.

In rotavirus vaccine trials, endpoints are defined as clinical diagnosis of severe AGE together with presence/absence of rotavirus in the stool and, if present, the viral serotype and genotype. Primary efficacy outcomes are stated in terms of vaccine-related reduction in rates of rAGE, serotype-specific rAGE and overall AGE. The vaccines contain multiple antigens that cover the major rotavirus serotypes.

Results on incidence of rAGE reported in 2008 from a Phase III vaccine trial of GSK's vaccine Rotarix conducted in Latin America [28] demonstrate relatively high levels of efficacy (around 80%), which are greater than those observed in trials conducted in developing countries throughout Africa and Asia but less than those in the developed world. Vaccine efficacy to prevent serotype-specific rAGE ranges from below 40% to over 80%. Moreover, the frequency distribution of serotypes was observed to shift considerably over the two-year follow-up period of the trial. These shifts from year to year may be due to natural variation in circulating strains of virus, may be by differential efficacy of the vaccine across serotypes and may be due to interactions amongst the different serotypes and their relation to vaccine-induced immune responses. Thus, the specificity provided by the biomarker annotation of clinical endpoints allows more precise focus on the specific vaccine effects on clinical outcomes and also raises questions about how to define endpoints and design trials that will deal with heterogeneity in efficacy across types, temporal variation in the distribution of types and the potential interaction between the two.

Example 2: There are 30–40 different types of human papilloma virus (HPV) that are sexually transmitted and infect epithelial cells in the cervix. Most (90%)

infections in young females are naturally cleared within 2–3 years but when persistent infection occurs with any one of about 14 "oncogenic" types, there is a high risk for development of precancerous lesions that can then progress to cervical cancer over a 10- to 20-year time period. There are two licensed HPV vaccines containing antigens from HPV 16 and 18 which are two of the oncogenic types and are associated with approximately 70% of all cervical cancers. Because the time course is so long to observe cervical cancer outcomes, the surrogate endpoint of precancerous lesions has been used as the primary endpoint in vaccine efficacy trials. Specifically, the clinical endpoint used in vaccine efficacy trials was a histological diagnosis of cervical intra-epithelial neoplasia of grade 2 or higher (CIN2+) annotated with presence/absence and type of HPV DNA in the cervical lesion.

Women were enrolled in an efficacy trial of the GSK vaccine Cervarix regardless of their HPV DNA status, HPV serostatus and cytology at baseline. The trial was conducted in 14 countries, the trial outcomes were reported in a subset of women who were HPV16/18 negative at baseline and vaccine efficacy was assessed relative to rates of HPV16/18-associated CIN2+, any CIN2+ and non-vaccine HPV type-specific CIN2+. Estimates of overall vaccine efficacy for types 16 and/or 18 were 87–92% depending on the specific combination of VT HPV in the lesion [29]. When considering all oncogenic HPV types (both VT and NVT), the efficacy ranges from 37 to 62% depending on the pattern of co-infection. As you might expect, the lower levels of efficacy are associated with lesions that contain any oncogenic HPV type except for HPV16/18. Vaccine efficacy also depends on baseline patterns of co-infection across the various HPV types.

In addition to age and the complexity of type-specific infection, absolute risk of CIN2+ depends strongly on the duration of persistence of HPV infection. The vaccine is highly efficacious in reducing rates of persistent HPV 16/18 infection (over 6 and 12 months) and has variable efficacy (from 0% to 60%) for non-16/18 oncogenic types [30]. Given the vagaries of histological diagnosis of CIN2, questions have been posed (but not yet answered) about whether persistent infection with oncogenic-type HPV is a better prognostic biomarker than a diagnosis of CIN2 for cervical cancer risk and maybe a better surrogate endpoint than CIN2 for vaccine trials.

4 Summary

Biomarkers are an integral component of clinical vaccine research and development. Two central classes of biomarkers are immune response to vaccine and presence/identity of pathogens associated with clinical endpoints. They are used as endpoints in Phase I/II trials to guide early clinical development and as components of clinical endpoints to increase sensitivity to detect vaccine effects. They are also used as the basis for explanatory analyses when there are multiple etiologies of the clinical outcome, and/or there is important antigenic variation in the pathogen. Both biomarkers are used in more controversial ways involving surrogate biomarker-based endpoints to predict efficacy in settings where no direct evaluation of vaccine efficacy is available. The most promising use of these biomarkers is in the generation of hypotheses for improving designs of partly protective vaccines in a program of iterative vaccine development. Concepts of causal inference and analytic methods for the evaluation of surrogate endpoints are directly applicable to this work and are active areas of methodologic research. The integration of multiple scientific disciplines (immunology, structural biology, genomics, microbiology, statistics) is resulting in novel approaches to sieve analyses that lend additional power and specificity especially when directly linked with analyses of immune correlates of risk and surrogates of protection.

References

1. Gustafsson L, Hallander HO et al (1996) A controlled trial of a two-component acellular, a five-component acellular, and a whole-cell pertussis vaccine. N Engl J Med 334(6):349–355
2. Arnou R, Eavis P et al (2010) Immunogenicity, large scale safety and lot consistency of an intradermal influenza vaccine in adults aged 18–60 years randomized, controlled, phase III trial. Hum Vaccin 6(4):346–354
3. Pfister M, Kursteiner O et al (2005) Immunogenicity and safety of BERNA-YF compared with two other 17D yellow fever vaccines in a phase 3 clinical trial. Am J Trop Med Hyg 72(3): 339–346
4. Campbell JD, Chambers CV et al (2011) Immunologic non-inferiority of a newly licensed inactivated trivalent influenza vaccine versus an established vaccine A randomized study in US adults. Hum Vaccin 7(1):81–88
5. Block SL, Nolan T et al (2006) Comparison of the immunogenicity and reactogenicity of a prophylactic quadrivalent human papillomavirus (types 6, 11, 16, and 18) L1 virus-like particle vaccine in male and female adolescents and young adult women. Pediatrics 118(5):2135–2145
6. Keam SJ, Harper DM (2008) Human papillomavirus types 16 and 18 vaccine (Recombinant, AS04 adjuvanted, adsorbed) [Cervarix (TM)]. Drugs 68(3):359–372
7. Sullivan NJ, Martin JE et al (2009) Correlates of protective immunity for Ebola vaccines: implications for regulatory approval by the animal rule. Nat Rev Microbiol 7(5):393–400
8. Rappuoli R, Black S et al (2011) New Decade of Vaccines 2 Vaccine discovery and translation of new vaccine technology. Lancet 378(9788):360–368
9. Qin L, Gilbert PB et al (2007) A framework for assessing immunological correlates of protection in vaccine trials. J Infect Dis 196(9):1304–1312
10. Prentice RL (1989) Surrogate endpoints in clinical-trials – definition and operational criteria. Stat Med 8(4):431–440
11. Frangakis CE, Rubin DB (2002) Principal stratification in causal inference. Biometrics 58(1):21–29
12. Follmann D (2006) Augmented designs to assess immune response in vaccine trials. Biometrics 62(4):1161–1169
13. Daniels MJ, Hughes MD (1997) Meta-analysis for the evaluation of potential surrogate markers. Stat Med 16(17):1965–1982
14. De Gruttola VG, Clax P et al (2001) Considerations in the evaluation of surrogate endpoints in clinical trials: summary of a National Institutes of Health Workshop. Control Clin Trials 22(5):485–502
15. Hughes MD (2002) Evaluating surrogate endpoints. Control Clin Trials 23(6):703–707

16. Levin MJ, Oxman MN et al (2008) Varicella-zoster virus-specific immune responses in elderly recipients of a herpes zoster vaccine. J Infect Dis 197(6):825–835
17. Oxman MN, Levin MJ et al (2005) A vaccine to prevent herpes zoster and postherpetic neuralgia in older adults. N Engl J Med 352(22):2271–2284
18. Weinberg A, Zhang JH et al (2009) Varicella-zoster virus-specific immune responses to herpes zoster in elderly participants in a trial of a clinically effective zoster vaccine. J Infect Dis 200(7):1068–1077
19. Gilderman LI, Lawless JF et al (2008) A double-blind, randomized, controlled, multicenter safety and immunogenicity study of a refrigerator-stable formulation of Zostavax. Clin Vaccine Immunol 15(2):314–319
20. Gilbert PB, Self SG et al (1998) Statistical methods for assessing differential vaccine protection against human immunodeficiency virus types. Biometrics 54(3):799–814
21. Gilbert PB, Lele SR et al (1999) Maximum likelihood estimation in semiparametric selection bias models with application to AIDS vaccine trials. Biometrika 86(1):27–43
22. Gilbert P, Self S et al (2001) Sieve analysis: methods for assessing from vaccine trial data how vaccine efficacy varies with genotypic and phenotypic pathogen variation. J Clin Epidemiol 54(1):68–85
23. Gilbert PB (2000) Large sample theory of maximum likelihood estimates in semiparametric biased sampling models. Ann Stat 28(1):151–194
24. Gilbert PB (2001) Interpretability and robustness of sieve analysis models for assessing HIV strain variations in vaccine efficacy. Stat Med 20(2):263–279
25. Sirskyj D, Diaz-Mitoma F et al (2011) Innovative bioinformatic approaches for developing peptide-based vaccines against hypervariable viruses. Immunol Cell Biol 89(1):81–89
26. Correia BE, Ban YEA et al (2010) Computational design of epitope-scaffolds allows induction of antibodies specific for a poorly immunogenic HIV vaccine epitope. Structure 18(9): 1116–1126
27. Reimer U, Reineke U et al (2011) Peptide arrays for the analysis of antibody epitope recognition patterns. Mini Rev Org Chem 8(2):137–146
28. Linhares AC, Velazquez FR et al (2008) Efficacy and safety of an oral live attenuated human rotavirus vaccine against rotavirus gastroenteritis during the first 2 years of life in Latin American infants: a randomised, double-blind, placebo-controlled phase III study. Lancet 371(9619):1181–1189
29. Paavonen J (2010). "Efficacy of human papillomavirus (HPV)-16/18AS04-adjuvanted vaccine against cervical infection and precancer caused by oncogenic HPV types (PATRICIA): final analysis of a double-blind, randomised study in young women (vol 374, p 301, 2009)." Lancet 376(9746):1054
30. Rodriguez AC, Schiffman M et al (2010) Longitudinal study of human papillomavirus persistence and cervical intraepithelial neoplasia grade 2/3: critical role of duration of infection. J Natl Cancer Inst 102(5):315–324

Part II
Biomarkers: Issues in Individualized Therapy

Recent Developments in the Use of Clinical Trials to Support Individualizing Therapies: A Regulatory Perspective

Robert T. O'Neill

Abstract This chapter covers a broad range of issues centered around the topic of optimizing therapies for individuals and the role of the clinical trial in reaching that goal. We describe how the clinical trial has been increasingly relied upon to provide the evidence for the patient level or patient marker level differential benefit or risk of therapies and how the study design choices can change depending upon the various study objectives. We consider the definition and role of prognostic and predictive classifiers or markers in the different clinical trial designs used for selecting and evaluating enriched study populations, and the difference between the retrospective and prospective approaches to evaluating differential treatment effects among marker subgroups. Some examples are given to illustrate the issues. Two of the most challenging aspects of identifying and validating a predictive marker are the simultaneous need to quantify the performance characteristics (sensitivity and specificity) of the classifier and the choice of whether the study design should include all comers or selection of the marker positive only subgroup. The motivation for these clinical trial approaches to individualizing therapy is to maximize the benefits and minimize the safety risks of therapies for patients.

1 Introduction

The interest in development of new therapies, particularly new drugs tailored to address an individual patient's needs and characteristics, sometimes expressed as personalized medicine, is increasing the expectations for a clinical trial to fulfill that evidentiary standard. We have seen growth in targeted therapies in oncology and a renewed interest in the use of biomarkers not so much as surrogate markers,

R.T. O'Neill (✉)
Office of Biostatistics, FDA Center for Drug Evaluation and Research,
10903 New Hampshire Avenue, Silver Spring, MD 20993-0002, USA
e-mail: Robert.ONeill@fda.hhs.gov

T.R. Fleming and B.S. Weir (eds.), *Proceedings of the Fourth Seattle Symposium in Biostatistics: Clinical Trials*, Lecture Notes in Statistics 1205, DOI 10.1007/978-1-4614-5245-4_4, © Springer Science+Business Media New York 2013

but as classifiers of a patient's potential response to a treatment. The regulatory interest in this area is focused on the development of evidence of efficacy and safety of medical products, primarily through controlled clinical trials, so that these products can be labeled with indications for use that optimizes the benefit and risk profile of a product. This emerging interest in optimization of product exposure may involve differential recommendations or warnings that depend upon the individual characteristics of a subpopulation or of an individual in the subpopulation exposed to the product.

As advances in genomics and cell biology increase, so have the opportunities for the rational design of targeted therapies to inhibit or enhance the function of specific molecules with the result that targeted therapies may offer a patient improved efficacy or, as selectivity increases, less toxicity. The randomized controlled clinical trial is the primary experimental vehicle to establish the efficacy and safety of new medical products; so it is necessary that the clinical trial be designed to provide the necessary evidence to support individualization of medical product use.

This article covers a broad range of issues centered around the topic of optimizing therapies for individuals and the role of the clinical trial in reaching that goal. The article is organized into ten sections, the second section dealing with a conceptual definition of individualized therapy. Sections 3 and 4 cover the distinction between prognostic and predictive markers; Sect. 6 provides several current examples of clinical trials whose results bear on individualizing therapy. Section 5 points out the relationship of individual therapy optimization to the generalizability of clinical trial results conducted globally. Sections 7 and 8 are about individual treatment response as a subgroup type problem with issues like replication of evidence in subgroups and imbalances in prognostic factors in subgroups. Section 9 briefly addresses a trial design challenge when time-dependent genetic changes may occur, and finally in Sect. 10 there is a brief summary of current targeted therapy clinical trial designs that have been proposed in the literature.

2 A Definition of Individualized Therapy

We will focus on new drugs and pharmaceutical agents in this article. Every pharmaceutical compound whether it be a biological or a chemical compound has a structure and makeup that contributes to the intended and unintended effects on a patient exposed to that compound. There are properties of the compound itself, and characteristics of the patients, each of which can interact and contribute to a variety of different patient responses observed or experienced. For example, if a patient cannot metabolize a drug taken through a route of administration, then generally the drug will not have its intended pharmacological effect(s) and such a patient may not be able to benefit from the drug, yet may share any risks or side effects associated with the exposure. Depending upon a patient's genetic makeup, he/she may be a slow, intermediate, or fast metabolizer of a drug, in which case, some individuals may or may not respond to the drug at the assigned dose. Depending upon the patient's individual ability to metabolize a drug, the same dosage level administered to three patients with differential metabolizer characteristics may provide three different blood levels thereby yielding three different clinical responses simply because patients are on different parts of the dose response curve. If the target for the drug is resistant or nonresponsive to the therapy, then the intended therapeutic effect is neutralized or minimized, such as is the case with some tumors in oncology. If a patient possesses a genomic marker that has been identified as predictive of clinical response to the drug, then a patient with the marker, now called a predictive marker, may have a better response to the drug than a patient without the marker. These are simply a few examples to help define the concept of individualized therapy targeted to an individual's characteristics or to the characteristics of a subgroup to which that person belongs or is classified. Thus, the concept of individualized therapy as it is being used in clinical trials is about the relationship of relative treatment response or treatment effect to a patient's covariates, and not as much about the prognostic relationship of patient outcomes related to covariates in a nontreated cohort.

3 A Rich Statistical History of Modeling and Identifying Risk Factors Associated with Differential Outcomes: Response Or Risk

Over the years there has been an extensive statistical literature developed on the methods for modeling and identifying factors associated with an individual's probability of having an outcome. This literature has been developed within the context of long-term single cohort follow-up studies and within the context of randomized clinical trials evaluating differential subgroup responses. Armitage and Gehan [1] in 1974 proposed statistical methods for the identification and use of prognostic factors; in 1980 Byar and Green [2] and Byar and Corle [3] proposed methods to choose treatment for cancer patients based on covariate information. In 1989, Gail et al. [4] proposed a model for projecting individualized probabilities of developing breast cancer for white females who are being examined annually, an approach that was eventually used as entrance criteria for clinical trials and eligibility for treatment. In 2003, Pepe et al. [5] considered the limitations of the odds ratio metric in gauging the performance of a diagnostic, prognostic, or screening marker. In 2006, Ware [6] reinforced this concept by discussing the limitations of risk factors as prognostic tools in a comment on Wang et al. [7], who considered whether multiple biomarkers for the prediction (note: term prognostic should have been used) of first major cardiovascular events and death might be an improvement over single biomarkers. All of these approaches and strategies are about relating a patient's outcomes to a function of that patient's covariates, usually considered as prognostic markers or factors. However, the problem we are facing today with the use of clinical trials to establish differential efficacy or safety in prespecified marker populations is somewhat different, as discussed below.

4 Prediction and Predictive Factors in Randomized Clinical Trials

Prediction of a patient's response to a particular treatment, as it is considered in the design and analysis of controlled clinical trials, requires that we distinguish between which markers associated with a subject are prognostic of disease outcome and which are predictive of treatment effect. Generally, the term prognostic has been used to imply an association with an outcome in a single cohort, as, for example, elevated blood pressure or cholesterol levels being prognostic of 5-year cardiovascular events. The term predictiveness is associated with the treatment effect, a relative concept, requiring a comparison of the treatment group with a control group with the same covariates or in the same subgroup. So one way to think about the distinction between prognostic and predictive biomarkers is to characterize the former as a single sample non-comparative problem, and the latter as a two-sample comparative problem where the prediction is with regard to a relative treatment effect, not just an outcome event or a response.

Considered in this way, a biomarker or classifying factor could be both prognostic and predictive at the same time. With regard to the impact of these concepts on the design, analysis, and inferences from clinical trials, proposals for clinical trial enrichment designs are emerging where the clinical trial is being enriched with subjects who are classified as having a marker expected to be predictive of enhanced treatment effect or benefit. This concept introduces a variety of eligible study designs. In addition, adaptive designs, which can prospectively adapt the mix of patient types selected into the trial depending upon patients' treatment response during the trial and thereby to change the sample size of the trial accordingly, are also being considered. Within these two frameworks, the emphasis seems to focus on type 1 error control in a controlled trial to account for the multiple subgroup hypotheses and the different strategies for declaring a trial successful. The genomic revolution has also contributed to using the clinical trial to search for and identify biomarkers which are predictive of treatment response so that the identified marker can be used to classify subjects into subgroups which the form the basis for the multiple subgroup hypotheses for treatment effects that are then considered. Biomarkers are not always well defined in advance of conducting a study; or, their sensitivity and specificity characteristics are not well known or studied prior to the conduct of a clinical trial. So the additional task of validation or qualification of the biomarker may be a new important feature of the design of a clinical trial, especially when this information is not known or well characterized prior to the trial being conducted. This issue raises a very interesting dialogue regarding retrospective vs. prospective study designs and validation strategies.

For the newer targeted therapy designs, the statistical framework seems to have changed from using covariates as prognostic factors for outcomes where the design and analysis of the trial incorporates a plan to adjust for them and where subgroups identified by these covariates are evaluated for heterogeneity of treatment effects using statistical tests of interactions that are known to have very low statistical power to detect differential treatment effects. Rather the statistical framework seems to have moved towards planning for differential treatment effects as functions of predictive factors and towards the trial including multiple hypotheses associated with each subgroup wherein each of these subgroup hypotheses has an acceptable "win" criteria achieved by allocation of the overall study type 1 error to these multiple hypotheses in a prospective statistical analysis plan in the protocol. For example, the acceptable win criteria might be for a demonstration of treatment effect in the enriched subset of patients only, or in the overall all comers (i.e., an unselected population) population, in a nested subset of a super enriched population or some other combinations. These potential inferences raise interesting considerations for the study design for sample sizing the trial, for planned detection of treatment effect sizes overall and in the enriched subset, and for the minimum sample size in the marker negative groups to rule out that a treatment effect does not exist in that subgroup.

5 A Related Topic: Dealing with Differential Treatment Response Associated with Ethnic Factors: The Role of the ICH E5 Guidance on Acceptance of Foreign Clinical Data

While not well known outside of the regulatory environment, since 1991 regulators and the pharmaceutical industry representatives from the European Union, Japan, and the USA have been working to harmonize procedures worldwide to make global drug development more efficient and predictable. One aspect of this effort relates to the acceptability as well as generalizability of clinical trial data and results of efficacy evaluations of therapies studied in these clinical trials when they are submitted to regulators in different regions of the world. Of particular relevance to the question of generalizability or extrapolation of treatment effects to different subpopulations is the concept of intrinsic and extrinsic ethnic factors and their impact on differential treatment responses and treatment effects, as discussed in depth in the Guidance on Ethnic Factors in the Acceptability of Foreign Clinical Data [8].

The ICH E5 guidance discusses the exploration of treatment effect differences as a function of both intrinsic factors and extrinsic factors. Intrinsic factors could be genetically based, gender based, or individual person level covariate based. Extrinsic factors could be the medical environment in which the trial was conducted or other geographically related behavioral practices or diet differences among countries or regions that would impact observed treatment effects. In a Questions and Answers addendum to the Guidance, the concept of a multiregional clinical trial to support evidence of efficacy and safety in different regulatory regions was introduced as a mechanism to support bridging data from one ethnic or regional location to another. A multiregional clinical trial is a multicenter clinical trial that is conducted in several regulatory regions of the world using a common study design and protocol (e.g. outcomes and entrance criteria) that is followed by all investigators and study participants. The multiregional clinical trial is intended to provide evidence of efficacy of a treatment that would satisfy the requirements of each regional regulatory body. Thus, it is reasonable to ask how much heterogeneity in regional treatment effects may be considered acceptable.

The objectives for a multiregional clinical trial, as described in ICH E5 impact the clinical trial design and its analysis in ways that have yet to be fully appreciated, discussed, or implemented. For example, as stated in ICH E5 the objectives of such a study are to (1) show that a treatment is effective in the region where the trial was conducted and (2) compare the results of the study between regions with the intent of establishing that the treatment is not sensitive to ethnic factors so that the data could be extrapolated or bridged to the new region. The primary endpoints of the study are to be defined and acceptable to the individual regions and data on all primary endpoints are to be collected in all regions under a common protocol.

Advice in the guidance on the analysis of such a trial is minimal but it focuses on providing efficacy and safety results by region, and seeks to examine consistency of results across regions. Advice on the evaluation of the results of the study is not as simple. The guidance recognizes that it would be difficult to generalize what study results would be judged persuasive. Instead, the guidance provides a "hierarchy of persuasiveness" of evidence ranging from statistically significant standalone results of efficacy demonstrated in each region to no statistically significant regional efficacy results yet similar results across all regions that contribute to an overall positive study result. These evaluation criteria have implications for study sample sizes, stratification strategies within regions, metrics of acceptable heterogeneity or similarity of effects, etc.

With the increasing use of the multiregional clinical trial and the increase in foreign clinical trial data in global regulatory submissions, it would seem that there is now a need to place more emphasis at the study design stage of multiregional trials to prospectively anticipate acceptable levels of heterogeneity. Additionally, it would seem appropriate to anticipate when intrinsic or extrinsic factors contribute sufficient systematic variability that the individual or personal treatment effect decisions cannot be ignored. Therefore, for those study endpoints or outcomes that are likely to be systematically related to region, country, or investigator training, or might be ethnically sensitive such as patient reported outcomes, it would be advisable to plan for such anticipated differences and to design the multiregional trial accordingly.

6 Some Recent Examples of Treatment Effects Related to Individual Or Patient Level Covariates

The drug clopidogrel (Plavix) is a platelet inhibitor with several cardiovascular uses and benefits. Recently, there have been three clinical trials of this drug which serve to illustrate how individual patient considerations play a role in whether to take the drug or how to take the drug and whether there is evidence of its effectiveness under certain individual circumstances. These examples also illustrate the need for caution in drawing causality conclusions.

The first example is about whether there is a genetic interaction between a patient's genetic profile and the response to the drug. Shuldiner [9] et al. report that they found an association between the cytochrome P450 2C19 genotype with diminished platelet response to clopidogrel treatment as well as poorer cardiovascular outcomes in such patients. These investigators examined only the clopidogrel arm of the randomized trial for this conclusion. Mega et al. [10] report on their study of patients treated with clopidogrel who, if carriers of a reduced function cytochrome P450 polymorphism (CYP2C19 allele), had significantly lower levels of the active metabolite of clopidogrel, diminished platelet inhibition, and a higher rate of major adverse cardiovascular events, including stent thrombosis, than did noncarriers of the allele. Both of these examples are essentially uncontrolled single cohort studies of exposed patients where the association has been observed. In contrast, Pare et al. [11] report the results of a randomized controlled clinical trial of clopidogrel and placebo in patients with acute coronary syndromes or arterial fibrillation, in which the effect of clopidogrel as compared with placebo is consistent, irrespective of the CYP2C19 loss of function carrier status, illustrating perhaps that inferences on subgroup treatment effects associated with a marker should not be made from noncomparative randomized studies, or from the treatment only arm of a randomized trial.

The second example concerns the results of clinical studies on the effect of clopidogrel when taken with the drug omeprazole (Prilosec, Prilosec OTC). The FDA, in an information alert [12] to health-care professionals, alerted the public to new safety information concerning an interaction between clopidogrel, an anti-clotting medication, and omeprazole, a proton pump inhibitor used to reduce stomach acid. The data showed that the effectiveness of clopidogrel is reduced when taken with omeprazole. Patients at risk for heart attacks or strokes who used clopidogrel to prevent blood clots will not get the full effect of this medicine if they also are taking omeprazole. Thus, this example illustrates the interaction between two drugs and the patient level choice that needs to be made to avoid differential benefit or perhaps risk from taking these drugs alone or in combination. This finding was not identified in the initial randomized clinical studies of clopidogrel that supported marketing. Rather, randomized clinical studies performed post-approval demonstrated the individual differences in response as a function of exposure to a concomitant therapy, but the exposure to omeprazole was not randomized.

The third example concerns clopidogrel's use as a control in a randomized multiregional trial of the investigational drug ticagrelor in patients with acute coronary syndromes [13]. In this study called PLATO, the effect of ticagrelor was observed to be better than clopidogrel overall, in the randomized study population, but the treatment effect was not seen in the US population studied. The results for the primary endpoint were actually reversed in the US subpopulation, raising the question as to the reasons why and to whether the reversed effect was real or due to chance. The study results were brought to an FDA advisory committee for advice and to consider whether differential use of aspirin doses in different regions of the study might be a plausible explanation [14]. At the time of this manuscript preparation, no regulatory decision has been made on the results of this study; but this example illustrates the difficulties in drawing conclusions with regard to subject or subpopulation specific effects from a randomized clinical trial when the trial was not prospectively designed for the goal, and also illustrates the role of intrinsic and extrinsic factors as addressed in the ICH E5 Guidance discussed above, as they impact on the evaluation of individual treatment effect differences in different regulatory regions.

It is of interest to consider some of the questions about the PLATO study results posed by FDA to its Cardiovascular Advisory Committee at a publically held meeting during its evaluation of the evidence.

(http://www.fda.gov/downloads/AdvisoryCommittees/CommitteesMeeting Materials/Drugs/CardiovascularandRenalDrugsAdvisoryCommittee/UCM221380. pdf)

Question 4 to the Committee was "Do you believe that the difference in clinical outcomes between the US and the rest of the world is attributable to:"

(a) The play of chance? There is only one country out of 43 whose results fall outside the 95% confidence limits for a region having the observed number of events. If you think that chance is the most likely explanation, are you sufficiently sure of that to take the overall results to be applicable to the USA?
(b) A difference in dosing of aspirin, which is generally higher in the USA?
(c) How do you explain the apparently different effect of aspirin dose on ticagrelor and clopidogrel?

7 Replication of Results of Differential Treatment Effects in Enriched and Non-Enriched Subpopulations: Why?

Given the different clinical study designs and strategies that have been proposed to evaluate marker (enriched)-based differential treatment effects, it is important to recognize that much of our current experience deals with retrospective strategies and to a lesser extent with prospective study designs which have specific subset differences as the objective. Moreover, those issues related to the performance characteristics of the classifier used to create or identify the enriched subpopulation have not yet been fully explored in these study design proposals, and it is important to assure that any results of enhanced treatment effects associated with marker status are truly reflective of truth, and can be replicated in other independent studies. The history of observing differential subgroup findings in clinical studies that subsequently are determined to be false is well known. Replication of subgroup findings in independent studies is an important scientific principle and is especially relevant to the situation where the performance characteristics of the patient level classifier are poorly known or quantified from prior experience or prior to the conduct of the current clinical trial. Sometimes, the approach has been to collect baseline marker data on a subset of the randomized population so that one is not certain that the benefits of randomization still apply. Lack of demonstrated appropriately high sensitivity and specificity of a classifier can lead to observed attenuation of real marker treatment effect differences between marker positive and negative subgroups. Moreover, the ability to replicate a marker-specific treatment effect in a follow-on study may be impaired when doing so is a function both of the patient marker prevalence in the follow-on study and the markers' poor sensitivity and specificity performance, all of which prevents true replication of a treatment effect in an independent study. For multivariate markers whose algorithms often search for optimal cutoffs, this can lead to many false positive findings that are not able to be replicated.

Moye and Deswal [15] discussed how fragile some cardiovascular clinical trial results are because the findings are often not associated with pre-specified hypotheses for which such findings would be considered confirmatory. Specifically, they discuss examples of clinical trials whose findings were reversed upon completion of second study planned to specifically test the hypothesis generated in the first study. Some of the explanations for the unexpected findings in the initial study are that the analysis plan changed after observing the data or the investigator, after observing the study results, placed a new emphasis on a non-planned subgroup finding or on a secondary endpoint not initially intended to be primary. These practices led to false discovery claims that were not replicated in follow-up independent clinical trials. Three examples dealing with the drugs, vesnarinone, amolodipine, and losartan illustrate the issue. Ioannedes [16] as well as others [17, 18] have also put forth the provocative hypothesis that most published research findings are false and cannot be replicated, particularly discussing circumstances surrounding genomic screening studies and microarray findings that may be overstatements of the truth.

8　Potential Impact of Prognostic Factor Imbalances in Retrospectively Identified Treatment/Marker Subgroups

Current practice in many clinical trials is to routinely collect blood samples of clinical trial participants for future genotyping in order to test associations that may later be suggested by emerging data. Usually the clinical trial subject has to separately consent to this sample collection, and sometimes the sample is collected on only a subset of subjects in the trial, either because those subjects consent or because of other convenience or compliance considerations. When these samples are collected only on a subset of patients randomized to each treatment groups, this becomes a non-randomized subset of patients whose baseline prognostic profile may differ either between the consenters and the non-consenters, and/or between the treatment groups within each marker classifier category, as these patient profiles are determined by a combination of the prevalence of the marker in the trial population, the distribution of prognostic baseline factors and the proportion of subjects consenting for testing in each treatment group. The issue for analysis and predictive treatment effect inference is whether the comparison groups are balanced with regard to potential prognostic factors, as an imbalance of these alone between treatment groups could explain any observed treatment effects if the prognostic factors are strong indicators of outcome, regardless of treatment assignment. The concern for the impact of prognostic factor imbalance seems to be most for small sample sizes and for when there is a small percentage of subjects in the entire clinical trial population who have consented for blood samples. The combinations of both can impact inferences. Wang, O'Neill and Hung [19] explored this problem for four case studies and proposed a range of minimal sample sizes to minimize the probability of baseline imbalance in one or more prognostic factors. For example, for 20 subjects per treatment arm in a consented subsample, were the true prevalence of an important strong prognostic factor between 30% and 50% in each treatment group, there would be close to a 25% chance that one would observe an absolute 20% difference in the prevalence among the two treatment arms, possibly sufficient to explain an apparent treatment effect that could be observed. Once the sample sizes in each treatment arm and marker subgroup approach 100, it appears unlikely that such imbalance would be observed were there in fact no true differences in these baseline factors among the subsets. More research on this topic is needed.

9   Genetic Changes Over the Course of Treatment Or Disease Progression: Impact on Inferences and Design

The idea that one can classify a subject into some predefined response category at a particular point in time in a clinical trial, say at pretreatment baseline status, and that that classification category remains constant throughout the course of the clinical trial, especially at the molecular level is receiving some attention and exploration. In the area of oncology, the assumption that a tumor can be classified based on a single biopsy taken at a point in time, usually at the time of diagnosis may be questionable. If tumors respond to treatment exposure, even different therapies, then these changes over time may need to be taken into account especially if treatment resistance may begin to occur. It is beginning to be appreciated that both the patient and the disease (e.g., virus) may have separate genetic profiles, and it may be the interaction of both, and the time course of any changes that determines clinical outcomes. The potential need for repeat biopsies to evaluate molecular changes throughout the course of a disease or treatment has important implications for the clinical study design and analysis.

10 Study Designs to Evaluate Targeted Therapy

Clinical trial designs for targeted therapy have been receiving considerable attention in the last few years. Several authors have compiled a variety of study designs or strategies, the majority of which seem to be motivated by drug or biological development in oncology. These clinical trial designs can generally be categorized as exploratory or confirmatory, the latter category being considered for evidence in registration trials. Mandrekar and Sargent [20] discuss and evaluate various clinical trial designs and strategies for the validation of biomarker-guided therapy, covering predictive marker validation in retrospective RCTs and in prospective RCT designs. The prospective designs fall into the categories of all comers (include all disease patients unselected for marker), enrichment designs (select for marker only), hybrid designs (randomize only some subjects selected), or adaptive designs (modify design during study conduct). Friedlin, McShane and Korn [21] describe a range of study designs for biomarker evaluation, concluding that in most settings randomized biomarker stratified designs should be used to obtain rigorous assessment of the biomarker clinical utility.

Several novel designs have been proposed which intend both to identify the marker during the course of the study and to evaluate the predictiveness of the marker to make targeted personalized therapy decisions. Friedlin and Simon [22], and Friedlin, Jiang and Simon [23] have particularly been leading these efforts with a design called the adaptive signature design and the cross-validated adaptive signature design. The experience with such designs is limited but the intent is to accomplish in a single study the identification of the marker and the confirmation of the treatment effect in the marker subgroup. When one is also searching in those designs for the optimal cutoff point that will serve as the binary indicator of the marker subgroup to which a subject is classified, this design has been called a signature "threshold" design (Jiang [24]). Wang, O'Neill and Hung [25] have expanded this exploration of designs for genomic subjects into the adaptive design areas, where sample sizes may be modified, either in a marker subset or in the entire study population, but under the condition that prospective plans be in place. Some of these designs are being considered in various drug development programs.

Exploratory trials are more flexible inferentially in that often the goal is to explore many design combinations and outcome possibilities so as to choose regimens matched to patient's profile or responses that can be further evaluated in subsequent confirmatory clinical studies whose design parameters are then more focused and limited. These designs would be used in early discovery and proof-of-concept trials. The focus may be on selection of design parameters or estimation of response probabilities. Such an example is provided by I-SPY 2 [26], which is an adaptive breast cancer trial design in the setting of neoadjuvant chemotherapy. This trial is an adaptive phase II clinical trial design to target rapid, focused clinical development of paired oncologic therapies and biomarkers.

A subset of these trials that is of particular regulatory interest involves the co-development of a drug and a device, usually a diagnostic, that is used to classify or select the subjects into the study who are more likely to benefit or respond to treatment. The challenge to these trials, in addition to demonstrating efficacy of the drug in the study for the planned marker type population or subpopulation, is the additional need to characterize the performance of the diagnostic that classifies subjects in the preferred target category. The metrics of interest for the diagnostics are the sensitivity and specificity of the classifier that place subjects into subgroups likely to be responders or super responders, and the positive and negative predictive value of the classifier. Whether fully characterizing the performance of the classifier can be accomplished in a single study or rather in a sequence of studies is a topic under discussion but this is an important practical consideration for the level of evidence needed to both support evidence for biomarker classifiers used in clinical trials and their use in stratify patients into potential treatment responder groups, and finally use in clinical practice to select patients for targeted treatment. As Simon and Maitournam [27, 28] have discussed, the sensitivity and specificity of the classifier are critical measures that drive the efficiency of a classifier enriched design (sample size) as well as the choice of which design is optimal. Diagnostic products often have an additional prediction objective at the level of an individual patient's outcome in contrast to the population risk set or subset that an individual is classified into.

Some examples of the use of diagnostic tests in clinical studies are the Her 2 IHC and Her2FISH/CISH tests which appear in the product label because they were used to select the patients into the clinical trials. The indication for the Her 2 test does not state that it is a predictive marker (i.e., that it predicts differential treatment response). MammaPrint is an approved test as a "prognostic" marker for breast cancer patients for risk of distant metastases.

The example of K-ras, a marker identified as potentially predictive of treatment response of two products in patients with metastatic colorectal cancer (mCRS), illustrates how retrospective use of markers identified pre-randomization was used to infer lack of treatment response to two currently marketed cancer treatments, cetuximab and panitumamab. The strength of the predictiveness with regard to positive treatment response was less than the strength of the predictiveness with regard to lack of treatment response. In this example, the results of six clinical trials were used to make the case for the predictiveness of K-ras of treatment effect. The strength of the predictiveness was not the same for survival as for progression-free survival, and the lack of 100% ascertainment of the K-ras status of each subject in each of the trials limited the ability to make stronger statements with regard to the predictiveness of the K-ras marker as it was obtained on subsets of patients in each of the six trials with different proportions of ascertainment as well as balance of other baseline factors that would lend to comparable baseline factors allowing an unbiased comparison of response treatment.

11 Summary

The goal of this article is to describe how the clinical trial has been increasingly relied upon to provide the evidence for the patient level or patient marker level differential benefit or risk of therapies and how the study design choices can change depending upon the various study objectives. Two of the most challenging aspects of identifying and validating a predictive marker are the simultaneous need to quantify the performance characteristics (sensitivity and specificity) of the classifier and the choice of whether the study design should include all comers or selection of the marker positive only subgroup. For those studies that select all comers, i.e. Marker positive and negative subjects, an unsettled issue is how large the marker negative subgroup should be in order to conclude that there is a lack of effect in that marker negative subgroup so that one does not rule out a modest treatment effect but perhaps not the desired larger treatment effect in the marker positive subgroup.

References

1. Armitage P, Gehan EA (1974) Statistical methods for the identification and use of prognostic factors. Int J Cancer 13:16–36
2. Byar DP, Green SB (1980) The choice of treatment for cancer patients based on covariate information: application to prostate cancer. Bull Cancer (Paris) 67(4):477–490
3. Byar DP, Corle DK (1977) Selecting optimal treatment in clinical trials using covariate information. J Chronic Dis 30(9):445–459
4. Gail M, Byar et al (1989) Projecting individualized probabilities of developing breast cancer for white females who are being examined annually. J Natl Cancer Inst 81(24):1879–1886
5. Pepe MS, Janes H et al (2004) Limitation of the odds ratio in gauging the performance of a diagnostic, prognostics, or screening marker. Am J Epidemiol 159(9):882–890
6. Ware JH (2006) The limitations of risk factors as prognostic tools. N Engl J Med 355(25): 2615–2617
7. Wang TJ (2006) Multiple biomarkers for the prediction of first major cardiovascular events and death. N Engl J Med 355(25):2631–2639
8. International conference on harmonization; guidance on ethnic factors in the acceptability of foreign clinical data. Federal Register, Vol 63, No 111/ Wednesday, June 10, 1998
9. Shuldiner AR, O'Connell JR et al (2009) Association of cytomchrome P450 2C19 genotype with the antiplatelet effect and clinical efficacy of clopidogrel therapy. JAMA 302(8):849–858
10. Mega JL, Close SL et al (2009) Cytochrome P-450 polymorphisms and response to clopidogrel. N Engl J Med 360(4):354–362
11. Pare G, Mehta SR et al (2010) Effects of CYP2C19 on outcomes of clopidogreal treatment. N Engl J Med 363(18):1704–14
12. FDA Information for Healthcare Professionals: update to the labeling go Clopidogrel Bisulfate (marked as Plavix) to alert healthcare professionals about a drug interaction with omeprazole (marketed as Prilosec and Prilosec OTS), November 17, 2009

13. Wallentin L et al (2009) Ticagrelor versus clopidogrel in patients with acute coronary syndromes. N Engl J Med 361(11):1045–1057
14. FDA Cardiorenal Advisory Committee, July 28, 2010
15. Moye LA, Deswal A (2002) The fragility of cardiovascular clinical trial results. J Card Fail 8(4):247–253
16. Ioannidis JPA (2005) Why most published research findings are false. PLoS Med 2(8):e124
17. Ioannidis JPA (2005) Microarrays and molecular research: noise discovery? Lancet 365: 454–455
18. Wacholder S, Chanock S, Garcia-Closas M, El Ghormli L, Rothman N (2004) Assessing the probability that a positive report is false: an approach for molecular epidemiology studies. J Natl Cancer Inst 96:434–442
19. Wang SJ, O'Neill RT, Hung HMJ (2010) Statistical Considerations in evaluating pharmacogenomics-based clinical effect for confirmatory trials. Clin Trials 7:525–536
20. Mandrekar SJ, Sargent DJ (2009) Clinical trial designs for predictive biomarker validation: theoretical considerations and practical challenges. J Clin Oncol 27(24):4027–4034
21. Friedlin B, McShane L, Korn EL (2010) Randomized clinical trials with biomarkers: design issues. J Natl Cancer Inst 102(3):152–160
22. Freidlin B, Simon R (2005) Adaptive signature design: an adaptive clinical trial design for generating and prospectively testing a gene expression signature for sensitive patients. Clin Cancer Res 11:7872–7878
23. Freidlin B, Jiang W, Simon R (2010) The cross-validated adaptive signature design. Clin Cancer Res 16(2):691–8
24. Jiang W, Freidlin B, Simon R (2007) Biomarker-adaptive threshold design: a procedure for evaluating treatment with possible biomarker-defined subset effect. J Natl Cancer Inst 99: 1036–43
25. Wang SJ, O'Neill RT, Hung HMJ (2007) Approaches to evaluation of treatment effect in randomized clinical trials with genomic subset. Pharm Stat 6:227–244
26. Barker AD, Sigman CC et al (2009) I-SPY 2: an adaptive breast cancer trial design in the setting of neoadjuvant chemotherapy. Clin Pharmacol Ther 86(1):97–100
27. Simon R, Maitournam A (2004) Evaluating the efficiency of targeted designs for randomized clinical trials. Clin Cancer Res 10:6759–6763
28. Maitournam A, Simon R (2005) On the Efficiency of targeted clinical trials. Stat Med 24: 329–339

Oncology Clinical Trials in the Genomic Era

Richard Simon and Jyothi Subramanian

Abstract Developments in genomics are providing a biological basis for the heterogeneity of clinical course and response to treatment that have long been apparent to clinicians. The ability to molecularly characterize human diseases presents new opportunities to develop more effective treatments and new challenges for the design and analysis of clinical trials.

In oncology, treatment of broad populations with regimens that benefit a minority of patients is less economically sustainable with expensive molecularly targeted therapeutics. The established molecular heterogeneity of human diseases requires the development of new paradigms for the design and analysis of randomized clinical trials as a reliable basis for predictive medicine.

We review prospective designs for the development of new therapeutics and predictive biomarkers to inform their use. We cover designs for a wide range of settings. At one extreme is the development of a new drug with a single candidate biomarker and strong biological evidence that marker negative patients are unlikely to benefit from the new drug. At the other extreme are phase III clinical trials involving both genome-wide discovery of a predictive classifier and internal validation of that classifier. We have outlined a prediction-based approach to the analysis of randomized clinical trials that both preserves the type I error and provides a reliable internally validated basis for predicting which patients are most likely or unlikely to benefit from a new regimen.

R. Simon (✉)
Biometric Research Branch, National Cancer Institute, Emmes Corporation, 9000 Rockville Pike, MSC7434, Bethesda, Rockville MD 20892-7434, USA
e-mail: rsimon@nih.gov

T.R. Fleming and B.S. Weir (eds.), *Proceedings of the Fourth Seattle Symposium in Biostatistics: Clinical Trials*, Lecture Notes in Statistics 1205, DOI 10.1007/978-1-4614-5245-4_5, © Springer Science+Business Media New York 2013

1   Introduction

This dominant paradigm for major clinical trials today involves using broad eligibility criteria and to randomly assign an experimental treatment or control to test a single null hypothesis that a single clinical outcome measure is on average unimproved by the experimental treatment. Although it is recognized that no two patients are identical, it is implicitly assumed that all have the same disease and that treatment benefit, if it exists, differs only in magnitude among subsets of patients. In this paradigm, subset analysis is viewed with suspicion and is considered only exploratory for purpose of hypothesis generation for future studies. All aspects of multiplicity are accounted for in the test of a single primary null hypothesis. Large sample sizes and multicenter participation are the rule in order to be able to detect small average absolute treatment effects.

The emphasis on broad eligibility criteria has been based on a concern that drugs found effective in clinical trials might subsequently be used in broader patient populations [1, 2]. Some clinical trials even abandoned formal eligibility criteria in favor of the "uncertainty principle" which stated that if the individual physician was uncertain about which treatment might be better for a patient, then that patient was eligible [3]. The focus on ignoring subset analysis unless the overall null hypothesis can be rejected is based on concern about data dredging, the assumption that qualitative interactions are unlikely [3, 4] and that drugs are inexpensive and without serious side effects. For oncology today, none of those assumptions are appropriate. Treating the majority for the benefit of the minority is no longer an effective public health strategy.

Randomized clinical trials have made important contributions to modern medicine and public health, but they have also led to the overtreatment of broad populations of patients, most of whom don't benefit from the increasingly expensive drugs and procedures shown to have statistically significant average treatment effects in increasingly large clinical trials. Fortunately the tools of biotechnology and genomics are providing the tools to identify the subsets of patients who benefit from treatments.

Developments in our understanding of the genomic basis of cancer have indicated that cancers of most primary sites (e.g., lung and breast) represent a heterogeneous collection of diseases that differ in pathophysiology, natural history, and sensitivity to treatment. Recent results have demonstrated that these diseases differ with regard to the mutations that cause them and drive their invasion. The new understanding of heterogeneous nature of tumors of the same primary site leads to new challenges with regard to clinical trial design. Today we are challenged to develop a new paradigm of clinical trial design and analysis that enables development of a predictive medicine that is science based and reliable. Physicians have always known that cancers of the same primary site were heterogeneous with regard to natural history and response to treatment. This understanding led to conflicts with statisticians over the use of subset analysis in the analysis of clinical trials. Although most statisticians expressed little interest in subset analysis methods [5], many practitioners rejected the results of clinical trials whose conclusions were based on average effects. Today we have powerful tools for characterizing the tumors biologically and using this characterization as a basis for the design and analysis of clinical trials.

Most oncology drugs are being developed for defined molecular targets but the traditional diagnostic classification schemes that are the basis for clinical trial eligibility criteria include patients whose tumors are and are not driven by deregulation of those targets. For many drugs, the targets are well understood and there is a compelling biological basis for restricting development to the subset of patients whose tumors are characterized by deregulation of the drug target. For other drugs there is more uncertainty about the target, and how to measure whether the target is driving tumor invasion in an individual patient [6]. It is clear that the primary analysis of the new generation of oncology clinical trials must consist of more than just treating the traditionally broad patient populations and testing the null hypothesis of no average effect. But it is also clear that the tradition of post-hoc data dredging subset analysis is not an adequate basis for predictive oncology. We need prospective analysis plans that provide for both preservation of the type I experiment-wise error rate and for focused predictive analyses that can be used to reliably select patients in clinical practice for use of the new regimen [7]. These two primary objectives are not inconsistent, and clinical trials should be sized for both purposes.

The following sections summarize some of the designs that have been developed for the new generation of cancer clinical trials. Developing new treatments with companion diagnostics or predictive biomarkers for identifying the patients who benefit does not make drug development simpler, quicker, or cheaper as is sometimes claimed. Actually it makes drug development more complex and probably more expensive. But for many new oncology drugs it is the only science-based approach and should increase the chance of success. It may also lead to more consistency in results among trials and has obvious benefits for reducing the number of patients who ultimately receive expensive drugs which expose them risks of adverse events but no benefit. This approach also has great potential value for controlling societal expenditures on health care.

The ideal approach is prospective drug development with a companion diagnostic [7]. This approach, which is being used extensively today in oncology involves (1) Development of a completely specified predictive classifier using preclinical and early phase clinical studies. The classifier may be based on a single gene or protein or a composite score incorporating the levels of expression of multiple genes. (2) Development of an analytically validated test for measurement of that classifier. Analytically validated means that the test accurately measures what it is supposed to measure, or if there is no gold-standard measurement, that the test is reproducible and robust. (3) Use of that completely specified classifier and analytically validated test to design and analyze a new clinical trial to evaluate the effectiveness of that drug and how the effectiveness relates to the classifier. The guiding principle is that the data used to develop the classifier should be distinct from the Phase III data used to test hypotheses about treatment effects in subsets determined by the classifier. This is in contrast to the typical paradigm in which multiple variables are measured using non-analytically validated tests and then performing an exploratory analysis that requires confirmation in a subsequent study. In the enrichment and stratified designs described below, biomarker discovery is performed prior to the phase III trial and a single completely specified classifier is used in the trial. We will also discuss designs and prospective analysis plans that incorporate multiple candidate classifiers or even broader classifier development and evaluation in the same clinical trial. But in all of these designs, the analysis plans are carefully pre-specified to ensure that treatment effects in classifier-based subsets are unbiasedly estimated and that overall type I error is preserved.

2 Targeted (Enrichment) Designs

Designs in which the eligibility criteria restrict the clinical trial to those patients considered most likely to benefit from the experimental drug are called "targeted designs" or "enrichment designs." With an enrichment design a diagnostic test is used to restrict eligibility for a randomized clinical trial comparing a regimen containing a new drug to a control regimen. This approach, was used for the development of trastuzumab in which patients with metastatic breast cancer whose tumors expressed HER2 in an immunohistochemistry test were eligible for randomization. Simon and Maitournam [8–10] studied the efficiency of this approach relative to the standard approach of randomizing all patients without using the test at all. They found that the efficiency of the enrichment design depended on the prevalence of test-positive patients and on the effectiveness of the new treatment in test-negative patients. When fewer than half of the patients are test positive and the new treatment is relatively ineffective in test-negative patients, the number of randomized patients required for an enrichment design is dramatically smaller than the number of randomized patients required for a standard design. For example, if the treatment is completely ineffective in test-negative patients, then the ratio of number of patients required for randomization in the enrichment design relative to the number required for the standard design is approximately $1/\gamma^2$ where γ denotes the proportion of patients who are test positive [10]. The treatment may have some effectiveness for test-negative patients either because the assay is imperfect for measuring deregulation of the putative molecular target or because the drug has off-target antitumor effects. Even if the new treatment is half as effective in test-negative patients as in test-positive patients, however, the randomization ratio is approximately $4/(\gamma + 1)^2$. This equals about 2.56 when $\gamma = 0.25$, i.e., 25% of the patients are test positive, indicating that the enrichment design reduces the number of required patients to randomize by a factor of 2.56.

The enrichment design was used for the development of trastuzumab and led to the approval of the drug for metastatic and primary breast cancer even though the test was imperfect and has subsequently been improved. The enrichment design enabled the drug to be evaluated in the patients for whom there was a biological rationale for expecting a benefit and to avoid exposing the others to a drug with serious toxicities. Simon and Maitournam also compared the enrichment design to the standard design with regard to the number of screened patients. Zhao and Simon have made the methods of sample size planning for the design of enrichment trials available on line at http://brb.nci.nih.gov. The web-based programs are available for binary and survival/disease-free survival endpoints. The planning takes into account the performance characteristics of the tests and specificity of the treatment effects. The programs provide comparisons to standard non-enrichment designs based on the number of randomized patients required and the number of patients needed for screening to obtain the required number of randomized patients.

The enrichment design is appropriate for contexts where there is a strong biological basis for believing that test-negative patients will not benefit from the new drug. In such cases, including test-negative patients may raise ethical concerns and may confuse the interpretation of the clinical trial. As described in the section on "stratification designs," if test-negative patients are to be included, then they must be included in sufficient numbers and the number of test-positive patients must be designed to provide adequate separate analysis of the two groups. Often this is not done and instead one sees a mixed population of patients in an inadequately sized trial leading to ambiguous conclusions.

3   Biomarker Stratified Design

When a predictive classifier has been developed but there is not compelling biological or phase II data that test-negative patients do not benefit from the new treatment, it is generally best to include both classifier positive and classifier negative in the phase III clinical trials comparing the new treatment to the control regimen. In this case it is essential that an analysis plan be predefined in the protocol for how the predictive classifier will be used in the analysis. The analysis plan will generally define the testing strategy for evaluating the new treatment in the test-positive patients, the test-negative patients and overall. The testing strategy must preserve the overall type I error of the trial and the trial must be sized to provide adequate statistical power for these tests. It is not sufficient to just stratify, i.e., balance, the randomization with regard to the classifier without specifying a complete analysis plan. The main value of "stratifying" (i.e., balancing) the randomization is that it assures that only patients with completed test results will enter the trial. Pre-stratification of the randomization is not necessary for the validity of inferences to be made about treatment effects within the test-positive or test-negative subsets. The test used in the pivotal clinical trial should be analytically validated; that is, previously demonstrated to be accurate, reproducible, and robust to sources of laboratory variation. If an analytically validated test is not available at the start of the trial but will be available by the time of analysis, then it may be preferable not to pre-stratify the randomization process but to perform the analytically validated assay later on tumor specimens collected prior to randomization.

The purpose of the pivotal trial is to evaluate the new treatment overall and in the subsets determined by the prespecified classifier. The purpose is not to modify or optimize the classifier. If the classifier is a composite gene expression-based classifier, the purpose of the design is not to reexamine the contributions of each gene. If one does any of this, then an additional phase III trial may be needed to evaluate treatment benefit in subsets determined by the new classifier. Several primary analysis plans have been described by Simon [7, 11, 12], and a web-based tool for sample size planning with these analysis plans is available at http://brb.nci.nih.gov. For example, if one does not expect the treatment to be effective in the test-negative patients unless it is effective in the test-positive patients, one might first compare treatment versus control in test-positive patients using a threshold of significance of 5%. Only if the treatment versus control comparison is significant at the 5% level in test-positive patients, the new treatment will be compared to the control among test-negative patients, again using a threshold of statistical significance of 5%. This sequential approach controls the overall type I error at 5% since a treatment ineffective in both test-negative and test-positive patients has a 5% chance of being found significant for test positives, and if that comparison is not significant, the comparison for the test negatives is not performed. To have 90% power in the test-positive patients for detecting a 50% reduction in hazard for the new treatment versus control at a two-sided 5% significance level requires about 88 events of test-positive patients, the same as for an enrichment design limited to test-positive patients. If at the time of analysis the event rates in the test-positive and test-negative strata are about equal, then when there are 88 events in the test-positive patients, there will be about $88(1 - \gamma)/\gamma$ events in the test-negative patients where γ denotes the proportion of test-positive patients. If 25% of the patients are test positive, then there will be approximately 264 events in test-negative patients. This will provide approximately 90% power for detecting a 33% reduction in hazard at a two-sided significance level of 5%. In this case, the trial will not be delayed compared to the enrichment design, but a large number of test-negative patients will be randomized, treated, and followed on the study rather than excluded as for the enrichment design. This will be problematic if one does not, a-priori, expect the new treatment to be effective for test-negative patients. In this case it will be important to establish an interim monitoring plan to terminate accrual of test-negative patients when interim results and prior evidence of lack of effectiveness makes it no longer viable to enter them. Most frequentist interim monitoring plans provide insufficient protection for test-negative patients in this circumstance and Karuri and Simon have recently developed a Bayesian design based on an informative prior that reflects the a-priori degree of confidence in the test [13]. The Karuri and Simon Bayesian design protects the chance of false positive conclusions for the study overall, and for the test-positive and test-negative patients separately.

In the situation where one has limited confidence in the predictive marker it can be effectively used for a "fall-back" analysis. Simon and Wang [14] proposed an analysis plan in which the new treatment group is first compared to the control group overall. If that difference is not significant at a reduced significance level such as 0.03, then the new treatment is compared to the control group just for test-positive patients. The latter comparison uses a threshold of significance of 0.02, or whatever portion of the traditional 0.05 not used by the initial test. If the trial is planned for having 90% power for detecting a uniform 33% reduction in overall hazard using a two-sided significance level of 0.03, then the overall analysis will take place when there are 297 events. If the test is positive in 25% of patients and the event rates in test-positive and test-negative patients are about equal at the time of analysis, then when there are 297 overall events there will be approximately 75 events among the test-positive patients. If the overall test of treatment effect is not significant, then the subset test will have power 0.75 for detecting a 50% reduction in hazard at a two-sided 0.02 significance level. By delaying the treatment evaluation in the test-positive patients power 0.80 can be achieved when there are 84 events and power 0.90 can be achieved when there are 109 events in the test-positive subset.

Wang et al. have shown that the power of this approach can be improved by taking into account the correlation between the overall significance test and the significance test comparing treatment groups in the subset of test-positive patients [15]. So if, for example, a significance threshold of 0.03 has been used for the overall test, the significance threshold for used for the subset can be somewhat greater than 0.02 and still have the overall chance of a false positive claim of any type limited to 5%. In the following descriptions of biomarker designs that use the fall-back analysis plan, we use the partition 0.03 overall analysis and 0.02 for subset analysis only for concreteness. Any partition that adds to 0.05 will preserve the type I error but sample size and power may vary substantially depending on the partition used. In many cases allocating most of the 5% to the subset analysis will be advantageous because having adequate sample size to achieve adequate power for the subset analysis is more constraining than obtaining adequate power for the overall analysis.

4 Designs That Evaluate a Small Number of Classifiers

The prospective drug and companion diagnostic test approach is being used today in the development of many new cancer drugs where the biology of the drug target is well understood. Because of the complexity of cancer biology, however, there are many cases in which the biology of the target is not well understood at the time that the phase III trials are initiated. We have been developing adaptive designs for these settings. The designs are adaptive, not with regard to sample size or randomization ratio, but rather with regard to the subset in which the new treatment is evaluated relative to the control.

For example with the adaptive threshold design [16] we assumed that a predictive biomarker score was prospectively defined in a randomized clinical trial comparing a new treatment T to a control C. The score is not used for restricting eligibility and no cut-point for the score is prospectively indicated. A fall-back analysis begins as described above by comparing T to C for all randomized patients using a significance threshold α_1, say 0.03, less than the traditional 0.05. If the treatment effect is not significant at that level, then one finds the cut-point s* for the biomarker score which leads to the largest treatment effect in comparing T to C restricted to patients with score greater than s*. Jiang et al. [16] employed a log-likelihood ratio measure of treatment effect and let L* denote the log-likelihood ratio of treatment versus control effect when restricted to patients with biomarker level above s*. The null distribution of L* was determined by repeating the analysis after permuting the treatment and control labels a thousand or more times. If the permutation statistical significance of L* is less than $0.05-\alpha_1$ (e.g., 0.02), then treatment T is considered superior to C for the subset of the patients with biomarker level above s*. Jiang et al. provided bootstrap confidence intervals for s*. They provided an approach to sample size planning for a trial based on this fallback strategy and also upon a more powerful strategy that does not utilize a portion of the total type I error for a test of the overall null hypothesis of average treatment effect.

The analysis plan used in the adaptive threshold design is based on computing a global test based on a maximum test statistic. For the adaptive threshold design, the maximum is taken over the set of cut-points of a biomarker score. The idea of using a global maximum test statistic is much more broadly applicable, however. For example, suppose multiple candidate binary tests, $B_1, \ldots, B_K$ are available at the start of the trial. These tests may or may not be correlated with each other. Let L_k denote the log-likelihood of treatment effect for comparing T to C when restricted to patients positive for biomarker k. Let L* denote the largest of these values and let k* denote the test for which the maximum is achieved. As for the adaptive threshold design, the null distribution of L* can be determined by repeating the analysis after permuting the treatment and control labels a thousand or more times. If the permutation statistical significance of L* is less than $0.05-\alpha_1$ (e.g., 0.02), then treatment T is considered superior to C for the subset of the patients positive for biomarker test k*. The stability of the indicated set of patients who benefit from T (i.e., k*) can be evaluated by repeating the computation of k* for bootstrap samples of patients.

5 Predictive Analysis of Clinical Trials

Freidlin and Simon [17] also published an adaptive signature design for settings where a single or small number of candidate classifiers are not available at the start of the phase III clinical trial. At the time of final analysis, one starts by comparing outcomes for the treatment group T to the control group C for all randomized patients. If this overall treatment effect is not significant at a reduced level α_1, the full set P of patients in the clinical trial is partitioned into training set Tr and validation set V. A prespecified algorithmic analysis plan is applied to the training set to generate a "predictive classifier" F(x;Tr) where x denotes the vector of variables available. This vector may include only candidate classifiers or may include variables with no a-priori credentials for predictive classification.

The design was originally proposed for settings where the x vector included gene expression values from a genome-wide expression measurement. A predictive classifier is a function that identifies the patients who appear to benefit from the new treatment T compared to the control C; $F(x;Tr) = 1$ means that a patient with covariate vector x is predicted to benefit from T whereas $F(x;Tr) = 0$ indicates that patient is not predicted to benefit from T. This is a predictive classifier based on comparing two treatment groups, not the more familiar kind of prognostic classifier for a single group. This classifier is developed based on analyzing outcome and covariates for the two treatment groups in the training set. Freidlin and Simon developed a weighted voting predictive classifier based on genes whose expression levels indicate an interaction with treatment in predicting outcome. Many other types of classifier development algorithms are possible and the design can be used broadly, not just when the covariates represent gene expression measurements. For example with survival data one could use a proportional hazards model

$$\log \frac{h(t;\underline{x},z)}{h_0(t)} = \alpha z + \underline{\beta}'\underline{x} + z\underline{\eta}'\underline{x}$$

where z is a treatment indicator $z = 0$ for C and $z = 1$ for T and $\underline{x}$ denotes the vector of covariates. This model can be fit on the training set by maximizing the penalized log partial likelihood with an L1 penalty on the components of the main effect vector β and the treatment by interaction vector η. The difference in log hazard for a patient with covariate vector $\underline{x}$ receiving treatment T compared to that same patient receiving treatment C is estimated by $\delta(\underline{x}) = \hat{\alpha} + \hat{\underline{\eta}}'\underline{x}$. This function can be used to classify or rank patients in the validation set. Patients with the most negative values of $\delta(\underline{x})$ are predicted to be the most likely to benefit from T relative to C. In order to classify patients in the validation set, a cut-point must be defined. This can either be a predetermined value such as zero, or a predetermined quantile of the distribution of $\delta(\underline{x})$ in the training set or used as an additional tuning parameter. All tuning parameters should be optimized by cross-validation within the training set.

An alternative classifier can be based on a generalization of the compound covariate method of Radmacher et al. [18]. The compound covariates are defined based on fitting single variable proportional hazards models

$$\log \frac{h(t;x_i,z)}{h_0(t)} = \alpha z + \beta_i'x_i + z\eta_i'x_i$$

for each variable $i = 1,2,\ldots,p$ where z denotes a treatment indicator $z = 0$ for C and $z = 1$ for T. One obtains estimates $\hat{\beta}_i$ and $\hat{\eta}_i$. The two compound covariates are defined as

$$v_1 = \sum \hat{\beta}_i x_i \text{ and } v_2 = \sum \hat{\eta}_i x_i$$

where the summations are over the variables for which the treatment by covariate interactions are nominally significant at level ξ in the corresponding univariate models. ξ is used as a tuning parameter. Prediction is based on the proportional hazards model involving only treatment and the two compound covariates:

$$\log \frac{h(t; v_1, v_2, z)}{h_0(t)} = \alpha z + \beta^* v_1 + z\eta^* v_2 \tag{1}$$

For predicting treatment the difference in log hazard for a patient with compound covariate values (v_1, v_2) receiving treatment T compared to that same patient receiving treatment C is estimated as $\hat{\alpha} + \hat{\eta}^* v_2$. This function can be used to classify or rank patients in the validation set. Patients with the most negative values of $\hat{\alpha} + \hat{\eta}^* v_2$ are predicted to be the most likely to benefit from T relative to C. For evaluating prediction accuracy one would classify patients in the validation set into quantiles based on their values of $\hat{\alpha} + \hat{\eta}^* v_2$ and examine the actual treatment effect within those quantiles.

A similar approach to that described above is to use a model like [1] for prediction but where v_1 is defined as the first supervised principal component of expression levels for the variables that are prognostic at nominal univariate significance level ξ and v_2 being the first principal component of expression levels of the variables that have nominal ξ level significant interactions. The level ξ is a tuning parameter [19].

Once a single completely specified classifier is defined on the training set, it is used to classify the patients in the validation set. These patients are classified as either "sensitive" to the new treatment, i.e., predicted likely to benefit from the new treatment T relative to C or not sensitive. Let S denote the set of sensitive patients in the validation set; i.e., $S = \{j \varepsilon V | F(x_j, Tr) = 1\}$. One then compares outcomes for sensitive patients in the validation set who received T versus sensitive patients in the validation set who received C. Let L denote the log-rank statistic (if outcomes are time-to-event) for this comparison of T vs C of sensitive patients in the validation set. The null distribution of L is determined by repeating the entire analysis after permuting the treatment and control labels a thousand or more times. If the permutation statistical significance of L is less than 0.05-α_1 (e.g., 0.02), then treatment T is considered superior to C for the subset of the patients predicted to be sensitive using the classifier developed in the training set.

Freidlin et al. [20] demonstrated that the statistical power of this approach can be substantially increased by embedding the classifier development and validation process in a K fold cross-validation. This idea is very powerful and much more broadly applicable than in the context described by Freidlin et al. [17] The concept is to prospectively define an algorithm A for classifying patients as likely or not likely to have better outcome on the new treatment T compared to the control C. This algorithm constitutes the entire preplanned subset analysis. In contrast to the usual subset analysis which results in a bunch of statements about statistical significance of treatment effects within multiple subsets, this algorithm results in a single completely determined predictive classifier. The predictive classifier partitions the space of covariate vectors into a region for patients who are predicted to benefit from the new treatment T and the complementary region for patients who are not predicted to benefit from T. This algorithm might, for example, be defined as indicated above by fitting a proportional hazards model involving treatment, main covariate effects and treatment by covariate interactions to the data and then defining the predictive classifier based on imposing a cut-point on the difference in log-likelihood for the predictive index computed if the new treatment is used minus if the control is used. With this approach the model could be fit to the high-dimensional data using penalized likelihood methods or univariate screening to find covariates with apparent interactions with treatment. Many other kinds of algorithms are possible. The algorithm A when applied to a dataset D defines a completely specified predictive classifier $F(x|D, A)$. The classifier that will potentially be used in the future is the one obtained by applying the algorithm to the full dataset (P), i.e., $F(x|P,A)$. But first it is necessary to evaluate the algorithm using cross-validation. It should be emphasized that the cross-validation procedure does not provide some abstract characteristic of the algorithm A, it provides an almost unbiased estimate of the predictive accuracy of the classifier $F(x|P, A)$ obtained by applying A to the full set of data D.

The cross-validation is performed in the following way. The full set (P) of patients in the clinical trial is partitioned into K disjoint subsets $P_1, \ldots, P_K$. The ith training set T_i consist of the full set of patients except for the ith subset; i.e., $T_i = P - P_i$. Let $F(x|T_I, A)$ denote the binary classifier developed by applying the algorithm A to training set T_i. Use this classifier to classify the patients in the omitted subset P_i. Let $v_j = F(x_j|T_i, A)$ denote the predictive classification for patients j in P_i. $v_j = 1$ if the patient is predicted to be sensitive to the new treatment T relative to control C, and zero otherwise. Since the patients in P_i were not included in the training set T_i used to train $F(x|T_i, A)$, this classification is predictive, not just evaluating goodness of fit to the same data used to develop the classifier. Since each patient appears in exactly one P_i, each patient is classified exactly once and that classification is done with a classifier developed using a training set not containing that patient.

Let S denote the set of patients j for whom $v_j = 1$, i.e., who are predicted to be sensitive to the new treatment. We can evaluate the predictive value of our algorithm by comparing outcomes of the patients in S who received treatment T to the outcomes for the patients in S who received the control C. Let L(S) denote a measure of difference in outcomes for that comparison; e.g., a log-rank statistic if outcomes are time-to-event. We can generate an approximation to the null distribution of L by repeating the entire analysis for thousands of random permutations of the treatment labels. This test can be used as the primary significance test of the clinical trial to test the strong null hypothesis that the new treatment and control are equivalent for all patients on the primary endpoint of the trial. Alternatively, it can be used as a fall-back test as described in the previous sections.

Having rejected the null hypothesis described above, the application of the algorithm A to the full dataset P provides a decision tool $F(x|P, A)$ that can be used by physicians for informing future treatment decisions for their patients. The classifier recommended for future use is the one obtained by applying the algorithm to the full dataset, i.e., $F(x;P,A)$. The K-fold cross-validation provides a proper statistical significance test and provides important information about this full sample classifier. Freidlin et al. showed that the hazard ratio for T vs C in the cross-validated set S is a conservative estimate of the hazard ratio for the sensitive set of the full sample classifier, i.e., for the set of future patients with covariate vectors for which $F(x|P, A) = 1$.

The effectiveness of the decision tool based on $F(x|P, A)$ depends on the algorithm used. Algorithms that over-fit the data will provide classifiers that make poor predictions. Algorithms based on Bayesian models with many parameters and non-informative priors may be as prone to over-fitting as frequentist models with many parameters. The effectiveness of an algorithm will also depend on the dataset, i.e., the unknown truth about how treatment effect varies among patient subsets. A strong advantage of the proposed approach, however, is that an almost unbiased estimate of the performance of a defined algorithm can be obtained from the dataset of a clinical trial itself. This can be compared to treating all patients or no patients based on the results of the conventional overall null hypothesis test. This is clearly preferable to performing exploratory analysis on the full dataset without any cross-validation, reporting the very misleading goodness of fit of the model to the same data used to develop the model, and cautioning that the results need testing in future clinical trials.

The approach described above can also be used in a clinical trial for which the overall treatment effect is significant. The approach permits one to identify, based on covariate profiles, the patients who do and do not benefit from the new treatment. Rather than just focusing on the patients predicted to be sensitive to the new treatment, one also compares treatment effects for the complementary subset defined by the cross-validated classifications. To illustrate this approach we have applied it to data from the gene expression profiling study conducted on pretreatment biopsy specimens from 181 patients with diffuse large-B-cell lymphoma (DLBCL) who received a standard chemotherapy combination called CHOP and 233 patients with this disease who received R-CHOP (CHOP plus the antibody Rituximab) was analyzed [19]. Unfortunately, this was not a randomized clinical trial, but the data will serve to illustrate the method of analysis.

The only clinical covariate considered for this analysis was the international prognostic index (IPI). For the purpose of this analysis the IPI was categorized into two groups—subjects with IPI scores of 0, 1, or 2 were categorized as "low" and subjects with IPI scores 3, 4, or 5 were called "high." For some of the subjects one or more of the variables that make up the IPI were missing. If for a given subject the value for the missing variable would not change the IPI group call (e.g., depending on the value of the missing variable the IPI value would be either 1 or 2), then the subject would be included as a member of that IPI group. However if the missing value could make a difference (e.g., between 2 and 3), then that subject was excluded from our analysis. Thirty-nine subjects were excluded because the IPI group could not be determined. Of the resulting 375 subjects 262 fell in IPI class "low" and 113 subjects were in IPI class "high." The end-point was overall survival (death from any cause). Prior to the start of analysis one subject who had a survival time of zero was removed, resulting in 374 subjects for this analysis.

Gene expression and clinical data were obtained from the Gene Expression Omnibus (acc. no. GSE10846). To account for the differences in microarray preprocessing between R-CHOP and CHOP samples, the expression values for each gene in the R-CHOP group was adjusted so that its median matched the median of

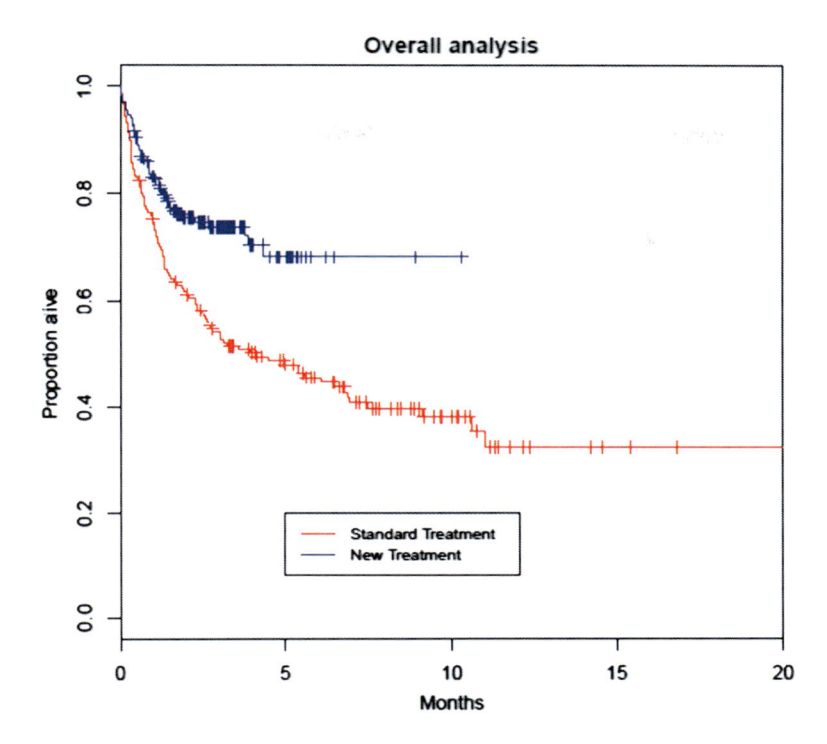

Fig. 1 Overall analysis. The value of the log-rank statistic is 14.1 and the corresponding p-value is 0.0002. The new treatment thus shows an overall benefit

the CHOP group [21]. For the predictive analysis the data were log2 transformed and the 1,000 genes with the highest variance were used.

A Cox proportional hazards (ph) regression model was developed using patients in both CHOP (standard treatment acronym of four chemotherapy drugs, C) and R-CHOP (new treatment consisting of standard CHOP plus antitumor antibody rituximab, E) groups. A 10-fold cross-validation was applied to estimate predictive accuracy. Univariate gene selection was used as the feature selection method. For each gene, a Cox ph model was developed in the training set using treatment, covariate (IPI), gene, and treatment by covariate and treatment by gene interactions. Ten genes with the lowest p-values for the treatment by gene interactions were selected for inclusion in the multivariate Cox ph model. The multivariate Cox ph model was again developed using treatment, IPI, 10 best genes, treatment by IPI and treatment by gene interactions. Gene selection and multivariate model development were all done within each cross-validation loop. In the multivariate Cox ph model, let δ = main effect of treatment, γ = vector of interaction coefficients. Then, for a patient in the test set with covariate vector X_{test} $F(X_{test}) = 1$ if $\delta + \gamma' X_{test} < c$ where c was fixed to be the median of the $F(X)$ values in the corresponding training set.

Figure 1 shows the results of the overall analysis. The results of applying the predictive algorithm in a ten-fold cross-validation loop are shown in Figs. 2 and 3.

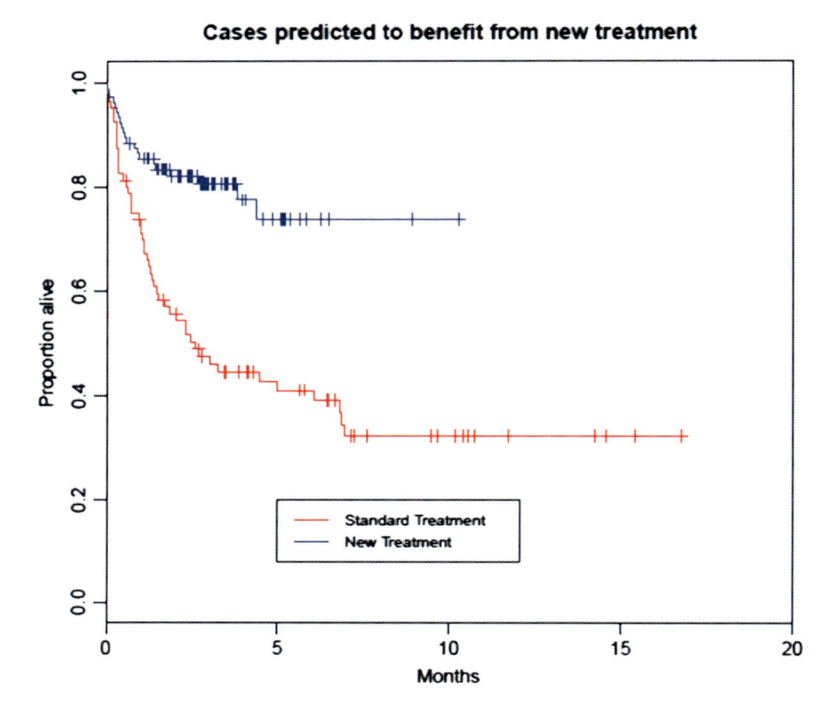

Fig. 2 Predictive analysis. Cross-validation was used to predict patients who would benefit or not from the new treatment. This figure shows the survival curves for patients predicted to benefit from the new treatment. The value of the log-rank statistic for the separation of the survival curves is 19.67 and the permutation p-value is 0.005 (200 permutations). The hazard ratio is -1.12 and the bootstrap-based 95% CI for the HR is $(-1.40, -0.125)$ (200 bootstrap samples)

For the sensitive subset of patients who appear to benefit from R-CHOP, the value of the log-rank statistic for the separation of the cross-validated survival curves is 19.67 and the permutation p-value is 0.005 (200 permutations). For this sensitive subset, the log hazard ratio is -1.12 and the bootstrap based 95% CI for the log HR is $(-1.40, -0.125)$ (200 bootstrap samples). For the complementary subset of patients who do not appear to benefit from R-CHOP, the value of the log-rank statistic for the cross-validated survival curves is 0.81 and the permutation p-value is 0.49 (200 permutations). The predictive analysis has thus identified a group of patients who are unlikely to benefit from the new treatment. Table 1 provides some information about the proportional hazards model developed on the full dataset. The p values listed are nominal p values conditional on including the 10 gene expression variables with the most nominally significant univariate interactions with treatment. Table 2 lists the genes that have more than 50% cross-validation support. The "%cv support" column indicates the proportion of the 10 loops of the cross-validation that the variable was selected for inclusion in the model.

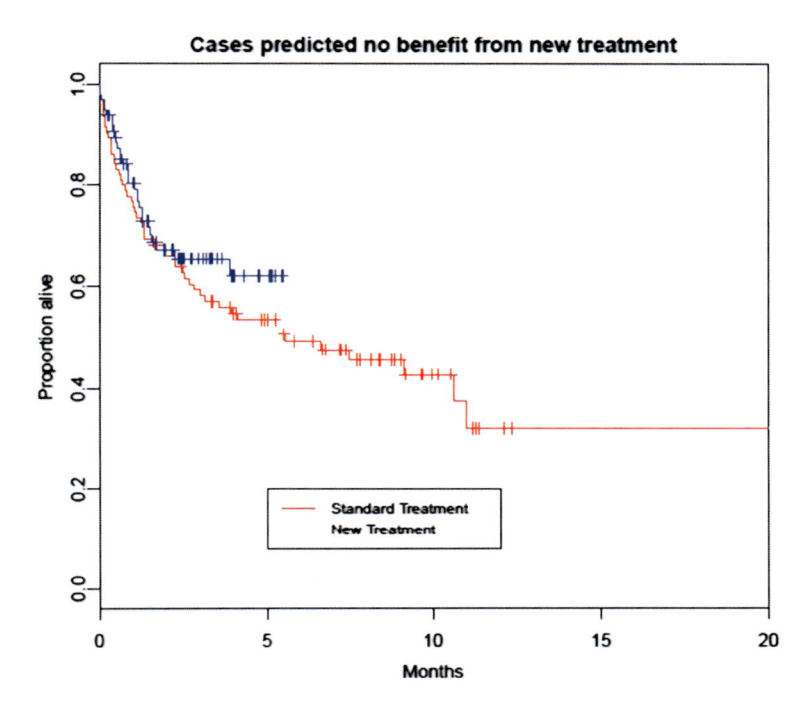

Fig. 3 Survival curves for cases predicted no benefit from new treatment. The value of the log-rank statistic in this case is 0.81 and the permutation p-value is 0.49 (200 permutations)

Table 1 The coxph model on applying the algorithm to the full dataset (for classifying future patients)

Variable	Coefficient	p-Value	Variable	Coefficient	p-Value
T	−1.69	0.27			
1552531_a_at	0.07	0.21	T*1552531_a_at	−0.15	0.06
210313_at	0.12	0.03	T*210313_at	−0.21	0.03
242334_at	−0.05	0.20	T*242334_at	−0.07	0.42
242107_x_at	−0.13	0.06	T*242107_x_at	0.35	0.002
231391_at	0.05	0.28	T*231391_at	−0.26	0.004
1565026_a_at	0.15	0.01	T*1565026_a_at	−0.34	0.0006
206413_s_at	−0.03	0.39	T*206413_s_at	0.11	0.08
203641_s_at	−0.18	0.008	T*203641_s_at	0.23	0.02
231898_x_at	−0.06	0.20	T*231898_x_at	0.20	0.007
243905_at	−0.06	0.28	T*243905_at	0.31	0.003
IPI	−1.6	<0.0001	T*IPI	0.29	0.43

T denotes treatment indicator. Variables with "at" suffix represent gene expression levels for Affymetrix probe sets. p-values are nominal values which ignore the effect of variable selection

Table 2 Genes with more than 50% cross-validation support (i.e., chosen as one of the 10 best genes in more than 5 CV loops)

Gene	% CV support	Name (symbol)	Molecular function
210313_at	100	Leukocyte immunoglobulin receptor, subfamily A, member 4 (LILRA4)	Receptor activity
1552531_a_at	100	NLR family, pyrin domain containing 11 (NLRP11)	Nucleotide binding, protein binding, ATP binding
242334_at	80	NLR family, pyrin domain containing 4 (NLRP4)	Nucleotide binding, protein binding, ATP binding
231391_at	80	Cortexin 3 (CTXN3)	Unknown
1565026_a_at	70	Orofacial cleft 1 candidate 1 (OFCC1)	Unknown
242107_x_at	70	Unknown	Unknown
206413_s_at	70	Unknown	Protein binding

6 Conclusion

Developments in genomics have increased the focus of biostatisticians on prediction problems. This has led to many useful developments for predictive modeling where the number of variables is larger than the number of cases. Heterogeneity of human diseases and new technology for characterizing diseased tissue presents new opportunities and challenges for the design and analysis of clinical trials. In oncology, treatment of broad populations with regimens that do not benefit most patients is less economically sustainable with expensive molecularly targeted therapeutics. The established molecular heterogeneity of human diseases requires the development of new paradigms for the use of randomized clinical trials as a reliable basis predictive medicine [1, 2]. We have presented here prospective designs for the development of new therapeutics with candidate predictive biomarkers. An approach to the Predictive Analysis of Clinical Trials (PACT) has also been presented. This approach preserves the type I error of the study and uses re-sampling to develop and validate a predictive classifier that can be used to inform treatment selection for future patients. This approach provides a statistically sound framework for bridging the gap between clinical trials and clinical practice that has long existed and may serve as a basis for clinical trials in the era of predictive medicine.

References

1. Simon R (2004) An agenda for clinical trials: clinical trials in the genomic era. Clin Trials 1:468–470
2. Simon R (2007) New challenges for 21st century clinical trials. Clin Trials 4:167–169
3. Peto R, Pike MC, Armitage P (1976) Design and analysis of randomized clinical trials requiring prolonged observation of each patient. I. Introduction and design. Br J Cancer 34:585

4. Peto R, Pike MC, Armitage P (1977) Design and analysis of randomized clinical trials requiring prolonged observation of each patient. II. Analysis and examples. Br J Cancer 35:1
5. Dixon DO, Simon R (1991) Bayesian subset analysis. Biometrics 47:871
6. Sawyers CL (2008) The cancer biomarker problem. Nature 452:548–552
7. Simon R (2005) A roadmap for developing and validating therapeutically relevant genomic classifiers. J Clin Oncol 23:7332–7341
8. Simon R, Maitournam A (2005) Evaluating the efficiency of targeted designs for randomized clinical trials. Clin Cancer Res 10:6759–6763
9. Simon R, Maitournam A (2006) Evaluating the efficiency of targeted designs for randomized clinical trials: supplement and correction. Clin Cancer Res 12:3229
10. Maitournam A, Simon R (2005) On the efficiency of targeted clinical trials. Stat Med 24: 329–339
11. Simon R (2008) Using genomics in clinical trial design. Clin Cancer Res 14:5984–5993
12. Simon R (2010) Clinical trial designs for evaluating the medical utility of prognostic and predictive biomarkers in oncology. Per Med 7(1):33–47
13. Karuri S, Simon R (2012) A two-stage Bayesian design for co-development of new drugs and companion diagnostics. Stat Med 31:901–914
14. Simon R, Wang SJ (2006) Use of genomic signatures in therapeutics development. Pharmacogenomics J 6:166–173
15. Wang SJ, O'Neill RT, Hung HMJ (2007) Approaches to evaluation of treatment effect in randomized clinical trials with genomic subset. Pharm Stat 6:227–244
16. Jiang W, Freidlin B, Simon R (2007) Biomarker adaptive threshold design: a procedure for evaluating treatment with possible biomarker-defined subset effect. J Natl Cancer Inst 99: 1036–1043
17. Freidlin B, Simon R (2005) Adaptive signature design: an adaptive clinical trial design for generating and prospectively testing a gene expression signature for sensitive patients. Clin Cancer Res 11:7872–7878
18. Radmacher MD, McShane LM, Simon R (2002) A paradigm for class prediction using gene expression profiles. J Comput Biol 9:531–537
19. Bair E, Hastie T, Paul D, Tibshirani R (2006) Prediction by supervised principal components. J Am Stat Assoc 101:119–137
20. Freidlin B, Jiang W, Simon R (2010) The cross-validated adaptive signature design for predictive analysis of clinical trials. Clin Cancer Res 16(2):691–698
21. Lenz G, Wright GW, Dave SS, Xiao W, Powell J, Zhao H et al (2008) Stromal gene signatures in large-B-cell lymphomas. N Engl J Med 359(22):2313–2323

Using SNPs to Characterize Genetic Effects in Clinical Trials

B.S. Weir

Abstract Characterizing the genetic basis of responses in clinical trials has been made substantially easier and more powerful through the use of single nucleotide polymorphism data. A million of more of these markers can now be scored cheaply with commercial SNP-chips and ten million or more additional SNPs can be inferred by imputation. These rich datasets offer a deep look at the human genome and they are likely to tag many of the response causal genes. It has already become common for SNP types to be included in drug box labels.

The ease and low cost of obtaining SNP profiles in clinical trials comes with the price of noisy data: it is common to have to reject data at 10% of the assayed SNPs. However, those SNPs that pass rigorous data cleaning protocols not only offer the chance of identifying the genes that affect response variables but also may reveal information about the genetic architectures of the trial participants and the populations to which they belong, as well as the relationships among the participants. Among novel applications of SNP profiles is the ability to determine HLA type without expensive sequencing.

1 Introduction

There is now clear evidence that at least some of the variation in individual response to pharmaceutical drugs has a genetic basis. Some of this evidence comes from genome-wide association studies (GWASs), [10] and a growing number of clinical trials (e.g., [7]). As a result of this activity, the FDA had, by October of 2011, added pharmacogenomic information to the labels of 111 drugs (see URL 3 below).

B.S. Weir (✉)
Department of Biostatistics, University of Washington, Box 357232, Seattle,
WA 98915-7232, USA
e-mail: bsweir@uw.edu

T.R. Fleming and B.S. Weir (eds.), *Proceedings of the Fourth Seattle Symposium in Biostatistics: Clinical Trials*, Lecture Notes in Statistics 1205, DOI 10.1007/978-1-4614-5245-4_6, © Springer Science+Business Media New York 2013

One of the best-documented cases for a genetic contribution to drug response concerns the anticoagulant warfarin (Roden et al. [20]). Dosing algorithms were originally based on clinical information and now use both clinical and genetic information. Initial GWAS showed an association of the gene VKORC1 (vitamin K epoxide reductase complex 1) with warfarin maintenance dose (Cooper et al. [8]), and subsequent studies [4, 22] found the effects of the cytochrome P450 genes CYP2C9 and CYP4F2. There have been mixed results from randomized clinical trials to determine if pharmacogenomic-based dosing will, in fact, improve anticoagulation control and clinical outcomes [1, 5] and other trials are in progress (see URL 2 below). The FDA 2011 drug label for warfarin provides genotype-specific dose ranges based on joint VKORC1–CYP2C9 genotypes (URL 3 below). There is good evidence for genotype-based dosing effects for the cardiovascular drug clopidogrel (sold as Plavix) and the CYP2C19 genotype for the cytochrome P450 gene [16].

Single nucleotide polymorphism (SNP) imformation in various genes is used in various genes that are used in warfarin or clopidogrel dosing algorithms, and other pharmacogenomic applications, and this chapter considers some aspects of the analysis and interpretation of SNPs. The chapter is informed by the author's involvement with SNP data in two consortia funded by the National Human Genome Research Institute: GENEVA ([9]; URL 5 below) is a collection of GWAS for several major human diseases, including atherosclerosis, cancers, and type II diabetes; GARNET is a series of GWAS of treatment response in randomized clinical trials that looks to identify genetic variants associated with response to treatments for conditions of clinical or public health significance (see URL 4 below). GARNET aims to utilize existing clinical trial data and sample resources to:

1. Identify genetic variants that influence an individual's response to treatment.
2. Determine whether specific treatments are more or less effective in groups defined by genotype.
3. Develop and disseminate innovative methods for adding genome-wide technologies to randomized clinical trials and interpreting the results in the context of a randomized treatment assignment.

The chapter will also point to the increased knowledge being gained about human genetic architectures, at both the individual and the population level, as a result of the recent explosion in the quantity of SNP data. These data may be collected from assays in targeted regions of the genome, or they may result from micro-array technology that allows up to five million SNPs across the genome to be studied with a "SNP-chip," or they may result from complete DNA sequencing of the genes in the genome, i.e. exome sequencing, or from whole genome sequencing. Each position in the complete human genomic sequence could, in theory, be occupied by one of the four nucleotide types. In practice, only a fraction of the sites show variation and then with only two different types, bases, segregating in the population. With individuals receiving one copy of the genome from each parent, there are three genotypes at each SNP and it is the frequencies of these three types that provide the building blocks for the genetic analysis of clinical trial data.

2 SNP Data

The amount of genetic information now available for use in clinical trials is vast, and the costs of generating these data have been steadily decreasing. The first large-scale survey of frequencies of SNP variants, alleles, in several populations was the International HapMap Project (see URL 6 below). The current version, HapMapIII, contains the genotypes of 1,396 individuals sampled from 11 populations, as shown in Table 1. Each individual is typed on at least 1.4 million SNPs. The geographic and ethnic diversity among the HapMap individuals allows a range of analyses to be conducted on SNP data collected in clinical trials, including the checking of self-reported ethnicity and relationship with other study members as described below.

A comprehensive search for SNPs is being undertaken by the 1000 Genomes Project (see URL 1 below). In a tutorial presented by Gabor Marth (see URL 1 below) in October 2011, it was reported that whole-genome sequencing with 20–50-fold coverage has been completed on 697 individuals from the CEU, CHB, CHD, JPT, LWK, TSI, and TRI populations of Table 1. The goal is to sequence 2,500 individuals from around the world and to locate 95% of all SNPs that have a minor allele frequency greater than 1% (and greater than 0.1% for SNPs in gene coding regions). This will avoid the ascertainment biases that characterized early SNP studies where SNPs were discovered by looking for variation among people of European ancestry. By October 2011, over 25 million SNPs had been discovered—over 17 million of them from the 1000 Genomes project. The locations of these 25 million are spread over the three billion nucleotide positions in the human genome.

An advantage of the large projects such as HapMapIII or 1000 Genomes is that they provide reference panels for genotype imputation (see GENEVA URL 5 below). Participants in a clinical trial could have SNP genotypes determined with a commercial platform that yields one million SNP genotypes and then have another ten million genotypes found by imputation. Genotype imputation is the process of

Table 1 HapMap III data

Population	SNPs	Total indivs.	Father, child pairs	Mother, child pairs	Father, mother child trios
ASW: African ancestry in Southwest USA	1,543,731	86	5	17	10
CEU: Utah residents of European ancestry	4,031,093	164	2	3	48
CHB: Han Chinese in Beijing, China	4,056,784	136			
CHD: Chinese in Metropolitan Denver, CO	1,312,343	108			
GIH: Gujarati Indians in Houston, Texas	1,409,510	100			
JPT: Japanese in Tokyo, Japan	4,055,077	112			
LWK: Luhya in Webuye, Kenya	1,527,403	109			
MEX: Mexican ancestry in Los Angeles, CA	1,453,659	85			30
MKK: Maasai in Kinyawa, Kenya	1,532,587	183			28
TSI: Tuscan in Italy	1,420,526	101			
YRI: Yoruban in Ibadan, Nigeria	3,985,822	203		2	54

inferring unobserved genotypes in a study sample based on the haplotypes (a region of one chromosome) observed in a more densely genotyped reference sample of similar genetic background. The GENEVA and GARNET consortia use imputation software in the BEAGLE package (Browning and Browning [2]). Imputed results are provided in two formats: (1) the expected allele dosage and (2) the probability of each of the three genotype states, reflecting the level of certainty in the genotype prediction. It is recommended that these probabilities be incorporated into any subsequent analyses, rather than taking the most likely imputed genotypes. Quality metrics are provided for each imputed SNP that can be used for filtering imputation results on a per-SNP level.

3 Cleaning SNP Data

3.1 SNP-Level Cleaning

High-throughput SNP genotyping is becoming low-cost, fast, and reliable but the inherent uncertainties in the current microarray technologies mean that 10% or more of the SNP genotypes may need to be discarded because of poor quality [13]. Apart from the difficulty sometimes in "calling" the SNP type from the signals provided by the typing systems, the sheer scope of the data can reveal low-frequency problems that used not to be an issue in genetic studies. The GENEVA and GARNET consortia examine SNP data with the criteria shown in Table 2. This table refers to results from a total of 4,936 female subjects selected from the Women's health initiative (WHI) hormone therapy (HT) trial (a trial of estrogen plus progesterone versus placebo) and genotyped on the Illumina HumanOmni1-Quad v1-0 B SNP array as part of the GARNET project. Complete details of the data cleaning are given at the URL 4 listed below, but the table summarizes the reasons SNPs may be excluded from a study. Over the eight data-cleaning steps, a total of 22.4% of the SNPs has to be excluded from further analyses because of data quality issues. The reason that excluded most SNPs was the requirement that minor allele frequencies exceed 0.02: this admittedly arbitrary threshold was to preserve the validity of subsequent association tests. Some of this loss may be avoided by refinement of the tests.

3.2 Individual-Level Cleaning

The genetic nature of SNP data offers several possibilities of detecting quality issues at the sample (individual) level as opposed to the SNP level. For example, indications of the presence of Y-chromosome SNPs in individuals annotated as female may indicate sample mix-up, incorrect annotation, or gender anomalies.

Table 2 FDA information about clopidogrel (see URL 3 below)

FDA drug safety communication: Reduced effectiveness of Plavix (clopidogrel) in patients who are poor metabolizers of the drug.

Data Summary

The liver enzyme CYP2C19 is primarily responsible for the formation of the active metabolite of Plavix. Pharmacokinetic and antiplatelet tests of the active metabolite of Plavix show that the drug levels and antiplatelet effects differ depending on the genotype of the CYP2C19 enzyme. The following represent the different alleles of CYP2C19 that make up a patient's genotype:

- The CYP2C19*1 allele has fully functional metabolism of Plavix.
- The CYP2C19*2 and *3 alleles have no functional metabolism of Plavix. These two alleles account for most of the reduced function alleles in patients of Caucasian (85%) and Asian (99%) descent classified as poor metabolizers.
- The CYP2C19*4, *5, *6, *7, and *8 and other alleles may be associated with absent or reduced metabolism of Plavix, but are less frequent than the CYP2C19*2 and *3 alleles.
- A patient with two loss-of-function alleles (as defined above) will have poor metabolizer status.

The pharmacokinetic and antiplatelet responses to Plavix were evaluated in a crossover trial in 40 healthy subjects. Ten subjects in each of the four CYP2C19 metabolizer groups (ultrarapid, extensive, intermediate and poor) were randomized to two treatment regimens: a 300 mg loading dose followed by 75 mg/day, or a 600 mg loading dose followed by 150 mg/day, each for a total of 5 days. After a washout period, subjects were crossed over to the alternate treatment. Decreased active metabolite exposure and increased platelet aggregation were observed in the poor metabolizers compared to the other groups. When poor metabolizers received the 600 mg loading dose followed by 150 mg daily, active metabolite exposure and antiplatelet response were greater than with the 300 mg/75 mg regimen. Health-care professionals should note that an appropriate dose regimen for patients who are poor metabolizers has not been established in clinical outcome trials.

Even randomly chosen individuals for a clinical trial may include some relatives and these should either be removed prior to subsequent analyses or those analyses modified to accommodate relatives. The usual procedure for identifying relatives with SNP data [18] has been to estimate a set of three probabilities, k_0, k_1, k_2, of two individuals sharing 0, 1, 2 pairs of alleles identical by descent. Unrelated pairs of people have $k_0 = 1$, parent–offspring have $k_1 = 1$, and identical twins have $k_2 = 1$. It is not unusual to find instances of full-sibs ($k_0 = 0.25, k_1 = 0.5, k_2 = 0.25$) or half-sibs ($k_0 = k_1 = 0.5$) in a clinical trial. It is sometimes convenient to summarize relatedness with the kinship or coancestry coefficient $\theta = k_2/2 + k_1/4$. This coefficient can be regarded as the probability that two alleles, one taken from each individual, are identical by descent, ibd. The analogous quantity for a single individual is termed the inbreeding coefficient.

There have been recent extensions (e.g., [12]) of relatedness estimation that distinguish among different classes of relatives with equal k values or that detect quite distant classes of relative. Individuals related as half-sibs or as uncle–nephew, for example, both have probability $k_1 = 0.5$ of receiving identical copies of an allele at any SNP from their most recent common ancestor. However, they have different probabilities of receiving the identical copies of the region between two SNPs because there has been no recombination between those SNPs in the paths of descent from the recent common ancestor: if c is the recombination fraction between two SNPs these probabilities are $(1 - c)^2/2$ for half-sibs and $(1 - c)^3/2$ for uncle–nephew. If identity by descent can be detected, then half-sibs will tend to have longer ibd regions than do uncle and nephew.

There are substantial computational challenges in determining the relatedness of all pairs of individuals in a study of 1,000 or more individuals, and even more challenges in determining ibd regions. Purcell et al. [18] use the method of moments which are fast but prone to large variances and problems when there are low minor allele frequencies. Maximum likelihood methods are preferred but the need for iterative solutions can make them prohibitively slow. All methods make use of allele frequencies, generally estimated from the data under study and any population structure or ethnic diversity in the study can make estimating the appropriate allele frequencies for a particular pair of individuals quite difficult.

Ethnicity can also be inferred from SNP profiles by reducing the high dimensionality of the number of SNPs to a small number of principal components. These components are for the matrix with dimensions equal to the total number of individuals in the study and with elements being estimates of one plus the inbreeding coefficient of the individuals on the diagonal and the coancestry coefficients of pairs of individuals off the diagonal. When individuals are plotted in two dimensions for pairs of the first few principal components they tend to cluster in populations (Novembre et al. [17]) in ways that often bear striking resemblances to geographic maps of population locations. Principal component analysis (PCA) can quickly identify individuals with outlier ethnicities in a study that may need to be removed from association analysis. Principal components can also be used as covariates when outcome variables are regressed on SNP genotype scores.

A novel finding of PCA is that chromosomal features such as inversions are revealed in samples from the same population. Tian et al. [23] reported the clustering into three groups of a sample of European-ancestry individuals corresponding to the genotypes of a cluster of highly correlated SNPs in chromosomal region 8p23, a region that contains a polymorphic inversion. SNPs in such structural elements may need to be removed from association analyses.

Another individual-level finding from whole-genome SNP studies is that of chromosomal aberrations whereby whole or parts of chromosomes may appear in other than two copies. Instead of an individual receiving one copy of each chromosome, other than X or Y, from each parent he or she may receive a copy from only one parent (a deletion), two copies from one parent and none from the other (uniparental disomy) or more than one copy from one parent and at least one from the other (duplication). These anomalies may be constitutive, having been present since conception, or they may be mosaic, having arisen during the lifetime of the individual by processes such as mitotic recombination. The anomalies are detected by examining features of the raw intensity data, rather than from called genotypes and details from the GENEVA consortium have been given by Laurie et al. [14]. Constitutive anomalies appear to be present in almost everyone, while mosaic anomalies occur in about 0.5% of the population up to age about 50, after which they increase to about 3%.

4 Association Testing

The search for SNPs $\mathbf{M}$ associated with outcomes in a clinical trial supposes that there are genetic loci $\mathbf{T}$ that affect that outcome, such as an adverse drug reaction or an elevated platelet reactivity. The evidence for a genetic basis may simply be that variation in response is found among individuals in a population, or there are differences in response rates among different ethnicities, or there is similarity of responses among relatives. There may be direct knowledge of the genes responsible for response to a drug, based on the known mechanism of drug action, in which case a candidate-gene approach can be used to identify SNPs that may be used to screen patients. If there is no prior knowledge, a GWAS may be used. The difference is mainly one of scale: in each case the observed SNP genotypes are coded as a marker variable $\mathbf{X}$ and evidence is sought for association between this and a response variable $\mathbf{Y}$, both measured on each individual in a clinical trial.

A simple model supposed that a measured response variable has a genetic component $\mathbf{G}$ and a nongenetic component E, with $\mathbf{Y} = \mathbf{G} + \mathbf{E}$. Although sophisticated analyses are used in practice, the essence of association testing can be seen by supposing that a test is made of the hypothesis that the observed variables $\mathbf{X}$ and $\mathbf{Y}$ are uncorrelated. If the mode of action for the response gene is additive, then it can be shown [24] that the square of the correlation coefficient between the two variables can be written as $\rho_{XY}^2 = \rho_{MT}^2 h_T^2$, where ρ_{MT}^2 (sample value r^2) is the linkage disequilibrium between marker and trait alleles M, T, and h_T^2 is the heritability of response from locus $\mathbf{T}$. Heritability is the additive genetic portion of the variance in response values. The SNP $\mathbf{M}$ with the highest correlation is likely to be the one closest to $\mathbf{T}$ in the genome, but that is less important in dose determination than in the utility of the $\mathbf{M}$ genotype to predict response. Shuldiner et al. [21] conducted a GWAS for clopidogrel response and found a cluster of 13 SNPs on chromosome 10 in the CYP2C18–CYP2C19–CYP2C9–CYP2C8 gene cluster with strong evidence for association with response. They showed that a guanine to adenine substitution in exon 5 of CYP2C19 (SNP rs 4244285, also known as CYP2C19*2) accounts for most or all of the association signal on chromosome 10. This $G \rightarrow A$ base substitution produces a nonfunctional truncated protein, and people with two copies of this allele are poor metabolizers of clopidogrel. Such findings are reflected in the FDA Drug Safety Communication about clopidogrel shown in Table 2.

5 HLA Typing

The discussion so far has centered on using SNP data for quality control measures, and then as biomarkers for outcomes in clinical trials. There are other uses of these markers. The human leukocyte antigen (HLA) region, located on human chromosome 6p21.3, is known to be highly polymorphic, and typing at classical HLA loci has been an essential tool for transplantation matching and detailed analyses of disease associations. Particular HLA types have also been shown to be associated with drug response: [6] noted that carbamazepine, an anticonvulsant and mood-stabilizing drug, is the main cause of the Stevens–Johnson syndrome (SJS) and its related disease, toxic epidermal necrolysis (TEN), in Southeast Asian countries. These authors found an association of SYS-TEN with the HLA B*1502 allele, and they used allele-specific assays in their study.

High-resolution HLA typing is expensive, especially in the context of clinical trials where the appropriate HLA type is to be determined, and there is interest in being able to predict HLA type from relatively inexpensive SNP types. The problem is complicated by the very large number of possible HLA types: the HLA-B locus, for example, has 2,069 alleles listed in the January 2011 release of the IMGT-HLA Database (see URL 7 below). To impute HLA types from multiple SNP markers, [15] used a hidden Markov model (HMM) based on coalescent theory to develop their LDMhc algorithm, and they used a leave-one-out cross-validation scheme for SNP selection. These authors [11] subsequently developed an integrated software "HLA*IMP" for imputing classical HLA alleles from SNP genotypes based on LDMhc, with a modification of SNP selection function that leads to pronounced increases in call rate. An alternative strategy, using an Attribute Bagging method [3] has been proposed by Zheng et al. [25]. This alternative method makes use of published haplotype frequencies from a training dataset, rather than requiring access to that dataset. A user does not have to provide a query SNP profile to a third party imputation provider. Imputed HLA types have been used in an association study by Raychaudhuri et al. [19].

6 Discussion

Characterizing the genetic basis of responses in clinical trials has been made substantially easier and more powerful through the use of single nucleotide polymorphism data. A million of more of these markers can now be scored cheaply with commercial SNP-chips and ten million or more additional SNPs can be inferred by imputation. These rich datasets offer a deep look at the human genome and they are likely to tag many of the response causal genes. It has already become common for SNP types to be included in drug box labels.

SNP typing in clinical trials offers much more than a source of potential biomarkers for response, however. By virtue of their genetic nature, they provide information about cryptic relatedness, an alternative to self-reported ethnicity or gender, and information about the detailed genetic structure of trial participants. Although whole-genome DNA sequencing is fast becoming practicable, even those complete datasets are likely to be reduced to SNP sets in the forseeable future.

Acknowledgements This work was supported in part by NIH grants GM 075091, HG 004464 and HG 005157.

URLs

1. 1000 Genomes: www.1000genomes.org/
   www.genome.gov/Pages/Research/DER/1000GenomesProjectTutorials/DataDescription-GaborMarth.pdf

2. Clinical Trials on Warfarin Dosing:
   clinicaltrials.gov/ct2/results?term=warfarin+dosing

3. FDA Table of Pharmacogenomic Biomarkers in Drug Labels:
   www.fda.gov/Drugs/ScienceResearch/ResearchAreas/Pharmacogenetics/ucm083378.htm
   For clopidogrel:
   www.fda.gov/Drugs/DrugSafety/PostmarketDrugSafetyInformationforPatientsandProviders/ucm203888.htm
   For warfarin:
   http://www.accessdata.fda.gov/drugsatfda_docs/label/2011/009218s107lbl.pdf

4. GARNET: Genomics and Randomized Trials Network:
   www.garnetstudy.org
   www.garnetstudy.org/docs/whi_qc_report_final.pdf

5. GENEVA: Gene Environment Association Studies:
   www.genevastudy.org
   www.genevastudy.org/Imputation_Reports

6. HapMap: The International HapMap Project:
   www.hapmap.org

7. HLA:IMGT-HLA Database:
   www.ebi.ac.uk/imgt/hla/

References

1. Anderson JL, Horne BD, Stevens SM, Grove AS, Bartion S, Nicholas ZP, Kahn SFS, May HT, Samuelson KM, Muhlsetein JB, Carlquist JF (2007) Couma-Gen 1. Randomized trail of genotype-guided versus standard warfarin dosing in patients initiating oral anticoagulation. Circulation 116:2563–2570
2. Browning B, Browning S (2009) A unified approach to genotype imputation and haplotype-phase inference for large data sets of trios and unrelated individuals. Am J Hum Genet 84:210–223

3. Bryll R, Gutierrez-Osuna R, Quek F (2003) Attribute bagging: improving accuracy of classifer ensembles by using random feature subsets. Pattern Recognit 36:1291–1302

4. Caldwell MD, Awad T, Johnson JA, Gage BF, Falkowski M, Gardina P, Hubbard J, Turpaz Y, Langaee TY, Eby C, King CR, Brower A, Schmelzew JR, Glurich I, Vidaillet HJ, Yale SH, Qi Zhang K, Berg RL, Burmester JK (2008) CYP4F2 genetic variant alters required warfarin dose. Blood 111:4106–4112

5. Caraco Y, Blotnik S, Muszkat M (2008) CYP2C9 genotype-guided warfarin prescribing enhanxcesthe efficacy and safety of anticoagulation: a prospective randomized controlled trial. Clin Pharmacol Ther 83:460–470

6. Chen P, Lin J-J, Lu C-S, Ong C-T, Hsieh PF, Yam C-C, Tai C-T, Wu S-L, Lu C-H et al (2011) Carbamazide-induced toxic effects and HLA-B*1502 screening in Taiwan. N Engl J Med 364:1126–1133

7. Cohen AL, Soldi R, Zhang H, Gustafson AM, Wilcox R, Weim BE, Chang JT, Johnson E, Spira A, Jeffrey SS, Bild AH (2011) A pharmacogenomic method for individualized prediction of drug sensitivity. Mol Syst Biol 7:513. doi:10.1038/msb.2011.47

8. Cooper GM et al (2008) A genome-wide scan for common genetic variants with a large influence on warfarin maintenance dose. Blood 112:1022–1027

9. Cornelis MC et al (2010) The Gene, environment association studies consortium (GENEVA): maximizing the knowledge obtained from GWAS by collaboration across studies of multiple conditions. Genet Epidemiol 34: 364–72

10. Daly AK (2011) Genome-wide association studies in pharmacogenomics. Nat Rev Genet 11:241–246

11. Dilthey AT, Moutsianas L, Leslie S, McVean G (2011) HLA*IMP: an integrated framework for imputing classical HLA alleles from SNP genotypes. Bioinformatics 27:968–972

12. Huff CD, Witherspoon DJ, Simonsen TS et al (2011) Maximum-likelihood estimation of recent shared ancestry (ERSA). Genome Res 21:768–774

13. Laurie CC, Doheny KF, Mirel DB, Pugh EW, Bierut LJ, Bhangale T, Boehm F, Caporaso NE, Cornelis MC, Edenberg HJ, Gabriel SB, Harris EL, Hu FB, Jacobs K, Kraft P, Landi MT, Lumley T, Manolio TA, McHugh C, Painter I, Paschall J, Rice JP, Rice KM, Zheng X, Weir BS for the GENEVA Investigators (2010) Quality control and quality assurance in genotypic data for genome-wide association studies. Genet Epidemiol 34:591–602

14. Laurie CC, Laurie CA, Rice K, Doheny KF, Zelnick LR, McHugh CP, Ling H, Hetrick KN, Pugh EW, Amos C, Wei Q, Wang L, Lee JE, Barnes KC, Hansel NN, Mathias R, Daley D, Beaty TH, Scott AF, Ruczinski I, Scharpf RB, Bierut LJ, Hartz SM, Landi MT, Freedman ND, Goldin LR, Ginsburg D, Li J, Desch KC, Strom SS, Blot WJ, Signorello LB, Ingles SA, Chanock SJ, Berndt SI, Le Marchand L, Henderson BE, Monroe KR, Heit JA, de Andrade M, Armasu SM, Regnier C, Lowe WL, Hayes MG, Marazita ML, Feingold E, Murray JC, Melbye M, Feenstra B, Kang JH, Wiggs JL, Jarvik G, McDavid AN, Seshan VE, Mirel DB, Crenshaw A, Sharopova N, Wise A, Shen J, Crosslin DR, Levine DM, Zheng X, Udren JI, Bennett S, Nelson SC, Gogarten SM, Conomos MP, Heagerty P, Manolio T, Pasquale LR, Haiman CA, Caporaso N, Weir BS (2012) Detectable clonal mosaicism from birth to old age and its relationship to cancer. Somatic mosaicism for large chromosomal anomalies from birth to old age and its relationship to cancer. Nat Genet 44:642–650

15. Leslie S, Donnelly P, McVean G (2008) A statistical method for predicting classical HLA 323 alleles from SNP data. Am J Hum Genet 82:48–56

16. Mega JL, Hochholzer W, Frelnger AL, Kluk MJ, Angiolilo DJ, Kereiakes DJ, Isserman S, Rogers WJ, Huff CT, Contant C, Pencina MJ, Scirica BM, Longtine JA, Michelson AD, Sabatine MS (2011) Dosing clopidogrel based on CYP2C19 genotype and the effect of platelet reactivity in patients with stable cardiovascular disease. J Am Med Assoc 306:2221–2228

17. Novembre J, Johnson T, Bryc K, Kutalik Z, Boyko AR, Auton A, Indap A, King KS, Bergmann S, Nelson MR, Stephens S, Bustamente CD (2008) Genes mirror geography within Europe. Nature 456:98–101

18. Purcell S, Neale B, Todd-Browne K, Thomas L, Ferreira MA et al (2007) PLINK: a tool set for whole-genome association and population-based analyses. Am J Hum Genet 81:559–575

19. Raychaudhuri S, Sandor C, Stahl EA, Freudenberg J, Lee HS, Jia X, Alfredsson L, Padyukov L, Klareskog L, Worthington J et al (2012) Five amino acids in three HLA proteins explain most of the association between mhc and seropositive rheumatoid arthritis. Nat Genet 44:291–296

20. Roden DM, Wilke RA, Kroemer KH, Stein CM (2011) Pharmacogenomics: the genetics of variable drug responses. Circulation 123:1661–1670

21. Shuldiner AR, O'Connell JR, Bliden KP, Gandhi A, Ryan K, Horenstein RB, Damcott CM, Pakyz R, Tantry US, Gibson O, Pollin TI, Post W, Parsa A, Mitchell BD, Faraday N, Herzog W, Gorbel PA (2009) Association of Cytochrome P450 2C19 genotype with the antiplatelet effect and clinical efficacy of clopidogrel therapy. J Am Med Assoc 302:849–858

22. Takeuchi F, McGinnis R, Bourgeois S, Barnes C, Eriksson N, Soranzo N, Whittaker P, Raganath V, Kumanduri V, McLaren W, Holm L, Lindh J, Rane A, Wadelius M, Deloukas P (2009) A genome-wide association study confirms VKORC1, CYP2C9 and CYP4F2 as principal genetic determinants of warfarin dose. PLoS Genet 5:e1000433

23. Tian C, Plenge RM, Ransom M, Lee A, Villoslada P, Selmi C, Klareskog L, Pulver AE, Qi LH, Gregersen PK, Seldin MF (2008) Analysis and application of European genetic substructure using 300K SNP information. PLoS Genet 4(1): article e4

24. Weir BS (2010) Statistical genetic issues for genome-wide association studies. Genome 53:869–875

25. Zheng X, Shen J, Cox C, Wakefield J, Ehm M, Nelson M, Weir B (2012) HIBAG - HLA genotype imputation with attribute gagging. Annual Meeting of the American Society of Human Genetics, Platform Abstract 290

Part III
Issues in Multi-Regional Clinical Trials

Why Is This Subgroup Different from All Other Subgroups? Thoughts on Regional Differences in Randomized Clinical Trials

Janet Wittes

Abstract Many Phase 3 randomized clinical trials are currently being conducted multinationally with too few participants from any individual country to allow reliable inference about the beneficial or harmful effects of the tested product using data from that country alone. Instead, the conclusions for a given country will come from the totality of the data. Insofar as "country" is just another subgroup defined by baseline variables, this strategy is defensible. On the other hand, in cases where "country" stands as a surrogate for country-specific variables that importantly influence the benefits and harms of an intervention, inferring from the study population at large to specific countries may be less appropriate. Such variables may include the nature of the disease being studied, the country-specific standard of care, the patterns of safety reporting, and the extent of adherence to study protocol. This paper presents four examples of studies where the observed treatment effect in the USA differed considerably from the effect observed elsewhere. It argues that the problem is in some sense intractable because a study large enough to provide precise estimates of effect sizes within specific countries would likely be infeasible. Instead, although the paper recommends generally applying the overall result to the participating countries, it provides suggestions for strategies in the design and analysis phase to mitigate potential inferential ambiguities.

1 Introduction

A subgroup in a clinical trial is a group of participants characterized by at least one common baseline characteristic. Subgroups may be defined by any baseline variable or set of variables, for example, demographic variables (e.g., males, females over

J. Wittes (✉)
Statistics Collaborative, Inc., 1625 Massachusetts Ave., NW; Suite 600,
Washington, DC 20036, USA
e-mail: janet@statcollab.com

T.R. Fleming and B.S. Weir (eds.), *Proceedings of the Fourth Seattle Symposium in Biostatistics: Clinical Trials*, Lecture Notes in Statistics 1205,
DOI 10.1007/978-1-4614-5245-4_7, © Springer Science+Business Media New York 2013

65), physiologic variables (e.g., ejection fraction over 30%), use of medications (e.g., prior use of chemotherapy, or current use of an antihypertensive agent), or, in the case this paper discusses, country or geographic region in which the participant lives. Anyone who has been involved extensively in randomized clinical trials has probably struggled with interpretation of subgroups. Many papers have warned of the treacherousness of taking seriously an effect in a subgroup that differs from effects in the totality of the trial [1–6]. The problem is most serious when the subgroup is defined after looking at the data because that smacks of betting on the horse after the race is over [7], but inference even from subgroups defined a priori can be incorrect because subgroups are often small and therefore estimates from them are subject to large variability. This is, of course, not to say that individual people all respond the same way to an intervention; it is simply a warning that relying on a surprising discordance in magnitude or direction of effect among subgroups in a randomized clinical trial has a high probability of leading the credulous observer down the primrose path. Instead, the seasoned trialist discounts apparent discrepancies among subgroups and argues, as Yusuf et al. [7] have commented, "We believe the prudent stance is to rely more on the overall results to indicate the likely 'true' effect in a particular subgroup, rather than on the actual observations, unless the trial was specifically designed to have sufficient power within subgroups of interest." Sometimes the argument against taking an observed subgroup effect seriously is purely statistical: given a true effect Δ that is constant across all elements in a population, the effect observed in a subgroup of size n will have an expectation of Δ but a standard error proportional to $1/n^{1/2}$. Therefore, relative to the effect size $\widehat{\Delta}$ observed in the trial as a whole, the effect size observed in a small subgroup has a high probability of being much less than, or much greater than, Δ. Lighting on a surprisingly modest, or surprisingly large, effect size in a small subgroup and declaring that the treatment does not work in some people or works marvelously well in others may reflect not a true finding, but an exaggerated effect due to the play of chance. The smaller the subgroup, the more likely the observed effect will fall far from the true value (even though on average the observed effect will be equal to the true value).

When $\widehat{\Delta}$ is the observed effect in a trial, one can expect that the observed effect in subgroups will likely hover around $\widehat{\Delta}$, but for very small subgroups the observed effect size may be considerably larger or considerably smaller than $\widehat{\Delta}$. An illustration of this phenomenon comes from the Systolic Hypertension in the Elderly Program (SHEP), which was a randomized clinical trial that studied the effect of reducing blood pressure in elderly people with systolic blood pressure at least 160 mm Hg but diastolic pressure less than 90 mm Hg. SHEP showed that reducing blood pressure led to a sizeable decrease in the rate of stroke, the primary outcome, and of cardiovascular events. For the latter, the relative risk was 0.68 with nominal 95% confidence interval (0.58, 0.79) [8]. If, however, one dichotomizes each baseline variable and looks at the effect size for cardiovascular events in the resulting pairs of subgroups (see Fig. 1; Byington R, private communication), one sees that among the smallest subgroups, while most of the estimated effect sizes fall close to 0.68, some are considerably larger than 0.68 and some considerably

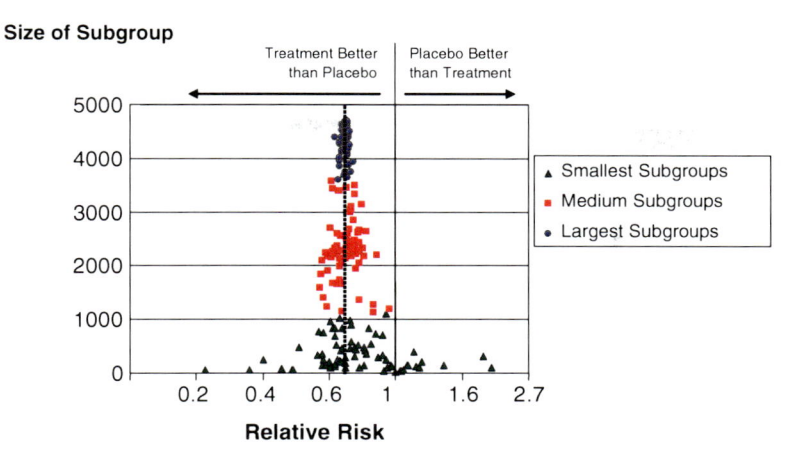

Fig. 1 Relative risk for fatal and nonfatal cardiovascular disease events by subgroup size. Overall, the relative risk of a cardiovascular event in SHEP was 0.68, which is indicated by the *vertical dotted line*. Two hundred eighty-nine (289) of the 2,365 treated and 414 of the 2,371 placebo participants experienced at least one cardiovascular event defined as fatal and nonfatal myocardial infarction, sudden cardiac death, rapid cardiac death, coronary artery bypass graft, angioplasty, fatal or nonfatal stroke, transient ischemic attack, aneurysm, or endarterectomy. Analysis and figure courtesy of Robert Byington

smaller. A few subgroups even show an observed *adverse* effect of reduction in systolic blood pressure. A researcher not familiar with the intrinsic variability in effect size might interpret these observed differences as reflecting true differences in the effect of reduction in systolic blood pressure; however, I would interpret these differences as the inevitable consequence of variability as a function of sample size, and I believe most experienced trialists would agree.

This paper deals with a specific type of subgroup, one defined by a country or geographic region in which the trial is conducted. In particular, it deals with the USA as a region of interest; however, readers more concerned with inference from another region can replace the words "United States" with the name of the region of interest. The general concerns expressed above about subgroups are relevant to interpretation of differences in effect size observed in such geographic regions. If we consider a geographic subgroup to act like any other subgroup, then investigators, sponsors, regulators, or treating clinicians who are interested in the effect of a treatment in a specific region should not be surprised with a study that overall shows a strong beneficial effect but that reports a point estimate in the region of interest with much smaller benefit or, worse yet, an estimate that sits in the direction of harm. Several trials have shown such a pattern, which is illustrated by the schematic forest plot in Fig. 2. Many people would view the discordance as most likely having arisen by the play of chance; however, for reasons amplified later in this paper, others consider geographic subgroups to hold a special place in the panoply of subgroups, a place that requires special consideration.

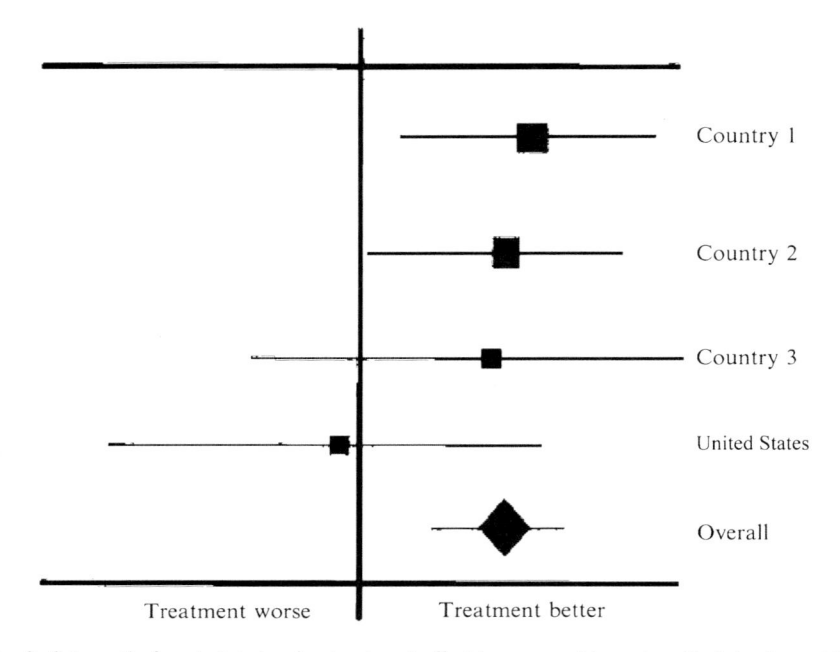

Fig. 2 Schematic forest plot showing treatment effect by geographic region. Each *horizontal line* in the plot shows the mean (*square* for each country-specific mean and *diamond* for the overall mean) and the 95% confidence limits for the estimated effect size. The area of the *square* or *diamond* is proportional to the information (the inverse of the variance) contained in the estimate

The statistical literature, the medical literature, and even the popular press have noted discordances in estimated treatment effects by geographic regions and have addressed the problem of making inference from trials conducted outside the USA to treatment of patients in the USA. One example from each type of paper shows the general concern. A 2010 paper written by a group of statisticians proposes a series of methods useful for assessing whether treatment effects are consistent across regions [9]. A paper in the medical literature published in 2011 by Kim et al. [10] warns, "Cardiovascular [randomized controlled trials] sponsored by the National Heart, Lung, and Blood Institute have substantial rates of international enrollment, particularly coronary artery disease trials. Given questions of applicability and ethical and financial considerations, [international participation] in U.S. clinical trials deserves further scrutiny." A 2011 article in Vanity Fair decries the enrollment of patients from developing countries in clinical trials that study treatments for use in the USA if the data from those trials are to form the basis of approval by the United States Food and Drug Administration [11].

The next section addresses why trials are often multinational. Focus then moves to the USA, first with a general discussion of interpreting observed differences between the USA and other countries. Four examples show how the FDA responded to trials when the observed effect in the USA was much smaller than in other countries. Subsequent sections briefly touch on how to classify countries when one is interested in the effect in the USA, issues regarding safety in multinational trials, and how data monitoring committees should look at interim data in light of the FDA's understandable regulatory discomfort approving products that have shown little or no effect in the USA. A short section distinguishes the inferential problems stemming from discordance between the results in the USA and other countries of the medically developed world from those when the results in the USA differ markedly from those in the developing world.

In some sense, the problem is intractable—to learn precisely the effect of a treatment in several specific geographic regions would require unfeasibly large sample sizes. In light of the likelihood that most observed country-specific differences result from the play of chance and the infeasibility of gaining a high degree of precision for country-specific estimates, the final section concludes with tentative answers to the question posed in the title. The section presents an argument that although countries, or geographic regions, or more specifically, the USA, is in some sense just another subgroup in a clinical trial, geographic classification serves as a surrogate for important factors that may in fact impinge upon the true balance of benefit and harms of a therapy. Therefore, the prudent trialist will consider strategies to increase the likelihood of being able to make reasonably accurate inference in specific countries.

2 Why Involve Participants from Many Countries?

Thus far, I have been deliberately coy about the phrase "treatment effect," for I have not defined the metric to be used. An appropriate metric will of course depend on the question the particular trial is asking. If the outcome is a mean, then the treatment effect is the difference in means divided by the standard deviation. Most of the trials discussed below, however, compare interventions either with respect to proportion of events or with respect to rates of events and use odds ratios, relative risks, or relative hazards as the metric of comparison.

If one believes—as I usually do—in near homogeneity of effect (if measured by a metric assessing relative risks or odds) across subgroups of patients who have no contraindications precluding them from taking the intervention under study, then recruiting participants from many countries will help fight the all-too-frequent problem of slow recruitment. Thus, the first reason to enter participants from more than one country is practicality—a multinational trial can recruit much more quickly than a trial that takes place in only one country. If the organization running the trial has the facilities to recruit participants in more than one country and the infrastructure to support high quality research in each participating country, so much the better. Another justification for multinational trials comes from appeal to distributive justice: "The principle of distributive justice requires that the trials be conducted with all groups to whom the treatment may apply" [12]. If an intervention is to be used in Country C, this argument implies that the trial should include residents of Country C. From a regulatory perspective, some countries will not approve a drug unless it has been studied in that country; holding separate trials in each country with such a requirement can satisfy these regulations, but it is often more efficient to conduct one or two large multinational trials rather than many smaller (or perhaps just as large if considerations of statistical power require large trials) country-specific trials. See Luo et al. [13] for an interesting proposal to ensure enough participants in countries that require representation of their residents before approving a drug.

These three reasons—a belief in homogeneity of effect, a commitment to distributive justice, and a desire to have a product approved in many countries—all lead naturally to multinational trials. Moreover, they allow hedging one's bet about the assumption of homogeneity: the absence of data from different countries or geographic regions precludes testing the assumption of homogeneity. Having different countries represented in a trial allows, at least theoretically, the possibility of testing for heterogeneity of effect. I say "theoretically" because the sample size within a country or region is likely to be too small to identify true differences in effect size, or, if a difference is seen, it may well have emerged by chance.

While the previous paragraphs in this section have provided reasons for multinational trials when the treatment effect is expected to be the same in many countries, some biologic or medical reasons argue strongly for multinational trials that limit recruitment to specific countries. For example, the distribution of the affected population in many genetic diseases reflects specific patterns of development of the genetic mutations and of patterns of migration. Thus, β—thalassemia, a blood disorder that reduces the production of hemoglobin, has a higher prevalence in countries bordering on the Mediterranean than elsewhere. A trial studying that disease would likely try to recruit patients from Italy, Greece, Northern Africa, and places—like the USA or Argentina—to which populations from these countries emigrated. If one is interested in learning about treating the disease, it makes sense to look for cases in the ethnic groups where it is found and to generalize across countries where those groups live. Another example is infectious disease. Just as Willie Sutton is purported to have said that he robbed banks because "that's where the money is," it makes sense to follow organisms if one is trying to cure or prevent infectious disease. For that reason, studies of influenza vaccine take place in the Southern Hemisphere—especially Latin America and South Africa—during their fall and winter and in the Northern Hemisphere during our fall and winter. There is no reason to believe that a vaccine effective against a specific strain of influenza in the Southern Hemisphere would not be effective against that same strain the following season in the Northern Hemisphere and thus in the USA.

Some practical considerations may lead to carrying out trials in specific countries. The cost of doing trials varies by orders of magnitude from country to country, leading to an incentive to carry out trials in countries where recruitment and services are inexpensive. Recruitment may be easier in countries where the benefits of participating in a trial and receiving care may be much more attractive than in wealthy countries, or wealthier parts of countries, where the population can afford high quality medical care. Adherence to therapies and willingness to attend clinic visits may also vary from country to country. Because low adherence and high loss to follow-up rates can wreak havoc on interpretation of data from clinical trials, designers of trials often try to select populations likely to adhere to the protocol. Still another important variable is access to concomitant medication. If investigators are studying a new drug for heart failure, for example, the effect of the experimental drug may be blunted if it is given on top of many other drugs for heart failure. Consider a design that compares a new drug to placebo on top of "local standard of care." If the local standard of care consists of no other drug, then the trial compares the new drug to placebo, both on top of no other treatment. If, on the other hand, the local standard of care includes several effective drugs, the new drug may show no benefit, or the benefit it does show may be much smaller than observed when it is the only drug prescribed. A drug company may want to test its drug in the setting most likely to show benefit, and therefore may choose to study it in a country whose population has limited access to other drugs. If such a study shows benefit of the tested drug, one can conclude that the drug is effective when used without other interventions. Applying the results without further testing to settings with a more aggressive standard of care assumes that the treatment will be effective in these settings as well.

3 Why Do Participants from Outside the USA Differ from Those in the USA?

The remainder of this paper deals with making inferences from multinational trials to patients in the USA. In addition to the reasons discussed in the previous section, participants from outside the US have some medically relevant characteristics that differ importantly from participants in the USA. The differences may be related to the characteristics of the participants themselves, the distribution and severity of the disease in the countries involved in the trial, or patterns of medical care. In chronic disease, what is called disease D in one country may be quite different from disease D in another. For example, wide access to Pap smears in the USA may translate to different relative frequency of stages of prevalent disease compared to countries like India where women have much less access to screening [14]. Thus, if one wants to study treatments for Stage IV cervical cancer, recruiting from India allows easier access to the disease than searching for late-stage disease in the USA. Similarly, early detection of breast cancer in the USA has led to a lower ratio of early stage to invasive disease in the USA than in some other countries. Another example comes from heart failure. Perhaps because of the generally more aggressive treatment of heart failure in the USA and Western Europe than in Russia and much of Eastern Europe, the mortality rates for heart failure, corrected for stage of disease, are generally lower in the former countries than in the latter.

For outcomes that assess prevention of invasive interventions (for example, time to dialysis or transplantation in trials of advanced kidney disease, or time to revascularization in trials of coronary disease), the threshold for intervention may vary considerably from country to country, and even from institution to institution within a country. These variations may results in variable event rates in the participating countries, leading to the need for a larger sample size to have enough events for adequate power. If, however, the outcome is a relative measure (e.g., hazard ratio, odds ratio, or relative risk) and the analysis is stratified by country or region, then the relative effects will often remain nearly constant. On the other hand, if the outcome is a difference in the proportion failing (e.g., the proportion of people who are dialyzed or receive a transplant within two years of randomization), the attributable risk will vary as a function of the underlying proportion and thus composition of the population may affect not only the underlying rate but also the effect size. The relationship of effect size to underlying risk is an argument for use of relative measures, rather than absolute measures, in multinational trials.

4 Some Examples: Are the Apparent Differences Real or Illusory?

This section describes four examples of Phase 3 trials where participants from the USA, or North America, showed less effect than did participants from the rest of the world: a trial of zanamivir (trade name Relenza) for the treatment of symptomatic influenza, MERIT-HF in heart failure, PLATO in patients with acute coronary syndromes, and the BLISS trials in lupus. In each case, the patients in the USA showed a smaller beneficial effect than did patients in the rest of the world, but in each case the Food and Drug Agency (FDA) granted approval for use in the USA. Because the four stories differ somewhat, it is interesting to review their results and describe the FDA's decisions. These examples are not meant to typify results from clinical trials; rather they are presented to illustrate how the FDA thought through decisions concerning approval in the face of discordant results between the USA and other countries.

Relenza. The case of zanamivir (Relenza), an antiviral drug for patients with influenza, highlights limitations in looking only at data from the USA. In February 1999, the FDA presented data to its Antiviral Advisory Panel showing that the drug had a very small observed effect in the USA but a statistically significant effect overall in reducing the number of days of illness. The Advisory Panel voted 13 to 4 against approving the drug without further study. The majority of the Panel contended that the trial showed very little evidence of an effect in the USA. The Panel members hypothesized that people in the USA were already taking over-the-counter medicines for symptomatic relief and most Panel members were not convinced that the small benefit observed was worth the potential harms of the drug. In spite of the lopsided vote of the Advisory Panel, the FDA approved the drug. Two quotations from the label are relevant:

The efficacy of RELENZA 10 mg inhaled twice daily for 5 days in the treatment of influenza has been evaluated in placebo-controlled studies conducted in North America, the Southern Hemisphere, and Europe during their respective influenza seasons. The magnitude of treatment effect varied between studies, with possible relationships to population-related factors including amount of symptomatic relief medication used . . . .

Principal Results: The definition of time to improvement in major symptoms of influenza included no fever and self-assessment of "none" or "mild" for headache, myalgia, cough, and sore throat. A Phase II and a Phase III study conducted in North America (total of over 600 influenza-positive patients) suggested up to 1 day of shortening of median time to this defined improvement in symptoms in patients receiving zanamivir compared with placebo, although statistical significance was not reached in either of these studies. In a study conducted in the Southern Hemisphere (321 influenza-positive patients), a 1.5-day difference in median time to symptom improvement was observed. Additional evidence of efficacy was provided by the European study [15].

MERIT-HF. The Metoprolol CR/XL (Controlled Release/Extended Release) Randomized Intervention Trial in Chronic Heart Failure, or MERIT-HF, was a randomized, double-blind, placebo-controlled trial studying patients with symptomatic heart failure. The dose of metoprolol used for those randomized to active drug depended on their New York Heart Association (NYHA) class. The trial randomized 3,991 participants, with roughly 2,000 per group. Participants came from the USA and 13 European countries, all of which can be considered developed in terms of access to, and sophistication of, medical treatments (Belgium, Czech Republic, Denmark, Finland, Germany, Hungary, Iceland, The Netherlands, Norway, Poland, Sweden, Switzerland, and the United Kingdom). The study had two co-primary outcomes: (1) time to death or (2) time to death or any hospitalization. A statistically significant improvement relative to placebo on either of these outcomes would lead the conclusion that metoprolol was beneficial in this patient population. The p-value was partitioned between the two outcomes in a way that protected the overall Type I error rate of the trial. Randomization began in February 1997 and ended on April 14, 1998. The study stopped at the second interim analysis (October 31, 1998) on a recommendation from the Independent Safety Committee. At that time, all participants had been randomized and half of the expected events had occurred (i.e., the information time was 50%); the mean follow-up time was one year; and the observed p-values for both primary outcomes were less than 0.001. When the study stopped, 145 participants in the metoprolol group and 217 in the placebo group had died. The estimated relative risk was 0.66 with a nominal 95% confidence interval of (0.53, 0.81). (The word "nominal" here reflects that the confidence interval is not corrected for the fact that the estimates came from an interim analysis.) The MERIT-HF Study Group has described the design of the study [16] and the primary results [17].

The large benefit seen, however, was limited to Europe where the observed relative risk was 0.55. In the USA, which randomized roughly one-quarter of the study cohort, the relative risk was 1.05; that is, in the USA slightly more deaths occurred in the metoprolol group than in the placebo group (see Table 1).

Table 1 Results from the MERIT-HF study: total mortality

Region	Relative risk	Nominal 95% confidence interval
Overall (n = 3,991)	0.66	(0.53, 0.81)
USA (n = 1,071)	1.05	(0.71, 1.56)
Europe (n = 2,920)	0.55	(0.43, 0.70)

Interaction p-value: 0.003. Data from descriptions of the MERIT-HF study [17–19]

In its review of the MERIT-HF study, the FDA addressed the discordance between the findings in the USA and elsewhere:

If the mortality endpoint is the most important among all endpoints, the US sub-population should be the most important subgroup in a multinational trial because the goal of the [New Drug Application] submission is to gain approval for marketing the drug in the US. The efficacy outcome in this population must be examined carefully as part of the evaluation of the totality of the evidence and possible extrapolation of the efficacy evidence from foreign population[s] to [the] US population [18].

An memorandum written at the FDA says,

Because of demographic differences or differences in concomitant care, a treatment might be beneficial overall but neutral or detrimental in some subpopulations. In particular, even though studies in the United States were not required for approval, evidence that a treatment is non-beneficial in United States patients (or even in some subpopulation among United States patients) must not be ignored. The observed mortality among United States patients receiving metoprolol was 105% of that seen in those receiving placebo.

How should this finding be interpreted? The finding of adverse United States mortality could of course be attributable to chance, but it could alternatively be a genuine finding, the result of US-differences in demographics or concomitant therapy (from an FDA memorandum [20]).

(Before proceeding, I cannot resist making a side comment. Although the memorandum speaks of patients "receiving" metoprolol and placebo, the data actually show results for patient *randomized* to metoprolol and placebo.)

The FDA handled the discordant finding by approving the drug but including in the label a forest plot showing the effects in various subgroups, including the discordant effect in the USA. See FDA [18] and Wedel et al. [21] for discussions of the differences between the observed effect of the drug in the USA and other countries.

PLATO (PLATelet inhibition and patient Outcomes trial) was a double-blind randomized controlled trial comparing ticagrelor (n = 9,333) against clopidogrel (n = 9,291) in patients with an acute coronary syndrome, with or without ST-segment elevation, with an onset of symptoms within the previous 24 hours. About 10% of the participants (n = 1,814) came from North America (the USA and Canada). Overall, the trial showed a 16% reduction in its primary outcome: time to the first occurrence of cardiovascular death, myocardial infarction, or stroke. The paper describing the results stated:

Table 2 PLATO: results for the primary outcome in the USA vs. other countries

Region	Ticagrelor (n/N)	Clopidogrel (n/N)	Hazard ratio (95% confidence interval)
Overall(n = 18,624)	9.8%(864/9,333)	11.7%(1,014/9,291)	0.84(0.77, 0.93)
Non-US(n = 17,211)	9.6%(780/8,626)	11.8%(947/8,585)	0.81(0.74, 0.90)
US(n = 1,413)	12.6%(84/707)	10.1%(67/706)	1.27(0.92, 1.75)

Nominal p-value for interaction: US vs. non-US: 0.0095
Source: Fiorentino and Zhang [24]

The results regarding the primary end point did not show significant heterogeneity in analyses of the 33 subgroups, with three exceptions: The benefit of ticagrelor appeared to be attenuated in patients weighing less than the median weight for their sex ($P = 0.04$ for the interaction), those not taking lipid-lowering drugs at randomization ($P = 0.04$ for the interaction), and those enrolled in North America ($P = 0.045$ for the interaction) [22].

In fact, the results in North America were not merely "attenuated"; they were in the opposite direction from the results elsewhere: a primary outcome occurred in 11.9% of those randomized to ticagrelor compared to 9.6% of those randomized to clopidogrel. The observed adverse effect, like the observed adverse effect in MERIT-HF, was not statistically significant. The difference might have been due to chance—a p-value of 0.045 for an interaction is hardly compelling evidence that a difference is real, especially given the post hoc nature of the test and the fact that many statistical tests were performed. It may, however, reflect a real phenomenon. The difference may have been due, at least in part, to a different approach in the USA to treatment with aspirin [23].

In its presentation to the Cardio-Renal Advisory Panel on June 28, 2010, the FDA reported on the United States cohort, which comprised about 80% of the North American cohort, and showed an even larger difference than reported in the published paper. The p-value for the interaction between North America and the rest of the world was 0.045, but the interaction p-value for the USA compared to the rest of the world was smaller, 0.0095, reflecting the observation that although the hazard ratio for Canada was 1.17, which was unfavorable to ticagrelor, lumping Canada into the non-US category and then testing the USA against all non-US countries decreased the p-value for the interaction from 0.045 to 0.0095 (see Table 2).

The FDA eventually approved ticagrelor in the USA, but the package insert includes the following language:

Results in the rest of the world compared to effects in North American (US and Canada) show a smaller effect in North America, numerically unfavorable to the control and driven by the US subset. The statistical test for the US/non-US comparison is statistically significant ($p = 0.009$) and the same trend is present for both CV death and non-fatal MI. The individual results and nominal p-values, like all subset analyses, need cautious interpretation, and they could represent chance findings. The consistency of the differences in both the CV and non-fatal MI comparisons, however, supports the possibility that the finding is reliable.

A wide variety of baseline and procedural differences between the US and non-US ... were examined to see if they could account for regional differences, but with one exception, aspirin maintenance dose, these differences did not appear to lead to differences in outcome [25].

Table 3 Subgroup analyses of the primary efficacy endpoint for the BLISS trials

	BLISS-76		BLISS-52	
		Belimumab		Belimumab
	Placebo (N = 275)	10 mg/kg (N = 273)	Placebo (N = 287)	10 mg/kg (N = 290)
Overall response:	93 (34%)	118 (43%)	125 (44%)	167 (58%)
Region				
USA/Canada	46/145 (32%)	47/136 (35%)	–	–
Western Europe/Israel	15/64 (23%)	38/75 (51%)	–	–
Eastern Europe	15/36 (42%)	16/30 (53%)	12/33 (36%)	23/31 (74%)
Americas (excluding USA/Canada)	17/30 (57%)	17/32 (53%)	71/145 (49%)	85/140 (61%)
Asia	–	–	40/103 (39%)	56/115 (49%)
Australia	–	–	2/6 (33%)	3/4 (75%)
Interaction P-value[a]	–	0.073	–	0.18
Interaction P-value[b]		0.15		

[a]For treatment by subgroup interaction effect from logistic regression as reported by the FDA.
[b]US/Canada vs. other, two sided calculated using StatXact [26]Source. FDA briefing document, 10-Oct-2010

So, as the FDA had done for the metoprolol, it approved ticagrelor for use in the USA, but it required that the label discuss the discordance between results in the USA and elsewhere. Moreover, the label expresses ambivalence about whether or not the findings reflect a true difference or a chance finding.

The BLISS trials. Two randomized double-blind trials compared belimumab (trade name Benlysta) to placebo in patients with systemic lupus erythematosus (SLE). In both trials, the primary outcome was a binary outcome measured at 52 weeks with success defined by an SLE Responder Index (SRI). BLISS-52 randomized patients from Asia, South America, and Eastern Europe; patients were to be treated for 52 weeks. Patients in BLISS-76 were treated for 76 weeks; participating centers came from North American and Europe. In its presentation to its advisory panel, the FDA pointed to a difference in the results from the USA and Canada and the remainder of the population: while the overall effect showed benefit, only a very small benefit was seen in the population from the USA and Canada. See Table 3 for some of the data the FDA presented. For simplicity, this table shows only the placebo and the high dose (10 mg/kg) group: the actual trials had included a 1 mg/kg arm.

While the briefing document showed a numerical difference between the effect in the four prespecified regions, the p-value cited by the FDA, derived from a logistic regression model (which I assume had three degrees of freedom), was 0.073, suggestive of, but not conclusive of, a difference among the regions. A one degree of freedom statistic comparing the USA and Canada to the rest of the world has an interaction p-value of 0.16, which is consistent with the effect in the USA and Canada being not different from the effect elsewhere. The FDA's analysis, however, went further; it examined the effect by race and required a label pointing out not the difference between the USA/Canada and the rest of the world, but to the difference between blacks and non-blacks.

Effect in Black/African-American Patients
Exploratory sub-group analyses of [the SLE Responder Index] response rate in patients of black race were performed. In [BLISS-52 and BLISS-76] combined, the [SLE Responder Index] response rate in black patients (N = 148) in the BENLYSTA groups was less than that in the placebo group (22/50 or 44% for placebo, 15/48 or 31% for BENLYSTA 1 mg/kg, and 18/50 or 36% for BENLYSTA 10 mg/kg). In [the Phase 2 trial], black patients (N = 106) in the BENLYSTA groups did not appear to have a different response than the rest of the study population. Although no definitive conclusions can be drawn from these subgroup analyses, caution should be used when considering BENLYSTA treatment in black/African-American SLE patients [27].

All four of these examples reflect common themes—a statistically significant benefit observed overall, a much smaller benefit—or, in MERIT-HF and PLATO, a point estimate in the direction of harm—in the USA (or the USA and Canada), an intellectual struggle with how to deal with the apparent discrepancies, but a resolution that led to approval of each drug with presentation of data in the package insert acknowledging the lack of consistency in the results and the uncertainty of whether to attribute the observed disparities to chance or to a true difference.

In MERIT-HF and PLATO, tests for interaction comparing the effect in the USA with other countries showed nominal statistical significance (again, the word "nominal" reflects that fact that these tests were not prespecified); in the BLISS trials, the nominal p-values for interaction were above 0.05. Tests for interaction, however, are notoriously hard to interpret. Tests performed after looking at the data, as the examples here were, lack clear probabilistic interpretation. Prespecified tests of interaction generally have low power. Thus, "statistically significant" unprespecified interaction has a high probability of being a false finding. On the other hand, failure to find a prespecified interaction may not be strong evidence of no interaction; it may simply be the result of low power. Moreover, the interaction tests usually performed ask the question, "Is the effect size constant over the subgroups investigated?" But that is not really the question of interest when we are looking at the difference between the USA and elsewhere—we do expect some variation in effect size so if the sample size is huge, the interaction test is highly likely to be statistically significant. The real question is whether in the USA the effect is in the direction of harm or if the effect size is so small that the product is not useful in the USA. Ultimately, the interpretation must come from a combination of statistical arguments and from consideration of the biological, medical, and regulatory milieu.

5　Against Whom Should We Compare the USA?

The four examples above suggest a taxonomic dilemma: how should one define geographic regions? In asking questions about the USA, should one compare the USA to the rest of world? That stance is consistent with the discussion about region in PLATO where the FDA disaggregated North America into the USA and Canada post hoc and in the FDA's discussion of the interpretation from MERIT-HF. Perhaps analysis should include only two categories—the USA compared to all other countries or the USA and other medically advanced countries in one category and other countries as the second. What about the USA and Canada compared to all others as in BLISS-76? Perhaps having three categories makes more sense: the USA, other medically advanced countries, and others. Or perhaps just a geographical split is desirable. In that case, should we lump Western Europe together and all Eastern Europe together? Should we gerrymander Eastern Europe so that Poland and the Czech Republic join Western Europe and other former Eastern Bloc countries join Russia? What about Israel? Australia? South Africa? Does Mexico belong with North America or should it be considered part of Central and South America? What constitutes Asia? Should it include only China, Japan, and Korea (and Taiwan and Hong Kong)? Does it include India? Where does Turkey go? Does Africa include the Mahgreb? Or should sub-Saharan Africa be split from Mediterranean Africa? And, who makes the decision? And is the decision made before or after looking at the data?

Perhaps this whole discussion is rather silly. After all, the USA itself is not homogeneous—our very motto, E pluribus unum, attests to our diversity. Moreover, the study population of a clinical trial is not representative of the population that will actually be treated, so fastidious classification of countries does not address the real question of interest to the FDA in deciding whether to approve a product or to treating physicians in the USA: is there convincing evidence that the benefit of the treatment under study outweighs the harm for patients in the USA? If this is the real question underlying a regional categorization (and I think it should be), then the choice of how to classify countries should depend on the particular study and the particular disease and chosen a priori.

6 Safety

The previous sections have addressed efficacy by asking how to interpret discordant conclusions regarding efficacy between the USA and other countries. The answer has been "it depends," for in the absence of adequate power, trials are unlikely to allow distinguishing a chance finding from a true one. But efficacy is only one face of the clinical trial die—another face is safety. Ultimately, the decision about whether to approve a medical product requires a judgment that the likely benefits exceed the likely harms. Most trials attempt to measure benefit carefully and precisely, with definitions that are constant across the trial and therefore constant across regions. The assessment of safety, on the other hand, is usually performed by unstructured reporting of adverse events, which then are coded into categories defined by a medical dictionary, the most common of which for regulatory reporting is currently the Medical Dictionary for Regulatory Activities, or MedDRA. The proportion of people experiencing each type of event is then reported across the entire clinical trial. This proportion is often called a "rate" though the estimates usually do not incorporate time. Typically the reporting is performed without stratification and rarely by geographic region. While efficacy is often measured in terms of relative benefit, most adverse event reporting compares treatments with respect to the difference between absolute risks in the treated and control groups. Therefore, if the reporting of adverse events differs considerably from region to region, the estimated difference in proportions may not reflect the actual risk of harm in the USA. I am not aware of published evidence for differences in reported risks by country; however, I have a strong belief, buttressed by a considerable amount of confidential data (trust me, dear reader) from many trials performed by many different public and private sponsors in a variety of therapeutic areas, that the reported proportions of adverse experiences differ dramatically from region to region. I suspect, but cannot prove, that depending on the event and the quality of the clinical center involved, the proportions of people experiencing many events are grossly underreported in certain cultures, and hence certain countries. Therefore, the estimated proportions of people experiencing specific adverse effects overall may or may not be relevant to the true proportions in the USA. Much as I am reluctant to recommend more data collection in Phase 3 trials, a few additional case report forms might alleviate the most serious aspects of this problem. For specific adverse events of special interest in a trial, either identified prior to the beginning of the trial or noted during the course of the trial, adding a structured case report form eliciting information about that event would be more likely to identify the occurrence of the event than the current method of passive reporting. Such active collection would remove the onus of categorizing reported events that are coded similarly, but not identically (e.g., when is a reported "myocardial infarction" not the same as a reported "acute myocardial infarction"?). The form would include relevant information to characterize the event. In addition, designers of large trials should consider including structured forms for collecting data on incident cancers and incident major cardiovascular events. I point to these events because the angst caused by seeing at the end of a trial even a small excess in cancers or major cardiovascular events can lead to failure to approve an otherwise promising drug. For a drug that is likely to affect immune function, a structured form to collect data on infections would be useful because classifying types of passively reported infections is a daunting task. Collecting accurate incidence of adverse events can help assess risks and benefits in a way that is very difficult if the data are reported at wildly different rates in different countries.

7 Hedging Bets in Design and Analysis

Realistically, studies will, and I believe should, continue to be performed globally. The questions sponsors and other designers must face is how best to design and analyze studies in a way that allows generalization to the country of interest, which here we assume is the USA. Thinking about how to generalize is best done prior to initiation of the trial. One approach, which is not likely to be used in large Phase 3 trials, is to minimize reliance on data from outside the USA; another is to write careful entry criteria to assure that patients outside the USA have a condition that is similar to the experience in the USA and treatments that would reflect what would happen in the USA. An alternative that I prefer is rather than limit the population by adopting extensive entry criteria, collect data that allow characterization of the population. Obviously, all studies should be conducted in way that provides reliable evidence regarding efficacy and safety.

Marschner [28] shows a graph depicting the expected magnitude of effect sizes when all regions have the same number of participants and when the true effect size in all regions is equal (Fig. 3). He recommends describing in the protocol or analysis plan the expected distribution of these order statistics. While his paper deals with equal size groups, his approach can easily be adapted to different sizes. His striking graph shows the wide variability in expected treatment sizes as the number of regions increases. This theoretical demonstration of the data shown in Fig. 1 can be applied not only to regional differences, but to other types of subgroups as well. Including such a graph in an analysis plan or a design paper, where the calculations are based on the actual sample sizes expected by region, would provide a warning to those designing the trial and those interpreting the data to expect variation in effect size.

The problem is more difficult if the treatment is likely truly to have different effects in different regions of the world, or if the treatment is less effective in the USA than it is elsewhere. The designers of a trial should think carefully, and honestly, about why the trial is global. They should think about the likely sources of variability and how that would affect the estimated efficacy and the reported safety. If, prior to designing the trial, the investigators believe or suspect or fear that the results in the USA may truly be substantially different from that in other regions, or if the investigators want to hedge their bets, a reasonable strategy is to select a sample size large enough in the USA alone that would give high power to see that the treatment effect is at least in the same direction as it is in the rest of the world. Such a calculation will likely increase the sample size.

More conservative approaches, which would lead to even larger sample sizes, would control the variability even more. One possible method would be to assume that the effect size δ is the same in all regions and to select a sample size such that the overall power is γ (e.g., 80% or 90%), but that the sample size in the USA is large enough to give a power of γ_{US} to show that the observed effect in the USA is above some value δ_{US}. An even more conservative approach, but one that is likely unfeasible, would be to select sample sizes in each region of interest large enough so that if the true difference were δ in all regions, the probability of finding a result in the opposite direction is controlled. Or, to be even more cautious (and even less feasible), to set the sample size in each region large enough to provide a bound for the probability of finding a result that is unacceptably smaller than the overall observed $\widehat{\delta}$. All of these strategies will necessarily increase the sample size, and, depending on the stringency of the control, the increase can be substantial. For trials that are unlikely to be replicated, a cautious approach to prespecification of likely

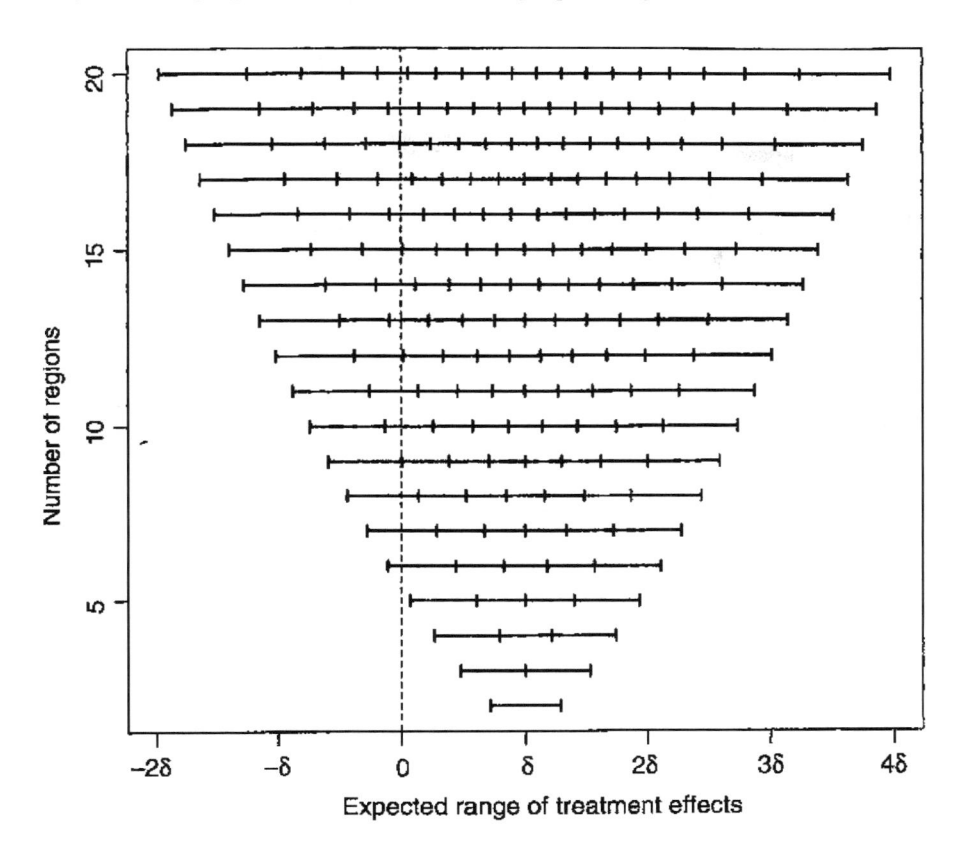

Fig. 3 Expected range of regional treatment effects in a trial with 80% power for a treatment difference of δ and a two-sided Type 1 error rate of 0.05. For each range, the *j*th tick mark from the *left* denotes the expected value of the *j*th largest regional treatment effect. (Figure from Ian C. Marschner [28]; Clinical Trials (Vol. 7, issue 2), page 150, copyright © 2010 by Sage Publishing. Reproduced by permission of SAGE)

variation in observed effect size should inform the design of the trial, even if it leads to a larger sample size (as long, of course, as the increase is feasible). Whatever decision is made, the trial designers would be wise to consider their options in the design phase of the trial, and do calculations that show the consequences of their choices.

8 Data Monitoring Committees

Thus far the discussion has dealt with thinking about studies during their design phase in a way that accounts for regional differences and then interpreting the data at the end of the trial. But of course trials have not only a beginning and an end; they also have a middle. An independent data monitoring committee (DMC) reviews data during the course of many trials. Each of the four trials discussed above did in fact have a DMC. As far as I am aware, there is no standard approach for DMCs to look at country-specific data on either efficacy or safety. Because of the frequent finding of disparate results on efficacy by region and my personal experience with even greater differences in safety, I routinely urge DMCs involved in multinational trials to look at region-specific analyses before recommending protocol changes or early termination either for efficacy or safety. For trials that will be used for regulatory submission to the USA, a prudent DMC will look at tables of the major efficacy variables and important safety variables from the USA alone and from other regions defined in a way that is sensible for the particular trial. Extra caution in recommending early stopping of a study when important subgroups are showing discordant results may prevent intellectual angst later. Once a trial stops, restarting is very difficult. I realize that this recommendation can lead a DMC to wring its hands when faced with a dramatic effect overall but a disturbing lack of consistency by region. Nonetheless, when a DMC observes large differences in effect size by region, it should examine whether the differences can clearly be explained by regional differences in concomitant medications, surgical therapies, demographic variables, and the degree of adherence to the protocol. Often the reasons for the differences in effect size will not be clear; after all, if the total sample size at the end of the trial is too small to allow reliable inference about subgroups, such inference is even more difficult during the trial when the sample size is smaller.

9 Topics Not Covered

Most of the previous discussion has dealt with Phase 3 trials and with countries that, like the United States, have populations with access to high quality medical care. Of course, in most countries, the USA included, some populations are grossly medically underserved. I have totally avoided one important issue and skirted a second. This brief section introduces those two topics. The topic avoided has to do with inference from Phase 2 trials. Many drugs have shown great promise in Phase 2 but disappointing results in Phase 3. Sometimes this lesser effect in Phase 3 may be due to regression toward the mean, sometimes it may be due to failure to recognize the variability in estimates from Phase 2 [29], but sometimes it may be due to studying a drug in a country where the patients and the therapies are so different from those in the USA that the conclusions from the Phase 2 studies are indeed not applicable to the USA. Articles in the financial press, for example Morrison [30], warn against using Phase 2 data from some foreign countries to provide estimates for results in Phase 3.

The skirted issue relates to use of data from developing countries where the data are of low quality, the patients are very different from those in the USA, and the drug company sponsor has no intention of marketing the drug in these countries. I have assumed throughout that the centers being used are of high quality. The Vanity Fair article referred to previously [11] addresses these problems; the authors cited many of the issues described earlier in this paper, and in addition stressed the huge gap in medical care in indigent populations of the developing world. The authors also questioned the ethics of conducting clinical trials of drugs that will be too expensive to be used in the countries in which they are being tested. This latter concern is the flip side of distributive justice—failure to include participants who would be eligible for the treatment is the topic addressed earlier in this paper, but inclusion of those who would not is the opposite problem.

10 Conclusion and Recommendations

Given my personal skepticism about interpreting effects from subgroups, I have entered the "region as subgroup" fray with reluctance convinced at the start that nearly all apparent regional differences in treatment effect are due to the play of chance. To my surprise I find myself suspecting that for many interventions the treatment effect may truly vary by country and may, in fact, often be smaller in the USA than in other countries. Am I being fooled by randomness? As my son says, "I used to be uncertain, but now I'm not so sure." The problem, of course, is that when one sees a difference between countries or regions, it is nearly impossible to know whether the difference reflects reality or simply the play of chance.

One answer to the question posed in the title is that region differs from other subgroups because it often serves as a surrogate for disease incidence, prevalence, and severity as well as a surrogate for standard of care. Another answer is that regulatory bodies are obligated by their legal mandates to make inferences about the effect of treatment for the country (or countries) for which they are responsible. Thus, they must look at country-specific data; how they interpret those data when estimate vary from country to country is part of regulatory art.

A few steps when the study is being designed may alleviate potential ambiguity when the study is over. First, the designers should carefully consider variables that are likely to affect the true treatment effect. If some characteristic of the patient population, the local standard of care, the quality of the centers in the various countries, or the projected country-specific adherence to protocol is likely to have a major influence on the true treatment effect, then the designers might consider recruiting from a more homogeneous group of countries. Sometimes, sponsors design two studies—one in more medically developed and one in less medically developed nations.

If, on the other hand, the effect size is assumed to be nearly constant across regions or countries, then the designers should prepare a document, perhaps as part of the statistical analysis plan, describing the expected country-to-country statistical variability. In any particular trial, if the proportion of participants from a given country is small, the data from that trial are unlikely to provide reliable insight into either the effect of treatment or the proportion experiencing harms within that country. For example, as seen in Table 4, if a trial has power of 80%, then a

Table 4 Power for a
geographic region as a
function of the region size

Percent of participants in the country of interest	Power for the study as a whole	
	0.80	0.90
100	0.80	0.90
90	0.76	0.87
75	0.68	0.80
50	0.51	0.63
25	0.29	0.37
10	0.14	0.17

country that has randomized 25% of the study cohort will have only 29% power to show a statistically significant benefit if the true benefit is the hypothesized effect size. Therefore, a prudent stance for trial designers interested in learning about a particular country is to calculate, prior to initiating the trial, what the power would be for the expected sample size along with the barely detectable difference for that size (i.e., the difference that can be detected with 50% power). If these values are unacceptable, then the sponsor might consider increasing the sample size in the countries of particular interest to maintain more desirable power [31].

In any case, the regions to be considered should be specified before looking at the data and the reasons for the classification described. The categorizations should be study-specific, taking into account the anticipated sources of variability that are likely to affect the magnitude of effect.

Metrics chosen should be those that are nearly invariant to country-specific rates; in general, relative measures of effect are more likely to be constant across countries than are attributable risks.

No matter what is done before the trial, the possibility of observing large differences by region or country is high in a multinational trial with many countries; ultimately, the interpretation will rest on balancing the likely contribution of chance and reality. Perhaps the best solution when reporting data is to assume that most of the variation is due to chance, but to report the data in the prespecified regions and to make the most scientific interpretation one can.

Acknowledgements Many thanks to Robert Byington for Fig. 1, Mark Schactman for insightful comments on an earlier draft of this paper, the referees for helpful suggestions, and Nancy L. Buc for a careful, critical reading.

References

1. Simon R (1980) Patient heterogeneity in clinical trials. Cancer Treat Rep 64(2–3):405–410
2. Simon R (1982) Patient subsets and variation in therapeutic efficacy. Br J Clin Pharmacol 14:473–482
3. Dixon D, Simon R (1991) Bayesian subset analysis. Biometrics 47(3):871–881
4. Oxman A, Guyatt G (1992) A consumer's guide to subgroup analysis. Ann Intern Med 116: 78–84

5. Lagakos S (2006) The challenge of subgroup analyses – reporting without distorting. N Engl J Med 354(16):1667–1669
6. Wittes J (2009) On looking at subgroups. Circulation 119(7):912–915
7. Yusuf S, Wittes J, Probstfield J, Tyroler H (1991) Analysis and interpretation of treatment effects in subgroups of patients in randomized clinical trials. J Am Med Assoc 266(1):93–98
8. The Systolic Hypertension in the Elderly Program (SHEP) Cooperative Research Group (1991) Prevention of stroke by antihypertensive drug treatment in older persons with isolated systolic hypertension: final results of the Systolic Hypertension in the Elderly Program (SHEP). J Am Med Assoc 265(24):3255–3264
9. Quan H, Li M, Chen J et al (2010) Assessment of consistency of treatment effects in multiregional clinical trials. Drug Inf J 44:616–632
10. Kim E, Carrigan T, Menon V (2011) International participation in cardiovascular randomized controlled trials. J Am Coll Cardiol 58:671–676
11. Bartlett D, Steele J (2011) Deadly medicine. Vanity Fair, January 2011
12. Soskolne CL (2006) Eliminating disparities in clinical trials (EDICT): The equitable inclusion of all populations into clinical trials from a distributive justice perspective. Baylor College of Medicine http://chronic.bcm.tmc.edu/edict/Distributive_Justice.pdf
13. Luo X, Shih W, Ouyang S, DeLap R (2010) An optimal adaptive design to address local regulations in global clinical trials. Pharm Stat 9:179–189
14. Nandakumar A, Anantha N, Venugopal T (1995) Incidence, mortality, and survival in cancer of the cervix in Bangalore, India. Br J Cancer 71(6):1348–1352
15. GlaxoSmithKline (2010) Package insert for Relenza
16. International Steering Committee on behalf of the MERIT-HF Study Group (1997) Rationale, design, and organization of the Metoprolol CR/XL Randomized Intervention Trial in Heart Failure (MERIT-HF). Am J Cardiol 80(Suppl 9B):54J–58J
17. MERIT-HF Study Group (1999) Effect of metoprolol CR/XL in chronic heart failure: Metoprolol CR/XL Randomized Intervention Trial in Congestive Heart Failure (MERIT-HF). Lancet 353:2001–2007
18. FDA (2000) Statistical review and evaluation (Amendment 1). NDA 19,962. May 30, 2000
19. FDA. Package insert for Toprol-XL
20. FDA memo as quoted by Moyé L (2000) Multiple Analyses in Clinical Trials. Springer, New York
21. Wedel H, DeMets D, Deedwania P et al (2001) Challenges of subgroup analyses in multinational clinical trials: experiences from the MERIT-HF trial. Am Heart J 142:502–511
22. Wallentin L, Becker R, Budaj A et al (2009) Ticagrelor versus clopidogrel in patients with acute coronary symptoms. N Engl J Med 361(11):1045–1057
23. Mahaffery KW, Wojdyla DM, Carroll K, et al (2011) Ticagrelor compared with clopidogrel by geographic region in the Platelet Inhibition and Patient Outcomes (PLATO) trial. Circulation 124(5):544–554
24. Fiorentino R, Zhang J (2010) NDA 22–433 Brinlinta (ticagrelor) Efficacy Review the Cardio-Renal Advisory Committee, July 28, 2010
25. AstraZeneca (2011) Package insert for Brinlinta (ticagrelor)
26. StatXact 9 [computer program]. Cytel, Cambridge, MA
27. Human Genome Sciences (2010) Package insert for Benlysta
28. Marschner IC (2010) Regional differences in multinational clinical trials: anticipating chance variation. Clin Trials 7(2):147–156
29. Lan K, Wittes J (2012) Some thoughts on sample size: a Bayesian-frequentist hybrid approach. Clin Trials. 1740774512453784, first published on August 3, 2012 as doi:10.1177/1740774512453784
30. Morrison T (2010) Lesson from an Alzheimer-drug failure: beware Russian clinical trial data (March 5, 2010). BNET, 2010
31. Quan H, Li M, Chen J et al (2010) Assessment of treatment effects in multiregional clinical trials. Drug Inf J 44:617–632

Part IV
Safety

Quantitative Risk/Benefit Assessment: Where Are We?

Christy Chuang-Stein

Abstract Pharmaceutical sponsors use a variety of approaches to make important benefit/risk decisions about their products internally. Benefit/risk assessment is equally important when regulators evaluate a product for marketing approval and payers evaluate it for reimbursement decision. Once a product receives marketing authorization, it is critical to communicate pertinent benefit and risk information to patients and health-care providers. All of the above can be made easier by the use of a common framework. In this paper, we review where we are in benefit/risk assessment. This includes endeavors by academic institutions, regulators, and the pharmaceutical industry. Despite concerns about quantitative benefit/risk assessment expressed by some, we argue that without a way to quantitatively incorporate the relative importance of factors impacting benefit/risk assessment, it will be hard to bring transparent decisions to questions such as "does the benefit of this product outweigh the risk."

1 Introduction

I saw a cartoon in the summer of 2010. The cartoon is a metaphor for a pharmaceutical developer who, like a hurdler, needs to cross a set of hurdles. The first hurdle is labeled quality, the second safety and the third efficacy. The fourth one is unlabeled, but looks menacing. The hurdle takes the form of a solid wall. There are sharp spikes coming out of the wall, facing the hurdler. The caption reads—There was general agreement that the fourth hurdle was the one to look out for.

I asked myself—Is the cartoon an exaggeration of the environment a product developer is in? If there is some truth to the cartoon, then what is this fourth hurdle?

C. Chuang-Stein (✉)
Statistical Research and Consulting Center, Pfizer Inc., Kalamazoo, MI 49007, USA
e-mail: christy.j.chuang-stein@pfizer.com

T.R. Fleming and B.S. Weir (eds.), *Proceedings of the Fourth Seattle Symposium in Biostatistics: Clinical Trials*, Lecture Notes in Statistics 1205, DOI 10.1007/978-1-4614-5245-4_8, © Springer Science+Business Media New York 2013

Is it benefit/risk? Is it relative effectiveness, a term frequently used in Europe? Is it comparative effectiveness, a term gaining momentum in the USA? Is it Health Technology Assessment, a cost-effectiveness evaluation pharmaceutical developers have to go through to have their products reimbursed in socialized health-care systems in Europe, Canada, and Australia? Or, is it all of the above plus other emerging value propositions?

I was told by a friend who was familiar with the origin of the cartoon that the cartoonist used the fourth hurdle as a symbol for health technology assessment. In an editorial in *Clin Pharmacology and Therapeutics*, Honig [1] described comparative effectiveness as the fourth hurdle in drug development. I cannot but feel that the cartoon could easily apply to benefit/risk evaluation because of the lack of a common approach for articulating the trade-off between benefit and risk to reach a transparent decision.

When preparing my presentation for the fourth Seattle Symposium, I checked the FDA Advisory Committee (AC) meetings from September to early November 2010 to see how the benefit/risk question was presented to the AC members. There were six AC meetings altogether. Among the six meetings, three were to decide whether approved products should remain on the market. One was to review a supplemental application of an approved product. Two were to review new molecular entities, one of which was lorcaserin hydrochloride (with diet and exercise) for weight management for obese patients on September 16th. The public meeting on lorcaserin attracted a lot of attention. The interest level for weight management is generally high. In this case, the interest was elevated by the diet drug subutramine that was reviewed the day before for possible regulatory actions including product withdrawal. On September 16th, the Endocrinologic and Metabolic Drugs AC was asked to vote on only one question. The question was whether available data demonstrated that the potential benefits of lorcaserin outweighed the potential risks to allow marketing approval.

There was a general agreement that lorcaserin's efficacy data met FDA's requirement, albeit marginally. Concerns were raised about lorcaserin's safety. These included the fact that lorcaserin is chemically similar to two weight-loss drugs that were withdrawn in 1997 due to their links to the valvular heart disease. In addition, two-year studies in rats reported an excess number of malignant mammary tumors in female rats. The cancer concerns were not confirmed in clinical trials. Nevertheless, it was felt that the duration of the trials might be too short and the study populations not diverse enough to allow a potential cancer risk to be detected.

When it was time to vote, the votes were five (36%) for approval and nine (64%) against approval. On October 22, 2010, FDA rejected lorcaserin for the proposed indication, signaling that, in the eyes of the agency, the safety concerns outweighed what the agency called lorcaserin's marginal effectiveness. Had the efficacy of lorcaserin been much better than what had been observed, would FDA approve lorcaserin for the indication sought? On August 2 2011, the Bloomberg news reported that lorcaserin's manufacturers announced that a newly completed study showed the concentrations of lorcaserin to be lower in human brains than in rat models. This finding helped ease concerns that lorcaserin may be linked to brain tumors. On July 22 2012 FDA granted marketing authorization to lorcaserin.

In general, how do we make decisions with opposing needs? A sensible approach is to adopt a framework where all relevant factors are first collected. This first step is then followed by articulating the relative importance of these factors, identifying a sensible way to combine factors with weights that reflect the relative importance of the factors, checking out the properties of the combination algorithms, settling on a decision rule and identifying conditions where the rule would lead to clear and unequivocal decision. Finally, make a decision and communicate the decision to individuals who have an interest in the outcome.

The rest of the paper is organized as follows. In Sect. 2, we discuss selected approaches to examine benefit and risk simultaneously. Some of these approaches combine benefit and risk into one measure for easy interpretation, while others consider benefit and risk jointly. Section 3 describes a benefit/risk framework developed by the Benefit Risk Action Team (BRAT) of the Pharmaceutical Research and Manufacturers of America (PhRMA). In Sect. 4, we discuss communicating benefit/risk to the public. Section 5 describes a report on current tools and processes for regulatory benefit–risk assessment issued by the Benefit–Risk Methodology Project of the European Medicines Agency. Section 6 describes briefly a recent FDA draft guidance on factors to consider when making benefit–risk determinations in medical device premarket review. We end this paper by acknowledging challenges of benefit/risk assessment of pharmaceutical products in general and offer some additional comments in Sect. 7.

2 Measures or Approaches to Assess Benefit and Risk Simultaneously

2.1 Quality-Adjusted Life Without Toxicity Q-TWiST

One of the earlier attempts to discount benefit by risk of cancer drugs was to calculate time without symptoms of disease and toxic effects (TWiST) [2]. This concept was further developed to form quality-adjusted TWiST (Q-TWiST) [3]. Q-TWiST was obtained by discounting survival by a utility weighting that reflected quality of life in different physical conditions. For example, the utility weighting could be different for days with toxic effects and days after disease progression. More recently, Hughes et al. [4] used quality-adjusted life-years within a decision-analytical framework.

While discounting survival by treatment-related toxicity and/or poor quality of life was intuitive, the discounting process could be subjective. As such, Irish et al. [5] suggested conducting a threshold utility analysis as a form of sensitivity analysis by comparing treatments across all combinations of the utility weightings for days with toxic effects and days after disease progression. Such sensitivity analysis allows researchers to observe how the comparison varies with different utility weightings. Variations of the threshold utility analysis are possible. For example, if data are available, one can incorporate patients' experiences or functions on days after disease progression instead of relying on utility weighting solely on such days.

The idea of discounting benefit by risk was also adopted by Chuang-Stein [6] who proposed a benefit-less-risk analysis. Under this analysis, benefit was discounted linearly by a risk measure via the use of a conversion factor. The conversion factor serves to convert benefit and risk to a similar scale to allow their integration into a single measure.

2.2 Clinical Utility Index

Pharmaceutical manufacturers regularly assess the benefit/risk profiles of their products. This applies to selecting a dose and making go/no go decisions. Regarding dose selection, some sponsors try to maximize benefit while keeping the risk at an (pre-specified) acceptable level. Alternatively, a pharmaceutical manufacturer can apply the concept of a clinical utility index (CUI) to facilitate dose selection. A clinical utility index is a composite measure that combines several measures (some of which may be desirable while others are not) into one to facilitate decision making.

Ouellet et al. [7] constructed a CUI when investigating the potential value of a new treatment for insomnia. Five efficacy endpoints had been used previously to evaluate benefit from an insomnia drug. They were latency to persistent sleep, wake after sleep onset, quality of sleep, and sleep architecture measured by the percentages of stage 1 and stages 3–4 sleep. An undesirable consequence of using an insomnia drug is the residual drug effect, which could make a user feel lethargic on the morning after taking the medication. Residual drug effect could be assessed by two measures from a commonly used Leeds questionnaire for insomnia research. If a withdrawal effect is a potential concern for an insomnia drug, it should be appropriately measured and included as a risk endpoint.

Faced with these seven endpoints recorded on different scales, Ouellet et al. first normalized the scales so that the endpoints were combinable. For example, a change of 25 min for wake after sleep onset was considered to be approximately equivalent to 15 min change in time to persistent sleep (see Table 1 in Ouellet et al. [7]). Next, they surveyed 581 physicians engaged in insomnia research and developed a weighting scheme to combine the seven endpoints into a CUI.

Using the CUI in a dose–response study, Ouellet et al. concluded that it would not be worthwhile to continue the development of the new compound for an insomnia indication.

2.3 Incremental Benefit/Risk Ratio

Assume that both benefit and risk could be described by a binary endpoint. We use pe_N and pe_C to denote the probability of experiencing the benefit in the new treatment and the control groups, respectively. We use pr_N and pr_C to denote the corresponding probabilities of experiencing risk. We will assume that the new treatment delivers more benefit, at the expense of more risk. If the new treatment delivers more benefit and less risk, then there is no need to discuss the benefit/risk tradeoff between these two treatments.

A measure frequently used in cost-effectiveness analysis is the incremental cost-effectiveness ratio, which looks at the increase in cost relative to every unit of increase in effectiveness. This concept could be used to form the incremental benefit/risk ratio (IBRR) in (1). As with any ratio-based measure, it is important to interpret (1) in conjunction with the magnitude of the numerator and the denominator that form the ratio. The construction of the ratio in (1) does not imply that the benefit and the risk are of equal clinical relevance.

$$IBRR = \frac{pe_N - pe_C}{pr_N - pr_C} \tag{1}$$

The IBRR in (1) could be re-expressed as in (2).

$$IBRR = \frac{\left(\frac{1}{pr_N - pr_C}\right)}{\left(\frac{1}{pe_N - pe_C}\right)} \tag{2}$$

The numerator in (2) is often interpreted as the number needed to treat to harm (NNTH) and the denominator is the number needed to treat to benefit (NNTB). So, if NNTH $= 10$ and NNTB $= 5$, then IBRR $= 2$. This ratio has the interpretation that, on the average, for each additional individual experiencing the adverse event under the new treatment, two more individuals will benefit from the new treatment compared to the control. Obviously, large IBRR values will make the new treatment more attractive. The question is—for the target patient population—is there an IBRR threshold beyond which the new treatment will be considered to have a more favorable benefit/risk profile (compared to the control)? If this threshold is not achieved in the entire target population, is there a clinically meaningful subgroup in which the new treatment is likely to have a more favorable IBRR?

The concept of IBRR was used in an FDA Cardiovascular and Renal Drugs Advisory Committee meeting on February 3, 2009. The committee was to evaluate prasugrel (an antiplatelet agent) for reducing cardiovascular events in patients with acute coronary syndrome (ACS) undergoing primary or delayed percutaneous coronary intervention. Data came from a single large trial TRITOM of 13,608 patients [23]. The primary endpoint was a composite endpoint of cardiovascular death, nonfatal myocardial infarction, and nonfatal stroke. Results from the study showed prasugrel to be more efficacious than the comparator clopidogrel, but at the expense of more bleeding. While some concerns were raised about a possible increase in malignancy risk associated with prasugrel, we will focus on bleeding here since bleeding is a common (and major) side effect of antiplatelet (and anticoagulant) agents.

By TIMI (Thrombolysis in Myocardial Infarction Trial) convention, bleeding was broadly classified as major, minor, or minimal. Figure 1 was extracted from an FDA presentation by Dr. Ellis Unger at the Advisory Committee meeting. In his presentation, Dr. Ellis Unger applied the ratio concept and showed the number of composite events prevented for each additional bleeding event with prasugrel. This ratio is represented on the y-axis. The x-axis notes number of days after the intervention. The bleeding events plotted in Fig. 1 correspond to serious events (the blue curve at the bottom), TIMI major bleeding events (the red curve on the top) or TIMI major and minor bleeding events combined (the black curve in the middle). The ratio was done in a cumulative fashion in that once an individual experienced an endpoint (a composite efficacy endpoint or a bleeding event), the individual was said to have experienced that endpoint at all subsequent time points. In other words, at a given number of days x after the intervention, pe_N and pe_C in (1) represent the probabilities that patients on prasugrel and control have not yet experienced the composite efficacy endpoint up to days x. As for pr_N and pr_C, they correspond to the probabilities that patients in these two groups have experienced a bleeding event by days x.

Figure 1 was used in an exploratory manner to help interpret the results from TRITON at the AC meeting. It is quite likely that the February 2009 meeting was the first time many AC members (as well as others in the audience) saw the use of IBRR. We will focus on the curve corresponding to major bleeding (the red curve on the top) in Fig. 1. The curve was high at the beginning. It gradually came down over time and eventually settled around a value of 3. Was 3 a good IBRR value in this case? There was no discussion of a minimum IBRR for prasugrel in order to receive marketing approval.

Prasugrel was approved on July 10, 2009 with a black box warning on bleeding risk. The black box warning also includes patient subpopulations for which prasugrel is contraindicated.

2.4 Graphic Display

Chuang-Stein et al. [8] proposed to use a multinomial random variable to capture efficacy (benefit) and safety (risk) outcomes simultaneously. The multinomial random variable Chuang-Stein et al. proposed has five outcome categories. They are *benefit and no serious adverse events, benefit and serious adverse events, no benefit and no serious adverse events, no benefit and serious adverse events*, and *side effects leading to withdrawal*. Here the term "serious adverse events" should be interpreted in the context of the patient population. They may not necessarily

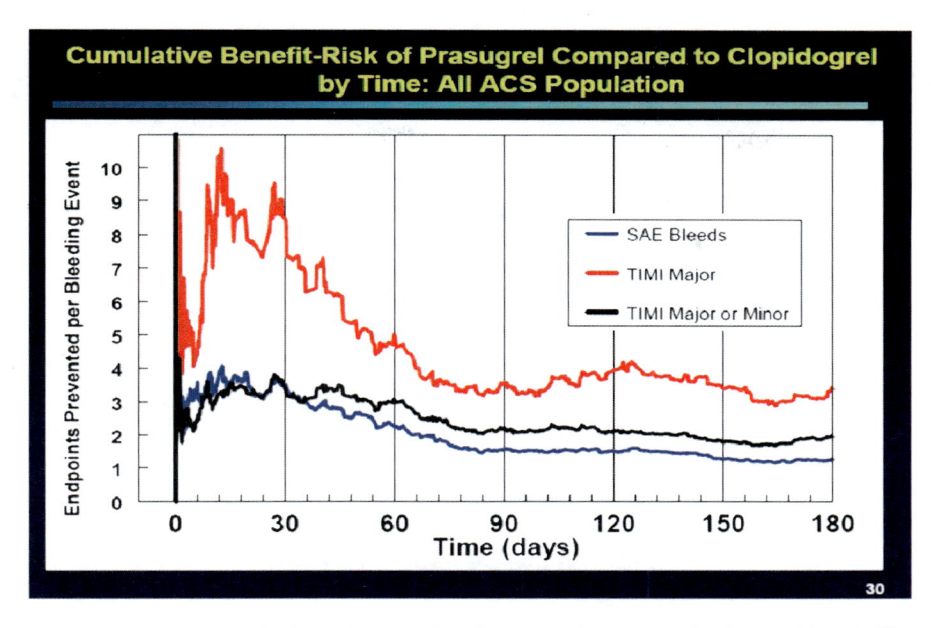

Fig. 1 Incremental benefit/risk ratio over time for comparing prasugrel with clopidogrel. The graph was taken from an FDA presentation at the February 3, 2009 Cardiovascular and Renal Drugs Advisory Committee Meeting

mean serious adverse events by the official regulatory definition. Chuang-Stein et al. proposed to use observed proportions of these categories, along with weights reflecting the desirability of these outcomes, to construct linear or ratio scores to compare treatments. Since weights reflect the clinical relevance of the categories, there is no need to assume that the categories are of equal relevance clinically. This idea was later extended by Entsuah and Gorman [9], Entsuah and Gao [10] and Pritchett and Tamura [11] to include more outcome categories in real-case applications. Entsuah et al. also discussed a simple case of sensitivity analysis to see how the comparison between two treatment groups could vary as a function of the chosen weights.

Norton [12, 13] used graphics to display the distribution of the five categories over time. Labeling the five outcomes as "Benefit Only," "Benefit + AE," "Neither," "AE only," and Withdraw", he plotted each individual's outcome category at each of the six post-randomization assessment points in a 12-week trial (Fig. 2). Individuals in Fig. 2 were arranged in such a way that dropouts were grouped together for easy visualization of the dropout pattern. Except for withdrawal, an individual could stay in or move to another response category from one assessment period to the next. In this sense, the graphic displays a snapshot in time on the response (i.e., not cumulative experience up to that point). Displaying response in this manner requires one to have access to observations on all patients at all assessment periods or until patients dropout of the study. Consequently, one needs to prespecify a

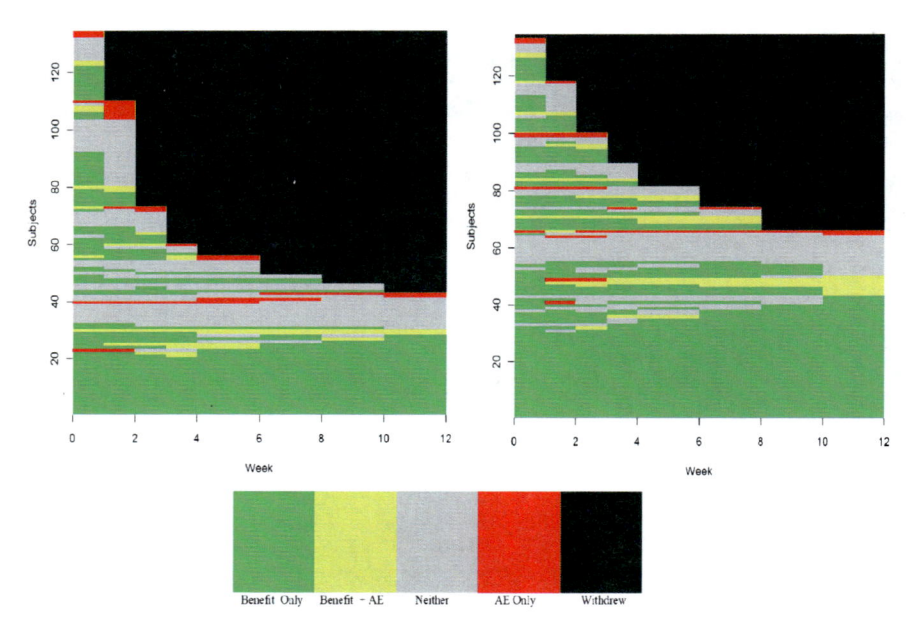

Fig. 2 Display of 5 (benefit, risk) outcomes over time. The *left panel* pertains to the control group while the *right panel* pertains to the investigational treatment group (Display is a courtesy from Norton [12].)

method to handle the situation where a patient missed a clinical visit between two completed ones. Possible approaches include carrying the last available response category forward or creating an extra category to represent the missing intermediate response.

The left panel in Fig. 2 corresponds to the control arm while the right panel corresponds to the investigational treatment group. There were no missing intermediate data in this example. Visual inspections of the figure reveal that compared to the investigational arm, the control group exhibited a higher and early dropout pattern. The graph shows clearly how the distribution of these five outcome categories changes over time and how the pattern differs between the two groups. One could compute the % of different colors (e.g., green) over a period of interest (e.g., weeks 8–12) to make a simple qualitative comparison between the groups. For both groups, Fig. 2 shows that some individuals derived benefit early and continued to do so without experiencing the adverse events.

The display in Fig. 2 could be extended to include more categories or multiple outcomes. For example, if positive outcomes on two equally important efficacy endpoints are twice as good as a single positive outcome on only one endpoint and that experiencing two distinct types of adverse events is twice as bad as experiencing only one, then one can form a net benefit/risk outcome by calculating (# of beneficial outcomes—# of untoward adverse events) for each individual. There are possible five values for the net outcome (i.e., 2, 1, 0, −1, and −2). One could plot the distribution of these five net outcomes over time. Implicit in this calculation is the assumption that one good outcome can offset one bad outcome, an assumption that may not be valid in many situations.

3 Benefit Risk Framework Developed by PhRMA

The Pharmaceutical Research and Manufactures of America (PhRMA) have long recognized the importance of and the need for a transparent benefit/risk assessment process. In 2006, PhRMA sponsored a Benefit Risk Action Team (BRAT). The objectives were to formulate a framework for the ideal benefit–risk approach and to provide greater structure to assist sponsor-regulator discussions. BRAT partnered with epidemiologists at the Research Triangle Institute Health Solutions on the task.

Before developing the framework, members of BRAT agreed that the framework should be considered as a set of processes and tools to guide decision makers. In addition, the framework should be flexible to handle different contexts. The proposed framework was required to go through three rounds of development and testing, using mock products in the statin, tumor necrosis factor, and triptan classes. Early experience with the BRAT framework has been published in Coplan et al. [14] and Levitan et al. [15]. In early 2011, the testing was completed and BRAT developed a software application to assist graphic displays of the framework as well as its output. BRAT offered the software tool to PhRMA member companies for internal pilots, hoping to receive additional comments on the framework and gain support for broad implementation.

The framework could be described as a series of six steps [14, 15]. They are: define decision context (step 1), identify outcomes (step 2), identify and extract source data (step 3), customize framework (step 4), assess outcome importance (step 5) and display and interpret key B-R metrics (step 6). These steps can be slightly modified to better fit a particular situation. Ideally, the six steps should be completed before a new drug application (or biologics license application) and that the first four steps should be completed before conducting the pivotal trials. In theory, the framework can be applied at any stage during product development or post-approval. One difficulty in establishing the framework after the outcome data are known is that the process could be influenced by the outcome, thus creating potential bias. This is usually not a problem for a mature field with well-articulated efficacy endpoints and classes of products with well-characterized side effects. For a product of novel mechanism, it might actually be necessary to rely on safety data from late-stage trials to help characterize product risk.

Steps 3 and 4 above involve identifying data sources (randomized clinical trials or observational studies) and assessing the relevance of the information. Step 6 discusses the display of benefit and risk summary. BRAT strongly encouraged displaying the summary graphically such as in a forest plot. The latter is illustrated in Coplan et al. [14] and Levitan et al. [15]. Fig. 3 shows a forest plot presented by the manufacturer of rivaroxaban at an FDA Cardiovascular and Renal Drugs

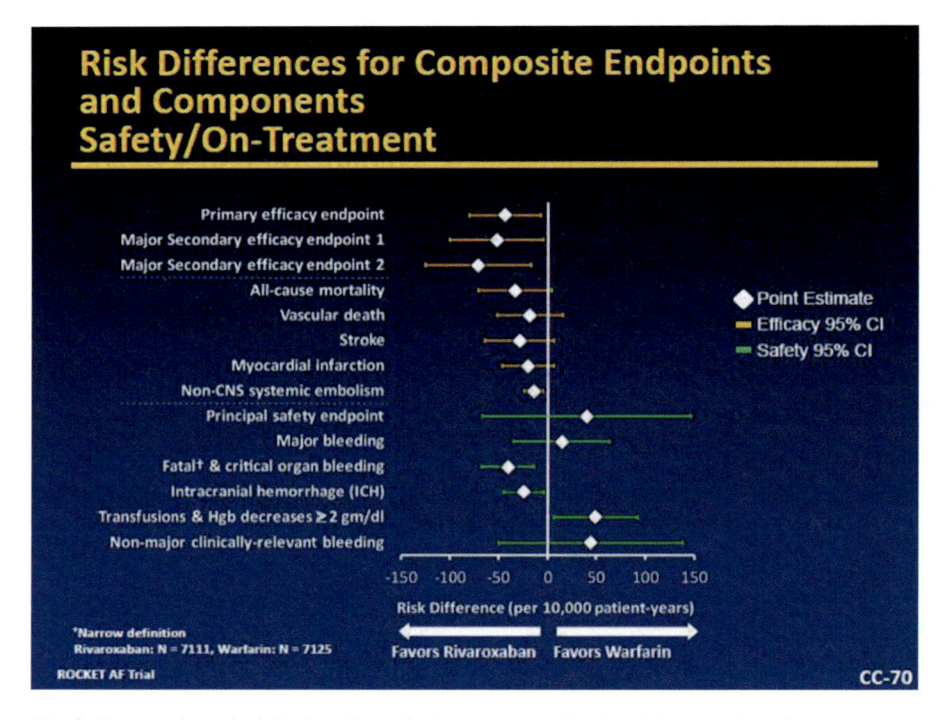

Fig. 3 Forest plot of eight benefit endpoints along with six risk endpoints for comparing rivaroxaban with warfarin, presented at the September 8 2011 Cardiovascular and Renal Drugs Advisory Committee meeting by the manufacturer of rivaroxaban

Advisory Committee meeting on September 8 2011. The meeting was to assess the benefit and risk of rivaroxaban against warfarin in preventing stroke and systemic embolism in patients with non-vascular arterial fibrillation. Details for the AC meeting could be found at the FDA website.

Fig. 3 displays results related to eight benefit and six risk endpoints. Some of the endpoints (e.g., all cause mortality, vascular death, stroke, MI) are components of a composite endpoint. For each endpoint, Fig. 3 shows the difference in the observed number of individuals/10,000 patient years who reported experiencing that endpoint. The difference is noted by a diamond in the plot with a companion 95% confidence interval. For all endpoints, the difference was calculated by subtracting the response in the warfarin group from that in the rivaroxaban group. Since all endpoints are undesirable, a difference that is greater than 0 will signal a better outcome for the warfarin group.

In general, point estimates and confidence intervals should be based on meta-analyses of relevant data sources. It is important that the data sources be systematically searched and critically appraised for inclusion so that the statistics in Fig. 3 are defendable.

In its initial work, PhRMA BRAT did not recommend any particular benefit/risk measure and did not promote the use of weights either. BRAT pointed out that data behind the forest plot in Fig. 3 could be used to support any chosen benefit/risk measure with weights chosen before seeing the data. In addition, getting into debates on weight selection early on could distract the team from focusing on the development of the framework. The decision probably also reflected a common concern that any effort to reduce multiple endpoints into a signal measure could result in information loss. In my opinion, without a mechanism to appropriately debate the roles the various benefit and risk endpoints play, without a way to quantitatively reflect the relative importance of these endpoints and how conclusion vary with the relative importance, answers to question such as "does the benefit of this product outweigh its risk" will continue to lack the transparency and structured deliberations we desire.

PhRMA transferred all work related to the BRAT framework to the Center for Innovation in Regulatory Science Ltd. for further development in January 2012.

4 Communication on Benefit/Risk to the Public

One major challenge in modern medicine is our ability to effectively communicate essential information about medicines to users. Surveys have repeatedly shown that many Americans don't understand the drugs they are taking. Lack of understanding often leads to noncompliance, contributing to medication errors, ineffective disease management, and considerable risks. The US FDA has a Risk Communication Advisory Committee. According to the information posted at the FDA web site, this Committee is to advise the Commissioner of the FDA or designee on methods to effectively communicate risk associated with products regulated by the FDA. The Committee reviews and evaluates strategies and programs designed to communicate with the public about the risks and benefits of FDA-regulated products. It also reviews and evaluates research relevant to such communication.

During a Committee meeting on February 26–27 in 2009, Steven Woloshin and Lisa Schwarz proposed to use a drug facts box to communicate the benefits and side effects of prescription drugs. The idea of the drug facts box was based on the successful implementation of a standardized nutrition facts box that is required of all packaged food sold publicly in the USA. Under Woloshin and Schwarz's proposal, the top panel of a drug facts box (Fig. 4) contains critical information on benefit while the bottom panel contains critical information on risk. The drug facts box can be viewed as a simplified tabular version of the forest plot display in Fig. 3 where data should come from all relevant sources and summarized in meta analyses.

Interestingly enough, the Patient Protection and Affordable Care Act H.R. 3590 (also known as the Health Care Bill) mentions a drug facts box. Specifically, it states that "*The Secretary of Health and Human Services … shall determine whether the addition of quantitative summaries of the benefits and risks of prescription drugs in a standardized format (such as a table or drug facts box) to the promotional labeling*

Prescription Drug Facts: AMCID (amoditine)

What is this drug for?	To relieve heartburn
Who might consider taking it?	Men and women bothered by heartburn or acid reflux disease
Who should NOT take it?	Women who are pregnant or breastfeeding
Recommended testing	None
Other things to consider doing	Eat frequent small meals; avoid fatty foods (and others which trigger your symptoms); excessive alcohol and eating close to bedtime; don't smoke; look into other medications.

AMCID STUDY FINDINGS BOX

500 people with bothersome heartburn were given AMCID
or a sugar pill for 2 weeks. Here's what happened:

What difference did AMCID make?	People given a sugar pill	People given AMCID (10 mg a day)
Did AMCID help? Fewer people taking AMCID had heartburn (17% fewer)	81% 810 in 1000	64% 640 in 1000
Did AMCID have side effects? *Life threatening side effects* No difference between AMCID and a sugar pill		None observed
Symptom side effects No difference in headache		About 5% in both groups 50 in 1000
No difference in diarrhea		About 2% in both groups 20 in 1000
No difference in dizziness		About 1% in both groups 10 in 1000

How long has the drug been in use?
Amcid was approved by FDA in 1991 - Studies show that most serious side effects or recalls of new drugs happen during their first 5 years of approval.

Fig. 4 An example of a drug facts box shown by Woloshin and Schwartz at the Feb 26–27 2009 FDA Risk Communication Advisory Committee meeting

or print advertising of such drugs would improve health care decision making by clinicians and patients and consumers.."

One cannot underestimate the power of a standardized format to assist public understanding of the facts about a drug. Because drug facts are typically more complicated than food, a drug facts box, if it becomes standardized, should have a drill-down option to offer additional summaries for individuals who desire more detailed information.

5 Report from EMA Benefit–Risk Methodology Project

On August 31, 2010, the Benefit–Risk Methodology Project sponsored by the European Medicines Agency (EMA) issued a report on current tools and processes for regulatory benefit–risk assessment (EMA/549682/2010). The report describes qualitative and quantitative approaches. It mentions ongoing work by PhRMA, the Center for Medical Research and the FDA. The latter are all classified as qualitative approaches by the report.

The report also describes 18 quantitative approaches and the view of the authors on each approach. Among the 18 quantitative approaches, the report comments that only three (Bayesian statistics, decision trees & influence/relevance diagrams, and multi-criteria decision analysis) incorporate the value or utilities of benefit and risk, along with probabilities representing the uncertainties of those effects, to numerically represent the benefit–risk balance.

The Bayesian statistics approach uses Bayes' Theorem to update the degree of prior belief as new information becomes available for incorporation. Prior belief may come from information related to similar products in the same class or opinions of key opinion leaders. In the latter case, it is important to ensure that the solicited prior belief is free of bias arising from the involvement of individuals with real or potential conflict of interest. The Bayesian approach calculates decision-relevant posterior probabilities. The decision trees & influence/relevance diagrams approach is derived from decision theory. It is based on three basic assumptions: (1) probabilities exist; (2) utilities exist; and (3) the action associated with the highest expected utility will be the most preferred. The multi-criteria decision analysis (MDCA) was developed by Mussen et al. [16, 17]. It was the prototype for the PhRMA BRAT framework. MDCA goes beyond the qualitative framework. It includes scoring and weighting. MDCA defines scoring as the process of measuring the value of options and uses weighting to ensure that the units of value on all the criteria are comparable to be combinable. The development of the clinical utility index (CUI) discussed in Sect. 2.1 is a simple case of applying these concepts.

The report acknowledges that any quantitative method requires a qualitative framework. On many occasions, utilizing qualitative and quantitative approaches in tandem can be useful. Since efforts to improve benefit/risk assessment are continuing at regulatory agencies, academic institutions and within the pharmaceutical industry, we can expect additional summary reports on this topic in the future.

6   FDA Draft Guidance on Factors to Consider When Making Benefit–Risk Determinations in Medical Device Premarket Review

On August 15, 2011, FDA issued a draft guidance, for public comment, on factors to consider when making a benefit–risk determination in medical device premarketing review. The agency hopes that a guidance on this topic can provide greater clarity for both the reviewers at the agency and the device industry. The document discusses three hypothetical examples in detail with likely assessment outcomes. The document also briefly describes six real cases and how the decision was made in each case.

The draft document contains a worksheet in the appendix. The worksheet offers users a systematic way to articulate factors that should be considered when making benefit–risk assessment. Major factor headings for the worksheet are: type of benefit, magnitude of the benefit, probability of the patient experiencing a benefit, duration of effect, severity and types of harmful events, probability and duration of a harmful event, risk of false-positive or false-negative for diagnostics, uncertainty, patient tolerance for risk, availability of alternative treatments or diagnostics, risk mitigation and novelty of technology.

The above factors reflect the core principles for benefit/risk assessment. They are (1) the risk of a product should be evaluated with respect to its potential benefit; (2) benefit/risk assessment should be conducted with respect to the target population and in view of available alternative therapies; (3) the strength of the supporting data (benefit and risk) is crucial to the evaluation.

In the draft guidance, FDA is hesitant to consider quantitatively weighting the factors because the appropriate weighting could change over time. We feel that this concern alone does not justify not using a quantitative approach if it can help make a better decision based on the available evidence at a particular point in time. Circumstances can indeed change and our priorities may shift over time. Temple [18] explained FDA's decision to remove terfenadine (a non-sedating antihistamine approved in the USA in 1985) from the market in 1998 when terfenadine's active metabolite fexofenadine became available. Terfenadine was linked to fatal ventricular arrhythmia *torsade de pointes* while fexofenadine was not. FDA's decision underscored a continuous benefit/risk assessment process that began in 1992 when *torsade de pointes* was first reported in patients taking terfenadine. When a new drug with a pharmacologically identical effect but without a major serious adverse reaction becomes available, the benefit/risk profile of the older product may no longer be considered favorable.

7   Discussion

It is well accepted that benefit/risk assessment is necessary for a new treatment. Over the past ten years, several workshops have been dedicated to this topic including the one sponsored by the Institute of Medicine entitled "*Understanding the Benefits and Risks of Pharmaceuticals*" on May 30, 2006. Our coverage on benefit/risk assessment in this paper was purposely kept simple. We did so to help readers gain some overall perspective on the benefit/risk assessment movement and not to get bogged down by technical details. In addition, we feel that any systematic approach for benefit/risk assessment needs to be intuitive, logical, and easy to understand to have a chance for broad uptake.

Many have pointed out the challenges of benefit/risk assessment [19, 20]. For one thing, while benefit might be realized shortly after initiating a treatment, serious risk might take a long time to surface. Randomized trials conducted during the premarketing phase are usually too short to observe long-term risk. As such, benefit/risk assessment needs to occur regularly after a product is available to the public. A product's benefit/risk profile could change over time with emerging post-marketing data and the availability of newer products. In the USA, the Drug Safety and Risk Management Advisory Committee plays an important advisory role to the FDA on this question.

Equally important is the need to quantify uncertainty in our estimates of benefit and of risk and therefore the chosen benefit/risk measures. Uncertainty affects the strength of the data. Figure 1 does not include any information concerning the variability around the reported incremental benefit risk ratio. One could apply the bootstrap methodology to construct confidence intervals and include them in the figure.

How can statisticians help? At a recent Joint Statistical Meetings, Hoerl and Snee [21] discussed the concept of "statistical engineering." They defined statistical engineering as the study of how best to utilize statistical concepts, methods, and tools and integrate them with other relevant sciences to generate improved results. The idea behind statistical engineering is that we have a list of statistical science parts. As statisticians, we need to assemble these statistical science parts to improve our systems and our processes. Hoerl and Snee claimed that statistical engineering could be applied to improve anything. I believe statistical engineering could help us develop a better process to conduct risk/benefit assessment also. To do this, we need to collaborate with other disciplines and bring alive the relevant statistical science parts on our list.

So, where are we now in terms of quantitative benefit/risk assessment? The good news is that we have started to see some concerted attention dedicated to this topic, both by the regulatory agencies and by the pharmaceutical industry. Several pharmaceutical companies piloted the BRAT framework within their organizations in 2011. Several references included in this paper describe the applications of benefit/risk assessment approaches to actual cases. Despite these, advancements are being made in small steps. There is no doubt that benefit/risk assessment is complicated and situation dependent. Many questions remain, some of which will not have easy solutions. For example, how do we address conflicting findings from different meta-analyses (or between observational studies and randomized trials) on the safety of a marketed product? How do we resolve conflicting recommendations from different branches within the same regulatory agency?

The last question in the above paragraph came into full focus during a joint meeting among three FDA Advisory Committees (Pediatric, Pulmonary-Allergy Drugs, Drug Safety and Risk Management) on December 11 2008. The three ACs along with FDA's Office of Surveillance and Epidemiology (OSE) and Division of Pulmonary and Allergy Products (DPAP) were to weigh the public health implications of real and serious but relatively infrequent occurrences of severe asthma exacerbations and asthma-related death against the asymptomatic benefits of bronchodilation and asthma control of long-acting beta-agonists (LABAs). During the FDA presentation, the Director of DPAP acknowledged differing views on how to manage LABA risk within the agency. While OSE preferred withdrawing asthma indication for all LABAs for the pediatric patients and removing asthma indication and contraindicating the use of single ingredient LABAs for all ages, DPAP preferred continued marketing of products containing LABAs and managing safety risk through labeling. Readers interested in this debate are referred to Kramer [22].

While we should continue to strive for the best approach possible, we should be mindful not to let the perfect become the enemy of the good. In my opinion, we should start experimenting with quantitative benefit/risk assessment using a common framework, sharing experience from these efforts collectively and deciding the next step among partnerships with academia, regulatory agencies, and the pharmaceutical industry.

Acknowledgements The author wants to thank Jon Norton for the use of Fig. 2. The author also wants to thank PhRMA BRAT, especially Bennett Levitan, Paul Coplan, Rebecca Noel, Marilyn Metcalf, and Diana Hughes, for BRAT-generated materials. In addition, the author wants to thank Leila Zelnick and Tom Fleming for their comments which have helped improve the quality of the paper.

References

1. Honig PK (2011) Comparative effectiveness: the fourth hurdle in drug development and a role for clinical pharmacology. Clin Pharmacol Ther 89(2):151–156
2. Gelber RD, Gelman RS, Goldhirsch A (1989) A quality of-life oriented endpoint for comparing treatments. Biometrics 45:781–795
3. Glasziou PP, Simes RJ, Gelber RD (1990) Quality adjusted survival analysis. Stat Med 9: 1259–1276
4. Hughes DA, Bayoumi AM, Pirmohamed M (2007) Current assessment of risk-benefit by regulators: is it time to introduce decision analyses? Clin Pharmacol Ther 82:123–127
5. Irish W, Sherrill B, Cole B, Gard C, Gledenning GA, Mouridsen H (2005) Quality-adjusted survival in a crossover trial of letrozole versus tamoxifen in postmenopausal women with advanced breast cancer. Ann Oncol 10:1458–1462
6. Chuang-Stein C (1994) A new proposal for benefit-less-risk analysis in clinical trials. Control Clin Trials 15:30–43
7. Ouellet D, Werth J, Parekh N, Feltner D, McCarthy B, Lalonde RL (2009) The use of a clinical utility index to compare insomnia compounds: a quantitative basis for benefit-risk assessment. Clin Pharmacol Ther 85:277–282

8. Chuang-Stein C, Mohberg NR, Sinkula M (1991) Three measures for simultaneously evaluating benefits and risks using a categorical data from clinical trials. Stat Med 10:1349–1359
9. Entsuah R, Gorman JM (2002) Global benefit-risk assessment of antidepressants: venlafaxine XR and fluoxetine. J Psychiatr Res 36:111–118
10. Entsuah R, Gao B (2002) Global benefit-risk evaluation of antidepressant action: comparison of pooled data for venlafaxine, SSRIs and placebo. CNS Spectr 7:882–888
11. Pritchett Y, Tamura R (2008) The application of global benefit-risk assessment in clinical trial design and some statistical considerations. Pharm Stat 7:170–178
12. Norton J (2010) A longitudinal model for medical benefit-risk analysis, with case study. Presented at the 19th Annual International Chinese Statistical Association Applied Statistics Symposium, Indianapolis, IN, June 20–23
13. Norton J (2011) A longitudinal model and graphic for benefit-risk analysis, with case study. Drug Inf J 45:741–747
14. Coplan PM, Noel RA, Levitan BS, Fergun J, Mussen F (2011) Development of a framework for enhancing the transparency, reproducibility and communication of the benefit-risk balance of medicines. Clin Pharmacol Ther 89:312–315
15. Levitan BS, Andrews EB, Gilsenan A, Ferguson J, Noel RA, Coplan PM, Mussen F (2011) Application of the BRAT framework to case studies: observations and insights. Clin Pharmacol Ther 89:217–224
16. Mussen F, Salek S, Walker S (2007) A quantitative approach to benefit-risk assessment of medicines – part 1: the development of a new model using multi-criteria decision analysis. Pharmacoepidemiol Drug Saf 16(Suppl 1):S2–S15
17. Mussen F, Salek S, Walker S (2007) A quantitative approach to benefit-risk assessment of medicines – part 2: the practical application of a new model. Pharmacoepidemiol Drug Saf 16(Suppl 1):S16–S41
18. Temple R (2007) Quantitative decision analysis: a work in progress. Clin Pharmacol Ther 82:127–130
19. Chuang-Stein C, Entsuah R, Pritchett Y (2008) Measures for conducting comparative benefit:risk assessment. Drug Inf J 42:223–233
20. O'Neill R (2008) A perspective on characterizing benefits and risks derived from clinical trials: can we do more? Drug Inf J 42:235–245
21. Hoerl RW, Snee RD (2010) Statistical engineering: an idea whose time has come? A discussion in honor of Gerry Hahn's 80th birthday. Presented at the Joint Statistical Meetings, Vancouver British Columbia, August 1–5
22. Kramer JM (2009) Balancing the benefits and risks of inhaled long-acting beta-agonists – the influence of values. N Engl J Med 360:1592–1595
23. Wiviott SD, Braunwald E, McCabe CH, Montalescot G, Ruzyllo W, Gottlieb S, Neumann FJ, Ardissino D, De Servi S, Murphy SA, Riesmeyer J, Weerakkody G, Gibson CM, Antman EM (2007) TRITON-TIMI 38 Investigators. Prasugrel versus clopidogrel in patients with acute coronary syndromes. N Engl J Med 357:2001–2015

Identifying and Addressing Safety Signals in Clinical Trials: Some Issues and Challenges

Thomas R. Fleming

Abstract Reliable evidence is needed from clinical research about whether the interventions used in clinical practice are safe as well as effective. Regarding risk, safety is not established by failure to establish excess risk, such as obtaining confidence intervals for the relative risk of safety events that include unity. Absence of evidence is not evidence of absence. Rather, safety is established if available data about safety are sufficiently favorable and reliable to rule out the threshold for unacceptable risk, where this threshold should be determined by considering the strength of the evidence for efficacy.

Important insights about safety usually will be provided before marketing through Phase 1, 2, and 3 clinical trials. These insights, especially regarding risks associated with long-term use of the intervention and risks of rare but clinically compelling events, are enhanced by post-marketing active and passive surveillance, and especially by large, long-term randomized trials that provide the most reliable approach for identifying and addressing safety signals. The integrity of these randomized trials is enhanced by preventing irregularities in the quality of trial conduct that would reduce their sensitivity to detecting clinically meaningful safety risks caused by the experimental regimen.

After considering approaches to identifying and addressing safety risks and discussing performance standards to improve the quality of conduct of safety trials, we will consider further the vulnerability to undetected safety risks when evidence for efficacy has been limited to documentation of effects on surrogate endpoints such as biomarkers, and then discuss important considerations regarding cardiovascular safety trials conducted in the setting of type 2 diabetes mellitus.

T.R. Fleming (✉)
Department of Biostatistics, University of Washington, Seattle, WA, USA
e-mail: tfleming@uw.edu

T.R. Fleming and B.S. Weir (eds.), *Proceedings of the Fourth Seattle Symposium in Biostatistics: Clinical Trials*, Lecture Notes in Statistics 1205, DOI 10.1007/978-1-4614-5245-4_9, © Springer Science+Business Media New York 2013

1 Introduction

When interventions are sufficiently potent to provide clinically significant benefits, it is plausible they have unintended effects that could meaningfully alter their benefit-to-risk profile. Hence, it is important to have reliable evidence about whether these interventions are safe as well as effective.

There are many examples where unintended effects would be problematic. Potent immunosuppressive treatments given to rheumatoid arthritis patients to treat symptoms and prevent the progression of disease may provide a clinically important increase in the risk of malignancy or opportunistic infections. Cox-2 inhibitors that provide analgesic relief to osteoarthritis and rheumatoid arthritis patients without inducing risk of gastrointestinal ulceration may have off-target effects such as increasing blood pressure that could induce increased risk of macrovascular complications, including cardiovascular death, myocardial infarction, or stroke. Agents that provide important antipsychotic symptomatic benefits may adversely impact cardiovascular markers, such as increasing weight or low density lipoprotein cholesterol, or decreasing high density lipoprotein cholesterol, where these effects could lead to increased risk of diabetes or major cardiovascular complications.

Figure 1 presents several settings where the benefit-to-risk profile of an intervention could be or in fact has been established to be meaningfully altered by harmful effects on measures of irreversible morbidity or mortality. One key setting arises where agents have been established to provide symptomatic benefits, such as analgesic, anti-asthmatic, or antipsychotic treatments. These benefits could be offset by harmful effects on the risk of major cardiovascular events, asthma-related death, torsade de pointes, or sudden death [1–3]. A second key setting arises where agents have been established to have favorable effects on a biomarker thought to be a surrogate for (and hence to provide indirect evidence of favorable effects on) measures of major morbidity or mortality. Examples include erythropoietin-stimulating agents that were accepted for use in renal disease or oncology patients based on normalization of hematocrit, or many therapeutic agents accepted for use in patients with type 2 diabetes mellitus based on reductions in levels of H_bA_{1c}, or selective estrogen receptor modulators considered for long-term use to prevent or treat osteoporosis based on their short-term effects on radiologic fractures or bone mineral density [4–13]. When evidence about clinical efficacy is available only indirectly though evidence about effects on biomarkers, judgment about whether the intervention's benefit-to-risk profile is favorable is strongly influenced when even just a signal for adverse effects on major morbidity/mortality emerges. For example, evidence that some selective estrogen receptor modulators have been associated with increased risk of venous thromboembolism or stroke, and evidence providing a signal that rosiglitazone increases the risk of fatal or non-fatal myocardial infarction in type 2 diabetes mellitus, as shown in Fig. 2, then raised concerns about their continued use [14].

In the remainder of this article, we will provide an overview of observational and clinical trial-based approaches to identifying and addressing safety risks

Class of Agents and Example members	Safety Event and Clinical Setting	Bkgd Rate /1000 PY	Relative ↑ In Safety Risk, r	Attrib Risk, #/1000 PY
Cox 2 inhibitors Celebrex, Vioxx , Bextra	CV Death / Stroke / MI RA, OA and Alzheimers	10	1.5	5
Long Acting β-Agonists Salmeterol, serevant	Asthma-related Death Severe Asthma	0.5	4	1.5
Anti-psychotics Ziprasidone	QTc related CV Events Schizophrenia	?	?	?
Tysabri	Progressive Multifocal Leukoenceph Multiple Sclerosis & Crohn'sDisease	0.001	1000	1
Rotavirus Vaccine	Intussusception High Risk for Rotavirus	0.1	>10	>1
Muraglitazar Rosiglitazone	CV Death / Stroke / MI Type 2 Diabetes	20	1.5 - 2	10-20
Erythropoietin Stimulating Agents	Death Renal Disease, Oncology	?	1.1-1.15	?
Ezetimibe/Simvastin	Cancer Incidence; Cancer Mortality Progression of Aortic-valve stenosis	20 5	1.1 1.5	2 2.5

Fig. 1 Illustrations where safety events meaningfully alter the benefit-to-risk profile of an intervention that has established effects on symptom endpoints or on biomarkers as replacement endpoints for direct measures of patient benefit. r is relative risk, PY is person years

Fatal or Non-fatal MI

- **NissenMeta-Analysis**

	MI	N
Rosiglitazone	86	15,565
Controls	72	12,282

Relative Risk: 1.43 ; 95% C.I.: (1.03, 1.98)

- **PROactive Trial**

	MI	N
Pioglitazone	164	2605
Controls	202	2633

Relative Risk: 0.82 ; 95% C.I.: (0.66, **1.00**)

Fig. 2 Cardiovascular safety of thiazolidinediones in patients with type 2 diabetes mellitus. *MI* is myocardial infarction, N is sample size per arm. With unity as the upper limit of the confidence interval, the PROactive trial rules out pioglitazone has adverse effects on MI

during both pre- and post-marketing phases. We then will discuss in greater detail how randomized clinical trials can be designed to reliably determine whether an intervention provides an unacceptable increase in safety risks, and will discuss performance standards that should be in place to improve the quality of conduct of such trials. We will consider the vulnerability to undetected safety risks that arises when evidence for efficacy has been limited to documentation of effects on surrogate endpoints such as biomarkers, and then discuss important considerations regarding cardiovascular safety trials conducted in the setting of type 2 diabetes mellitus.

2 Approaches to Pre- and Post-Marketing Evaluation of Safety

2.1 Pre-marketing Safety Evaluation

Enhanced insights about safety of interventions are provided by each phase of the clinical development plan. Phase 1 clinical trials often give insights about dose-limiting toxicities in addition to information about metabolism, bioavailability or acceptability of the experimental regimens. Often, in a Phase 1 trial, after a dose escalation stage, approximately 15–25 patients are given what is thought to be the "maximum tolerated dose" of the regimen in order to determine whether we can rule out that the true rate of important toxicities is at least 15–20%. To be specific, suppose 17 (respectively, 23) patients receive the experimental regimen at a targeted dose and schedule, and no events of a specified category are seen. Then with this preliminary evidence about that safety risk, based on the upper 97.5% one-sided confidence interval, one could rule out that the true probability of events of that specified category is 20% (retrospectively, 15%).

Phase 2 trials usually are designed to provide enhanced insights about safety, in addition to "proof of concept" information regarding efficacy. If 35 (respectively, 72) patients receive the intervention at a targeted dose and schedule and no events of a specific category would be seen, then one could rule out (at a 2.5% false positive error rate) that the true rate of that event is at least 10% (respectively, 5%).

While Phase 1 and 2 trials provide useful insights about safety and efficacy, much more reliable evidence usually is needed before a product could be used in non-research clinical settings. Such information typically is provided by prospective randomized Phase 3 trials. However, even when these Phase 3 trials yield sufficient evidence to justify marketing a product, there may be safety signals or inadequate insights about rare but clinically important events, or about safety in the (usually) broader population of people who will eventually receive the drug once its marketed, or there may be a need for an adequate understanding about the long-term safety profile, especially when there could be long-term use of an intervention in a chronic disease setting. These considerations motivate the need for evidence about safety from a Phase 4 post-marketing extended evaluation.

2.2 Post-marketing Safety Evaluation

There are several approaches for "post-marketing" evaluation of safety that may be implemented to pursue existing signals or as surveillance for new safety signals: passive surveillance systems, active surveillance systems, and larger or longer term randomized clinical trials. We will consider the strengths and weaknesses of these approaches.

Passive surveillance for safety risks is provided by an adverse event reporting system based on caregivers' *voluntary* submission of MedWatch forms for serious adverse events they believe might be related to a drug or biologic. Advantages of this approach include obtaining timely information from a reporting procedure that is uniformly implemented by caregivers. However, this information often is difficult to interpret due to (1) lack of a comparator group that usually would be needed to assess whether events are occurring more frequently than expected based on the patient's clinical condition, (2) lack of a "denominator" (i.e., the number of patients who has received the treatment), (3) inaccurate information about the "numerator" (i.e., the number with the safety event) due to underreporting caused by the voluntary nature of data submission, and (4) lack of information on important confounders.

Active surveillance systems, based on use of large prospective cohorts and linked databases, can provide better insights about the numerator and denominator. This system could be prospective, created by a sponsor's pharmaco-vigilance program or by linking automated databases from health maintenance organizations that provide access to data from hundreds of thousands of patients [15, 16]. This creates the possibility of having sensitivity to safety events that occur at a rate of less than 1 per 1,000 person years of exposure. Even with these improved features, active surveillance systems still have important shortcomings, including lack of randomization, inadequate information about important confounders, and inconsistent levels of sensitivity (i.e., whether all targeted events are being captured) and specificity (i.e., whether reported events truly are targeted events). Additional weaknesses of active surveillance systems include lack of a stable population (e.g., due to enroll/disenrollment), exposure misclassification (e.g., databases measure "prescriptions filled" not actual "drug taken"), and often constraints around combining data across multiple HMO sites due to privacy concerns (which can limit analytic possibilities).

The strengths of randomized trials when seeking a reliable assessment of efficacy also apply when evaluating safety. Caregivers and patients usually do not start or stop interventions "at random" in clinical practice. Therefore, when comparing a cohort of patients receiving an intervention with a non-randomized control group, estimates of the effect of treatment on either efficacy or safety measures will be confounded by imbalances between these two groups in important prognostic variables. Statistical procedures used to adjust for these imbalances have limited usefulness, since known and recorded covariates are only the "tip of the iceberg" of the factors that are confounding the estimates of treatment effect.

This confounding may not meaningfully compromise sensitivity to safety risks when the safety assessment is focused on the detection of very large effects on the risk of events, such as when treatment induces a tenfold or larger increase in important safety events. Examples of such large increases in Fig. 1 include the greater than tenfold increase in intussusception induced by the rotavirus vaccine, and the 1,000-fold increase in progressive multifocal leukoencephalopathy induced by natalizumab in patients with Crohn's disease or multiple sclerosis [17, 18]. In spite of their vulnerability to confounding, active and passive surveillance approaches might be sufficient in these settings because these approaches are able to detect such large increases in risk, and because these are settings where it might not be necessary to detect small to moderate increases in risk. To be specific, for the rotovirus vaccine, a doubling of an endpoint of moderate clinical relevance such as intussusception would be offset by the benefits of an effective vaccine and, for the setting of natalizumab, inducing a doubling of progressive multifocal leukoencephalopathy would correspond to an absolute increase of only one case per million person years of treatment, due to the extremely low risk of this event in patients who do not receive natalizumab.

The value of having safety data from randomized trials is high when interventions would have unacceptable safety profiles even if they induce only 1.1- to 2-fold increases in the relative risk of clinically important safety outcomes. This is true in several of the examples in Fig. 1. In these settings, passive and active surveillance could not reliably discern between interventions having no increase in risk and those inducing these small yet unacceptable increases in the risk of clinically important safety outcomes. One approach to reliably address this issue is to conduct large randomized clinical trials designed to evaluate effects on important prespecified safety measures. Through randomization, we can eliminate confounding due to systematically occurring imbalances between treatment and control groups in important prognostic factors. In these trials, to preserve the integrity of randomization, all patients in the treatment and control groups should be uniformly followed until a fixed time post-randomization or until a prespecified calendar time. Stopping follow-up after a patient stops randomized treatment or changes supportive care will lead to risk of substantial bias due to informative missingness.

The duration of follow-up in randomized safety trials should be influenced by the anticipated duration of use of the intervention in clinical care and by the likelihood that adverse effects of the treatment would be seen immediately or on a delayed basis. These safety trials often should be designed to follow patients for duration sufficient to provide sensitivity to safety risks that depend on cumulative exposure, such as cardiovascular risks arising with Adriamycin. Uniform long-term follow-up also is necessary to have sensitivity to safety risks that would be seen only after longer follow-up, such as risks for induction of malignancy. In clinical trials that have group sequential boundaries for monitoring efficacy data, such efficacy boundaries should be adequately conservative regarding early termination in settings where sensitivity to long-term safety risks is important [19].

One of the important advantages of having prospective cohorts for assessing safety risks, such as those arising in randomized clinical trials, is that procedures can be put in place to ensure sensitivity and specificity, by ensuring systematic and reliable capture of all targeted safety events, and by ensuring timely adjudication of these events, a process that would be particularly important in open label safety trials.

While the reliability of evidence is greatly enhanced when randomized trials are conducted to address safety risks, whether conducted in pre- or post-marketing settings, such trials typically will require large sample sizes and long timeframes to be completed. Suppose it is intended to have 90% power to rule out a threefold increase in safety risks when the intervention truly provides no increase in risk, using a statistical test having a (one-sided) 2.5% false positive risk of declaring safety when the intervention truly does induce the threefold increase in risk. When ruling out a difference of 1 vs. 3 events per 1,000 person years, as in the setting of evaluating the effect of long acting beta-agonists on asthma-related death or intubation, or evaluating the effect of type 2 diabetes mellitus drugs on pancreatitis, a randomized trial would need 20,000 person years follow-up. When the background rate of targeted safety events is 10 events per 1,000 person years, as in the adult setting when evaluating the effect of Cox-2 inhibitors or ADHD drugs on the risk of the composite endpoint, "cardio-vascular death, stroke or myocardial infarction," then assessing a threefold increase of 10 vs. 30 events per 1,000 person years would require a randomized trial with follow-up of only 2,000 person years. However, it likely would not be adequate to simply rule out 20 excess events per 1,000 person years when these events are major morbidity/mortality outcomes, especially when efficacy relates to symptom benefit or effects that have only been established on a biomarker. When the background rate is 10 events per 1,000 person years, to rule out an increase of 5 events, the randomized trial again would require 20,000 person years of follow-up. In the setting of type 2 diabetes mellitus where the background rate is 20 events per 1,000 person years, ruling out an increase of 5 events would require a randomized trial having 40,000 person years follow-up.

2.3 Interpreting and Addressing Safety Signals

The SEAS trial evaluating the efficacy of ezetimibe/simvastatin on slowing progression of aortic-valve stenosis illustrates the challenges in interpreting and addressing safety signals discovered in exploratory analyses [20]. While the SEAS trial was not designed to provide confirmatory evidence about malignancy, Fig. 3 presents evidence from exploratory analyses in SEAS suggesting ezetimibe/simvastatin provides an estimated 55% increase in cancer incidence, and a 78% increase cancer-related deaths, where 95% confidence intervals for relative risk exclude unity. While this meets a traditional standard for "statistical significance," the exploratory nature of this result should lead to caution about making inferential statements. Furthermore, the increase in risk likely is overestimated due to random high bias [21]. Such bias occurs because there are both true signal and random noise in every estimate of treatment effect, and when many analyses are conducted, the results that

- **SEAS Trial** 　　　N　　CA. Incidence　　CA. Deaths

	N	CA. Incidence	CA. Deaths
Vytorin	944	101	37
Placebo	929	65	20
Relative Risk:		**1.55**	**1.78**
95%C.I.:		(1.13,2.12)	(1.03.3.11)

- **IMPROVE-IT & SHARP Trials** 　　N　　CA. Incidence　　CA. Deaths

	N	CA. Incidence	CA. Deaths
Vytorin	10,391	313	97
Control	10,298	326	72
Relative Risk:		**0.96**	**1.34**
95%C.I.:		(0.82,1.12)	(0.98, 1.84)

Fig. 3 Cancer risk with ezetimibe/simvastatin (vytorin) in SEAS trial evaluating effect in slowing progression of aortic-valve stenosis, and in the confirmatory IMPROVE-IT and SHARP trials

appear to be most extreme tend to be at least partially due to random overestimates of the true effect.

Usually, conducting analyses such as these would be regarded as hypothesis generation rather than hypothesis confirmation. For efficacy or safety signals discovered in exploratory analyses to be viewed to be reliable, several important criteria may need to be simultaneously satisfied. *First*, the likelihood this safety signal could be explained by chance should be low, even when taking into account the sampling context of the exploratory analysis. For example, when three cases of progressive multifocal leukoencephalopathy occurred in several thousand patients receiving natalizumab, this event rate that is 1,000-fold higher rate than would be expected in natural history almost surely could not be attributed to chance, even when taking into account the exploratory context for this discovery. *Second*, there should be a biologically plausible linkage between the safety event and the intervention, based on its known mechanisms of action. For example, ezetimibe blocks the absorption of phytosterols and other phytonutrients linked to protection against cancer, which provides some biologic plausibility that the drug could have an effect on the growth of cancer cells [22–24]. *Third*, there should be independent evidence to confirm the observed association. While additional evidence regarding a safety signal could be provided within the trial generating that signal, such as obtaining data about whether there are increases seen not only in cancer mortality but also in cancer incidence, the ideal independent evidence would be provided by separate prospective trials.

After the discovery of cancer risks in the SEAS trial, the ongoing IMPROVE-IT and SHARP trials were used as an independent source of confirmatory evidence to better understand this finding [25, 26]. Figure 3 gives the data from these two trials and provides evidence that the findings of excess cancer risks from the exploratory analysis of SEAS data were overestimates, consistent with random high bias that results from such exploration of data. The estimates of the ezetimibe/simvastatin to placebo relative risk for cancer incidence from IMPROVE-IT and SHARP were 0.96 for cancer incidence and 1.34 for cancer death, where the 95% confidence intervals included unity in both instances. Peto et al. [27] stated, *"The available results from these 3 trials do not provide credible evidence of any adverse effect of Ezetimibe on rates of cancer."* However, safety is not established by obtaining confidence intervals for relative risk that include unity. That is, failure to establish excess risk is not sufficient to justify safety. Rather, safety is established by ruling out any level of excess risk that would be unacceptable [28]. The IMPROVE-IT and SHARP trials yield an estimated 34% increase in risk of cancer death, where the upper limit of the 95% confidence interval is 1.84. Since the data are consistent with ezetimibe/simvastatin causing as much as an 84% increase in cancer incidence, further study of the effect of this agent on cancer risk is needed.

3 Safety Trials Assessing Whether Unacceptable Excess Risk Can Be Ruled Out

Suppose there is an important signal from either pre- or post-marketing studies that an intervention induces unacceptable safety risks. This may arise when a therapy has been proven to have beneficial effects on direct outcomes of how a patient feels or functions, or on biomarkers that are surrogates for major morbidity/mortality outcomes, and yet a signal exists for adverse effects on measures of major morbidity/mortality. Examples of such measures are fulminant hepatic failure, asthma-related death, cardiovascular death, stroke, myocardial infarction, or risk of malignancy. If only small to moderate relative increases (such as relative risks in the range of 1.1–4.0) in the risk of these major safety events would result in an unfavorable benefit-to-risk profile of the intervention, then a prospective randomized safety trial may be needed. In this section, we will provide insights into the design of such a trial, with an illustration provided from the setting of use of cox-2 inhibitors in patients with osteoarthritis or rheumatoid arthritis.

Cox-2 inhibitors, such as celecoxib, provide analgesic benefit and, relative to NSAIDS, have reduced risk of inducing gastrointestinal ulceration. However, data from at least 50,000 patients who participated in randomized trials conducted across multiple disease settings have suggested that the class of cox-2 inhibitors meaningfully increases the risk of macrovascular complications [1]. This resulted in withdrawal of the drugs rofecoxib and valdecoxib from the market. Celecoxib remained on the market under agreement that a large prospective randomized safety trial would be conducted in a timely manner.

In the PRECISION trial, patients with osteoarthritis or rheumatoid arthritis were randomized to receive either celecoxib, or one of two control regimens, ibuprofen or naproxen [28, 29]. The size of the trial was based on the need to reliably estimate the relative risk for the composite endpoint, "cardiovascular death, stroke or myocardial infarction," for each pairwise comparison of celecoxib with a control regimen. Even though celecoxib provides important analgesic benefit and, relative to nonselective NSAIDS, an important reduction in the risk of gastrointestinal ulceration, it was judged it would be clinically unacceptable for the agent to induce more than 3 or 4 excess "cardiovascular deaths, stroke or myocardial infarction" events per 1,000 person years. Since the rate of this composite endpoint is approximately 10 events per 1,000 person years on the control arm, the PRECISION trial then was designed to determine whether a 1.333 relative increase in the rate of this composite could be ruled out. For each pairwise comparison of celecoxib with a control regimen, 508 patients would need to experience the composite endpoint for the trial to have 90% power to rule out a 1.333 relative risk when celecoxib truly provides no increase in the risk of the composite endpoint, when using a statistical test having a (one-sided) 2.5% false positive risk of declaring safety when celecoxib truly does induce a 33.3% increase in relative risk. Given the annual event rate of 10 composite endpoints per 1,000 person years follow-up, it follows that approximately 20,000 patients would need to be randomized for each pairwise comparison in the PRECISION trial and be followed for approximately 30 months in order to yield 508 events.

Figure 4 provides the interpretations for some of the possible results from the PRECISION safety trial. Focus is on the relative risk of the "CV death/MI/stroke" composite endpoint for the comparison of celecoxib to the naproxen control arm. The least favorable result that successfully rules out that celecoxib truly induces a 33% increase in the composite endpoint is given in scenario B, where the estimated relative risk is 1.12, corresponding approximately to celecoxib inducing an estimated increase of 1.2 "CV death/MI/stroke" events per 1,000 person years. In contrast, in scenario D, celecoxib has "inferior" cardiovascular safety to naproxen since the data with an estimated 1.9 additional "CV death/MI/stroke" events per 1,000 person years provide statistically significant evidence that rules out a 1.0 relative risk.

Scenario E presents an informative situation of a statistically overpowered trial having more than 1,000 (rather than 508) patients who have primary endpoint events. In such a trial, if the data yield an estimated 15% increase in the relative risk of primary endpoints, then that trial simultaneously would establish inferiority (by ruling out the 1.0 relative risk, corresponding to no increase) while establishing noninferiority of safety risk (by ruling out the 1.33 relative increase). This paradox is explained by recognizing that cardiovascular safety can be worse on celecoxib than on naproxen (i.e., corresponding to ruling out the relative risk of unity) while not being unacceptably worse (i.e., corresponding to ruling out the relative risk is greater than 1.33). Importantly, ruling out the 1.33 margin in scenario B does not allow one to conclude that celecoxib is at least as safe as naproxen with respect to cardiovascular risk; scenario A is the only one in Fig. 4 where such a conclusion holds. Rather, the conclusion justified by the data in scenario B is that the data rule out that the safety profile of celecoxib is unacceptably worse than that of naproxen. To justify that "positive" conclusion in scenario B, it is necessary that any increase

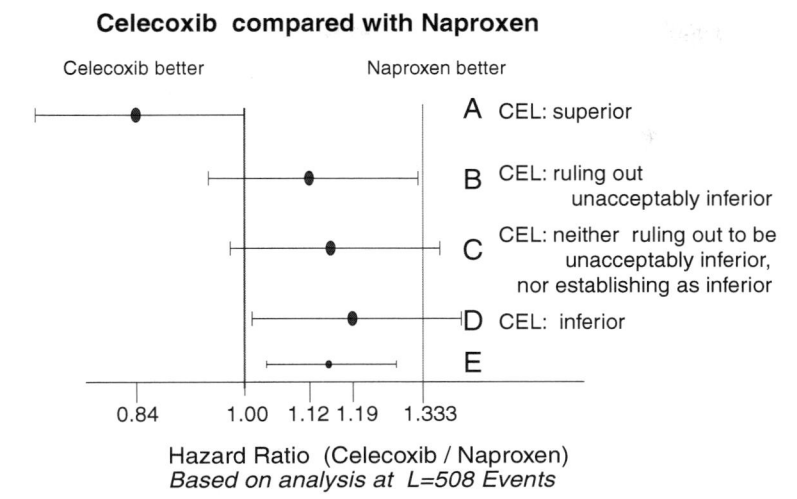

Fig. 4 Possible outcomes in the PRECISION trial for the celecoxib to naproxen hazard ratio for the safety endpoint, "cardio-vascular death/myocardial infarction/stroke." *Black circles* are point estimates, and the *horizontal lines* are the 95% confidence intervals CEL is celecoxib

in cardiovascular safety that is less than a 33% relative increase must be clinically acceptable in the context of the relative safety, acceptability, convenience, and cost of these two regimens.

4 Study Performance Standards for Safety Trials

For safety trials such as PRECISION that are designed to provide interpretable and reliable evidence regarding harm, irregularities in the quality of trial conduct can reduce the sensitivity to detecting clinically meaningful true differences in safety risks between the experimental and control regimens. These irregularities include failure to achieve timely enrollment of the targeted population in which excess risk from the experimental regimen is most plausible, failure to enroll patients who are at sufficiently high risk for the targeted number of primary safety events to be achieved, violations in eligibility criteria, lack of adherence to the experimental and control regimen at a level that matches best achievable in a real-world setting, cross-ins from one regimen to the other, and lack of achieving long-term retention in nearly all patients who undergo randomization [28, 30, 31]. These irregularities could lead to an increased likelihood of falsely ruling out unacceptable thresholds of risk in settings where the experimental regimen truly provides increased risks of clinically important harmful effects. As stated in [32]: "Many flaws on the design or conduct of the trial will tend to bias the results toward a conclusion of equivalence."

To address the concerns about these risks to trial integrity, performance standards regarding quality of trial conduct should be established. These should be specified either in the study protocol or in a separate performance standards document that is developed before the initiation of the clinical trial. For each of these performance standards, there should be specification of both targeted levels and minimally acceptable levels of performance, and specification of creative strategies that are being developed to maximize the ability to achieve these targeted levels. For illustration, consider the performance standard regarding retention. The targeted level of performance might be that no more than 2% of the randomized patients have incomplete capture of the primary endpoint information for reasons related to informative missingness, while the minimally acceptable level of performance might be an upper limit of 10% of patients with this irregularity. The creative approaches to achieve the targeted levels of retention might be similar to those specified in Fleming [30]. Finally, monitoring procedures should be in place during the trial to evaluate whether these performance standards are being met, with a plan for correction actions or even for trial termination if minimally acceptable levels of performance are not met.

5 Vulnerability to Undetected Safety Risks When Relying on Biomarkers as Surrogate Endpoints

In order to reduce the size and duration of Phase 3 clinical trials, it often is proposed to use biomarkers as replacement endpoints for measures that directly assess how a patient feels, functions, or survives [33–37]. For example, in type 2 diabetes mellitus, agents given to improve long-term microvascular or macrovascular disease endpoints might be assessed simply by evaluating their effect on changes in H_bA_{1c} at 6 months post randomization or, in end-stage renal disease, erythropoiesis-stimulating agents (ESAs) given to reduce the risk of myocardial infarction or death may be assessed simply by evaluating their effect on hematocrit [4–9].

Many agents have received regulatory approval for marketing based on small trials having short-term follow-up, where only the effects on a replacement endpoint such as a short-term intermediate endpoint or a biomarker have been assessed. For example, natalizumab received accelerated approval based on its effects on 1-year relapse rate in multiple sclerosis patients [18], while full regulatory approval was given to ESAs in chemotherapy-induced anemia and in hemodialysis in end stage renal disease based on effects on hematocrit, and full regulatory approval has been given to new agents in type 2 diabetes mellitus based on effects on HbA1c at 6 months post-randomization.

Strategies to use replacement endpoints such as biomarkers to reduce the size and duration of clinical trials lead to widespread marketing of interventions not only when efficacy data are limited, but also when safety data are limited. Hence, it should not be surprising in such settings when important off-target effects are discovered only after the product has already been widely used in clinical practice. In post-marketing settings, it was discovered that natalizumab induces progressive multi-focal leukoencephalopathy, ESAs induce thrombosis, and rosiglitazone appears to negatively impact the risk of macrovascular events in type 2 diabetes mellitus [37].

The hazards of reliance on replacement endpoints for regulatory approval are even worse when one recognizes that interventions are assessed based on their benefit-to-risk profile. The stronger the efficacy evidence, the greater the resilience regarding uncertainties about safety. Therefore, when post-marketing safety risks are detected in settings where efficacy has been established only on short-term replacement measures, there have been significant controversies about whether the product should continue to be used in the clinical practice. Natalizumab was removed from the market for some time, and the indications for use of ESAs and rosiglitazone have been substantially reduced. These controversial circumstances could have been avoided had trials been conducted pre- or post-marketing that provided reliable evidence about efficacy and safety. For example, the uncertainty about the clinical utility of natalizumab could have been addressed had long-term trials been conducted to assess its effects on measures of irreversible morbidity for multiple sclerosis patients, such as a delay in time to walking with a cane (i.e., Expanded Disability Status Scale Score = 6) or being wheelchair bound (i.e., Expanded Disability Status Scale Score = 7). Similarly, the uncertainty about the clinical utility of rosiglitazone in type 2 diabetes mellitus could have been avoided had this agent been studied in a trial similar to PROactive, a large-scale long-term clinical trial conducted in a high-risk patient population to reliably evaluate effects of another thiazolidinedione, pioglitazone, on measures of major morbidity and mortality (see Fig. 2) [38].

6 Illustration: Considerations for Cardiovascular Safety Trials in Type 2 Diabetes Mellitus

For many years, experimental regimens were approved for use in clinical practice in type 2 diabetes mellitus (T2DM) patients even though efficacy was evaluated only through an assessment of the effect of treatment on the biomarker, "H_bA_{1c} changes at 6 months." As discussed in the previous section, one of the consequences of this approach is the lack of reliable insights about important safety risks on measures of major morbidity and mortality.

A principal goal of effective management of T2DM is the reduction in risk of long-term complications that result in major morbidity and mortality. Clinical trials such as the DCCT [39] and the UKPDS 33 [40] provide evidence that sustained intensive blood-glucose control by using either sulfonylureas or insulin substantially decreases the long-term risk of microvascular complications, such as diabetic retinopathy, nephropathy, and neuropathy. However, sustained blood-glucose control has not been established to reduce the long-term risk of macrovascular disease, such as stroke, myocardial infarction, or death due to cardiovascular disease. Furthermore, while clinical trials of muraglitazar and rosiglitazone had established their positive effects on glucose control (specifically, on the outcome "HbA1c at 6 months"), recent overviews of available clinical trials strongly suggest these agents lead to increased major morbidity and mortality due to adverse effects on macrovascular complications [14, 41].

In late 2008, FDA's Division of Metabolic and Endocrine Drug Products, in response to advice received in July of that year from the FDA Endocrinologic and Metabolic Drugs Advisory Committee, determined that small- and short-term studies evaluating effects on H_bA_{1c} do not provide sufficiently reliable evidence about the benefit-to-risk profile of experimental products in patients with T2DM [42, 43]. The Agency took a significant step forward in its efforts to protect public health by deciding that long-term cardio-vascular (CV) safety trials would be required as part of the evaluation of new interventions in this clinical setting.

In these CV safety trials, patients with T2DM would be randomized to the experimental regimen against a standard of care therapeutic intervention. To ensure sensitivity to CV safety risks induced by the experimental regimen, evidence establishing CV safety should be required for any ancillary agents that would be administered more frequently in the standard of care control relative to the experimental arm of the trial. Examples of ancillary agents with such evidence include pioglitazone, metformin, sulfonylureas, or insulin. The trial would need to be of sufficient size and duration to allow reliable estimation of the relative risk for the composite CV endpoint, "cardiovascular death, stroke or myocardial infarction." Due to enhanced beneficial effects on microvascular complications provided by interventions that enhance glucose control, it was judged that a new regimen with improved effects on HbA1c would be acceptable as long as it induces no more than 5 or 6 excess "cardiovascular death, stroke or myocardial infarction" events per 1,000 person years. Since the rate of this composite endpoint is expected to be approximately 20 events per 1,000 person years on the control arm, the CV safety trial would be designed to determine whether a 1.3 relative increase in the rate of this composite could be ruled out. In the CV safety trial, 611 patients would need to experience the composite endpoint to have 90% power to rule out a 1.3 relative risk when experimental regimen truly provides no increase in the risk of the composite endpoint, when using a statistical test having a (one-sided) 2.5% false positive risk of declaring safety when the experimental truly does induce a 30% increase in relative risk. This CV safety trial would successfully rule out a relative risk of 1.3 if the estimated (experimental to control) relative risk, r, of "CV death, stroke, myocardial infarction" events is less than 1.11, corresponding to an estimate of approximately 2.2 excess major CV events per 1,000 person years. Given the annual event rate of 20 composite endpoints per 1,000 person years follow-up, it follows that approximately 6,000 patients would need to be randomized and followed for an average of approximately 60 months in order to yield 611 events.

Due to the size and duration of the CV safety trial, it was proposed at the July 2008 meeting of the FDA Endocrinologic and Metabolic Drugs Advisory

➤   Assume 2% per year rate of CVD/MI/Stroke

➤ Safety Trial:	Confirmatory	Screening
Rule out	**1.30**	**1.80 1.50 1.30**
• Excess Events per 1000 PY	6.0	16.0 10.0 6.0
• # Events	611	122
• Critical Value	1.11	1.262*

*Pr (Screening trial "+") is 0.90 (if r = 1)   &   0.025 (if r = 1.80)

&   0.17 (if r = 1.50)

&   0.44 (if r = 1.30)

Fig. 5 Illustration of sizes and properties of "screening" and "confirmatory" cardiovascular safety trials in type 2 diabetes mellitus patients. *CVD* is cardiovascular death, *MI* is myocardial infarction, *PY* is person years

Committee that the trial could be conducted in a pre-marketing "screening" stage and a post-marketing "confirmatory" stage [42]. If the data in the "screening" stage rule out that the true (experimental to control) relative risk, r, of "CV death, stroke, myocardial infarction" events is at least 1.8, then marketing approval followed by the post-marketing "confirmatory" stage would be considered. With 122 events in the screening stage, this would be achieved if the estimated relative risk is less than 1.262, corresponding to an estimate of approximately 5 excess major CV events per 1,000 person years. This "screening" stage would have 90% power for achieving favorable results that justify marketing approval for regimens with true relative risk, r, equal to unity, while having 97.5%, 83%, and 56% probability for screening out experimental regimens with true relative risk, r, equal to 1.80, 1.50, and 1.30, respectively, (see Fig. 5). To obtain 122 events in the screening stage, if approximately 2,500 patients would be randomized, they would need to be followed for an average of approximately 24 months.

The "confirmatory" stage can be separate from the "screening" stage, as in scenario #1 in Fig. 6 or can include the 122 events from the "screening" stage, as in scenario #2 in Fig. 6. In both scenarios, the 122 event dataset in the "screening" stage is used to test the "null hypothesis" that $r = 1.80$, at a traditional false positive error rate 0.025, where satisfying this CV safety criterion would allow marketing of the product. These data also can be used to test the "null hypothesis" that $r = 1.30$, the defined criterion for establishing CV safety. In scenario #1, the "null hypothesis" that $r = 1.30$ is tested at a traditional 0.025 false positive error rate. If the estimated relative risk is less than 0.91, a post-marketing "confirmatory" stage would not be

➤ Scenario #1: $L = 122$ "pre-marketing" events
   are *not* included in post-marketing safety evaluation

Pre-Marketing	Post-Marketing
$L = 122$	Additional $L = 611$

If est. $r = \mathbf{1.26} \Rightarrow$ Rule out 1.80   If est. $r = \mathbf{1.11} \Rightarrow$ Rule out 1.30
If est. $r = \mathbf{0.91} \Rightarrow$ Rule out 1.30

➤ Scenario #2: $L = 122$ "pre-marketing" events
   are included in post-marketing safety evaluation

Pre-Marketing	Post-Marketing
$L = 122$	Additional $L = 489$

If est. $r = \mathbf{1.26} \Rightarrow$ Rule out 1.80   If est. $r = \mathbf{1.11} \Rightarrow$ Rule out 1.30
If est. $r = \mathbf{0.53} \Rightarrow$ Rule out 1.30*

* Using an O'Brien-Fleming adjustment

Fig. 6 Issues regarding "interim analyses" of "confirmatory" CV safety trials in type 2 diabetes mellitus; L represents targeted number of events, r represents relative risk

needed; however, if the estimate is greater than 0.91, the "screening" stage data could not be used in the "confirmatory" stage due to multiplicity issues. In contrast, scenario #2 allows pooling of the "screening" and "confirmatory" stage data to test the "null hypothesis" that $r = 1.30$, by making a multiplicity adjustment (such as using an O'Brien-Fleming design [44], as illustrated in Fig. 6) when testing that hypothesis at the time of the analysis of the 122 event "screening" stage data.

7 Conclusions

It is important to have reliable evidence about whether the interventions used in clinical practice are safe as well as effective. Substantial insights about safety usually will be provided before marketing through Phase 1, 2, and 3 clinical trials. These insights, especially regarding risks associated with long-term use of the intervention and risks of rare but clinically compelling events, are enhanced by post-marketing active and passive surveillance, and especially by large, long-term randomized trials that provide the most reliable approach for identifying and addressing safety signals. To enhance the integrity of these randomized trials, it is important to prevent irregularities in the quality of trial conduct that reduce the sensitivity to detecting clinically meaningful true differences in safety risks between the experimental and control regimens.

The discovery and evaluation of the signals for cancer risks from use of ezetimibe/simvastatin to slow progression of aortic-valve stenosis illustrate important opportunities and challenges in the evaluation of safety, (see Fig. 3). Exploratory analyses of the SEAS trial provided a signal for increased risk of cancer incidence and cancer death [20]. However, due to the exploratory nature of the process leading to the discovery of this finding, p-values representing the strength of evidence for this safety signal are difficult to interpret, and estimates of the excess risk have random high bias. The IMPROVE-IT and SHARP trials provided important confirmatory evidence about the signal for cancer risk from exetimibe/simvastatin [25, 26]. While the confidence intervals for relative risk of cancer events from the meta-analysis of data from these two trials include unity, the failure to establish excess risk is not sufficient to justify safety. Rather, safety is established by ruling out any level of excess risk that would be unacceptable [28]. Since the data are consistent with ezetimibe/simvastin causing as much as an 84% increase in cancer incidence, further study of the effect of this agent on cancer risk is needed.

The use of the IMPROVE-IT and SHARP trials to address the safety signal from SEAS was appropriate. However, since these 2 trials were ongoing, the SEAS trial data should have been presented to the Data Monitoring Committees from IMPROVE-IT and SHARP, and the interim data from these 2 trials regarding cancer risks should have been released only when their Data Monitoring Committees judged the trials provided reliable answers to the questions they were designed to address. Unfortunately, rather than following this process, it appears the safety data from these two trials were prematurely released to the sponsor and others who were seeking rapid access to data informative about the safety signal from SEAS. Interim data prematurely released from IMPROVE-IT and SHARP regarding cancer risks are difficult to interpret due to the lack of a prespecified sampling context for such post-hoc interim analyses, and the lack of full access to peer-reviewed summaries of data from the two trials to address whether performance standards for safety trials have been met. Furthermore, the release of such interim data compromises the integrity of IMPROVE-IT and SHARP regarding the effect of ezetimibe/simvastin on the primary outcome measures these trials were designed to address.

A primary goal of clinical research is to obtain a timely and reliable assessment of the benefit-to-risk profile of an intervention. Benefit is established by clinical data providing substantial evidence of efficacy. Regarding risk, as discussed with ezetimibe/simvastin, safety is not established by failure to establish excess risk, such as obtaining confidence intervals for the relative risk of safety events that include unity. Absence of evidence is not evidence of absence. Rather, safety is established by determining the threshold for unacceptable risk, where this threshold should be dependent upon the strength of the evidence for efficacy, and then by obtaining safety data that rule out that threshold.

Acknowledgements The source of financial support for research described in this article is an NIH/NIAID grant entitled "Statistical Issues in AIDS Research" (R37 AI 29168). The author acknowledges New England Journal of Medicine as the source for Fig. 4. The author also acknowledges Jennifer Clark Nelson and Daniel L. Gillen for providing important insights.

References

1. Meeting Transcript of the joint Advisory Committee meeting of FDA's Arthritis and Drug Safety and Risk Management Advisory Committees, February 16–18, 2005. http://www.fda. gov/ohrms/dockets/ac/05/transcripts/2005-4090T1.htmhttp://www.fda.gov/ohrms/dockets/ac/ 05/transcripts/2005-4090T2.htmhttp://www.fda.gov/ohrms/dockets/ac/05/transcripts/2005-4090T3.htm
2. Nelson HS, Weiss ST, Bleecker ER, Yancey MS, Dorinsky PM, SMART Study Group (2006) The Salmeterol Multicenter Asthma Research Trial. Chest 129:15–26
3. Strom BL, Faich GA, Reynolds RF, Eng SM, D'Agostino RB, Ruskin JN, Kane JM (2008) The Ziprasidone Observational Study of Cardiac Outcomes (ZODIAC): design and baseline subject characteristics. J Clin Psychiatry 69(1):114–121
4. Pfeffer MA, Burdmann EA, Chen CY, Cooper ME, de Zeeuw D, Eckardt KU, Feyzi JM, Ivanovich P, Kewalramani R, Levey AS, Lewis EF, McGill JB, McMurray JJ, Parfrey P, Parving HH, Remuzzi G, Singh AK, Solomon SD, Toto R, for the TREAT Investigators (2009) A trial of darbepoetin alfa in type II diabetes and chronic kidney disease. N Engl J Med 361: 2019–2032
5. Singh AK, Szczech L, Tang KL, Barnhart H, Sapp S, Wolfson M, Reddan D, for the CHOIR Investigators (2006) Correction of anemia with epoetin alfa in chronic kidney disease. N Engl J Med 355:2085–2098
6. Drüeke TB, Locatelli F, Clyne N, Eckardt KU, Macdougall IC, Tsakiris D, Burger HU, Scherhag A, for the CREATE Investigators (2006) Normalization of hemoglobin level in patients with chronic kidney disease and anemia. N Engl J Med 355:2071–2084
7. Besarab A, Bolton WK, Browne JK, Egrie JC, Nissenson AR, Okamoto DM, Schwab SJ, Goodkin DA (1998) The effects of normal as compared with low hematocrit values in patients with cardiac disease who are receiving hemodialysis and epoetin. N Engl J Med 339:584–590
8. Center for Drug Evaluation and Research. Approval package: Avandia (rosiglitazone maleate) tablets. Company: SmithKline Beecham Pharmaceuticals. Application no. 21–071. Approval date: 5/25/1999. (Accessed 15 May 2007, at http://www.fda.gov/cder/foi/nda/99/21071_ Avandia.htm)
9. The Action to Control Cardiovascular Risk in Diabetes Study Group (2008) Effects of intensive glucose lowering in type 2 diabetes. N Engl J Med 358:2545–2559
10. Ettinger B, Black DM, Mitlak BH et al (1999) Reduction of vertebral fracture risk in postmenopausal women with osteoporosis treated with raloxifene: results from a 3-year randomized clinical trial. JAMA 282(7):637–645
11. Wooltorton E (2006) Osteoporosis treatment: raloxifene (Evista) and stroke mortality. CMAJ 175(2):147–148
12. Stefanick ML (2006) Risk–benefit profiles of raloxifene for women. N Engl J Med 355: 190–192
13. Mosca L, Grady D, Barrett-Connor E, Collins P, Wenger N, Abramson BL, Paganini-Hill A, Geiger MJ, Dowsett SA, Amewou-Atisso M, Kornitzer M (2009) Effect of raloxifene on stroke and venous thromboembolism according to subgroups in postmenopausal women at increased risk of coronary heart disease. Stroke 40:147–155
14. Nissen SE, Wolski K (2007) Effect of rosiglitazone on the risk of myocardial infarction and death from cardiovascular causes. N Engl J Med 356:2457–2471
15. Baggs J, Gee J, Lewis E et al (2011) The Vaccine Safety Datalink: a model for monitoring immunization safety. Pediatrics 127:S45–S53

16. Behrman RE, Benner JS, Brown JS et al (2011) Developing the sentinel system — a national resource for evidence development. N Engl J Med 364(6):498–499

17. Murphy TM, Gargiullo PM, Massoudi MS, Nelson DB, Jumaan AO, Okoro CA, Zanardi LR, Setia S, Fair E, LeBaron CW, Schwartz B, Wharton M, Livingood JR, for the Rotavirus Intussusception Investigation Team (2001) Intussusception among infants given an oral rotavirus vaccine. N Engl J Med 344:564–572

18. Assche GV, Van Ranst M, Sciot R, Dubois B, Vermeire S, Noman M, Verbeeck J, Geboes K, Robberecht W, Rutgeerts P (2005) Progressive multifocal leukoencephalopathy after Natalizumab therapy for Crohn's Disease. N Engl J Med 353:362–368

19. Emerson S, Kittelson J, Gillen D (2007) Frequentist evaluation of group sequential clinical trial designs. Stat Med 26(28):5047–5080

20. Rossebo AB, Pedersen TR, Boman K, Brudi P, Chambers JB, Egstrup K, Gerdts E, Gohlke-Bärwolf C, Holme I, Kesäniemi YA, Malbecq W, Nienaber CA, Ray S, Skjærpe T, Wachtell K, Willenheimer R, for the SEAS Investigators (2008) Intensive lipid lowering with Simvastatin and Ezetimibe in aortic stenosis. N Engl J Med 359:1343–1356

21. Fleming TR (2010) Clinical trials: discerning hype from substance. Ann Intern Med 153:400–406

22. Bradford PG, Awad AB (2007) Phytosterols as anticancer compounds. Mol Nutr Food Res 51:161–170

23. Assmann G, Kannenbert F, Ramey DR, Musliner TA, Gutkin SW, Veltri EP (2008) Effects of ezetimibe, simvastatin, atorvastatin, and ezetimibe-statin therapies on non-cholesterol sterols in patients with primary hypercholesterolemia. Curr Med Res Opin 24:249–259

24. Imanaka H, Koide H, Shimizu S et al (2008) Chemoprevention of tumor metastasis by liposomal β-sitosterol intake. Biol Pharm Bull 31:400–404

25. Cannon CP, Guigliano RP, Blaxing MA et al (2005) Rationale and design of IMPROVE-IT (IMProved Reduction of Outcomes: Vytorin Efficacy International Trial): comparison of ezetimibe/simvastatin versus simvastatin monotherapy on cardiovascular outcomes in patients with acute coronary syndrome. Am Heart J 149:464–473

26. Baigent C, Landry M (2003) Study of heart and renal protection (SHARP). Kidney Int 63(Suppl 84):S207–S210

27. Peto R, Emberson J, Landray M et al (2008) Analyses of cancer data from three ezetimibe trials. N Engl J Med 359(13):1357–1366. doi:10.1056/NEJMsa0806603

28. Fleming TR (2008) Identifying and addressing safety signals in clinical trials. N Engl J Med 359:1400–1402

29. Becker MC, Wang TH, Wisniewski L, Wolski K, Libby P, Lüscher TF, Borer JS, Mascette AM, Husni ME, Solomon DH, Graham DY, Yeomans ND, Krum H, Ruschitzka F, Lincoff AM, Nissen SE, for the PRECISION Investigators (2009) Rationale, design, and governance of Prospective Randomized Evaluation of Celecoxib Integrated Safety versus Ibuprofen Or Naproxen (PRECISION), a cardiovascular end point trial of nonsteroidal antiinflammatory agents in patients with arthritis. Am Heart J 157:606–612

30. Fleming TR (2011) Addressing missing data in clinical trials. Ann Intern Med 154:113–117

31. Fleming TR, Odem-Davis K, Rothmann MD, Shen YL (2011) Some essential considerations in the design and conduct of non-inferiority trials. Clin Trials 8:432–439

32. ICH E-9—International conference on harmonisation: statistical principles for clinical trials, published in the Federal Register of May 9, 1997, (62 FR 25712)

33. Fleming TR, DeMets DL (1996) Surrogate end points in clinical trials: are we being misled? Ann Intern Med 125(7):605–613

34. Fleming TR (2005) Surrogate endpoints and FDA's accelerated approval process. Health Aff 24(1):67–78

35. Temple RJ (1995) A regulatory authority's opinion about surrogate endpoints. In: Nimmo WS, Tucker GT (eds) Clinical measurement in drug evaluation. Wiley, New York

36. IOM (2010) Evaluation of biomarkers and surrogate endpoints in chronic disease. Washington DC, National Academies Press. http://www.iom.edu/Reports/2010/Evaluation-of-Biomarkers-and-Surrogate-Endpoints-in-Chronic-Disease.aspx

37. Fleming TR, Powers JH (2012) Biomarkers and surrogate endpoints in clinical trials. Stat Med doi:10.1002/sim.5403, 2012
38. Dormandy JA, Charbonnel B, Eckland EJA et al (2005) Secondary prevention of macrovascular events in patients with type 2 diabetes: a randomized trial of pioglitazone. The PROactive Study (PROspective pioglitAzone Clinical Trial In macroVascular Events). Lancet 366:1279–1289
39. The DCCT Research Group (1993) The effect of intensive treatment of diabetes on the development and progression of long-term complications in insulin-dependent diabetes mellitus. N Engl J Med 329:977–986
40. UKPDS Group (1998) Intensive blood-glucose control with sulphonylureas or insulin compared with conventional treatment and risk of complications in patients with type 2 diabetes (UKPDS 33). Lancet 352:837–853
41. Nissen SE, Wolski K, Topol EJ (2005) Effect of muraglitazar on death and major adverse cardiovascular events in patients with type 2 diabetes mellitus. JAMA 294:2581–2586
42. Meeting Transcript of the FDA Endocrinologic and Metabolic Drugs Advisory Committee and Drug Safety and Risk Management Advisory Committee, September 24, 2012/www.fda.gov/downloads/AdvisoryCommittees/CommitteesMeetingMaterials/Drugs/Endocrinologicand MetabolicDrugsAdvisoryCommittee/UCM 222628.pdf and UCM222629.pdf
43. Guidance for industry. diabetes mellitus — evaluating cardiovascular risk in new antidiabetic therapies to treat type 2 diabetes. http://www.fda.gov/downloads/Drugs/GuidanceComplianceRegulatoryInformation/Guidances/ucm071627.pdf
44. O'Brien PC, Fleming TR (1979) A multi-stage procedure for clinical trials. Biometrics 35:549–556

Past, Present, and Future of Drug Safety Assessment

Robert Temple

Abstract Adverse effects are an expected consequence of drug use, but how to detect them when they are rare or represent only a small increase over background rates remains a formidable problem. It is useful to review the past history of how important adverse effects were discovered so that we can improve our ability to detect them more rapidly.

We discover serious adverse effects in different ways, depending on how rare they are and whether they occur spontaneously (i.e., in the absence of a drug), and on how great the increase over background rate is. Depending on such factors we rely on spontaneous reports, epidemiologic data (if the risk increase is reasonably large), and on large controlled trials or meta-analyses (when the increase in risk is smaller).

These methods, the history of their use, and their usefulness in the future are considered.

1 Introduction

Developers and reviewers of drugs, as well as the patients and physicians who use them, are well aware that drugs have adverse effects, some of them serious. Common, non-serious adverse effects are seen with virtually all drugs and are generally readily detected in pre-marketing controlled trials (as long as the right questions are asked). Serious adverse effects, if frequent, are also readily detected as part of development, a common situation for cancer chemotherapy, where such serious risks may be acceptable in light of benefits. Detection of risks pre-marketing is described in FDA's Guidance, Pre-marketing Risk Assessment [1].

R. Temple (✉)
Center for Clinical Science, FDA Center for Drug Evaluation and Research, 10903 New Hampshire Avenue, Silver Spring, MD 20993-0002, USA
e-mail: Robert.Temple@fda.hhs.gov

T.R. Fleming and B.S. Weir (eds.), *Proceedings of the Fourth Seattle Symposium in Biostatistics: Clinical Trials*, Lecture Notes in Statistics 1205, DOI 10.1007/978-1-4614-5245-4_10, © Springer Science+Business Media New York 2013

In most cases, however, serious risks are not frequent and become apparent only after marketing, often surprising us, and often raising concern about how long it took to discover them. A question increasingly being raised, both within and outside FDA, is whether there are approaches that could lead to earlier detection of such serious adverse effects, ideally pre-marketing, but, if not, more rapidly post-marketing.

Risk is always weighed against benefit, and substantial rates of serious risks can be accepted when there is no safer alternative; examples include:

- Life-threatening risks of many oncologic drugs, older anti-HIV medications, and inflammatory disease modifiers
- A rate of agranulocytosis of about 1.5% with clozapine for use in people failing other antipsychotic treatment
- Serious bleeding, sometimes fatal, with anticoagulants (coumadin, dabigatran, riveroxiban, with rates of about 5% in atrial fibrillation) and platelet-inhibiting drugs (prasugrel, ticagrelor, clopidogrel, with rates of 3–5% with use in acute coronary syndrome, post-infarction)
- PML (progressive multifocal leukoencephalophy), a usually fatal viral encephalitis that occurs at a rate of about 1/1,000 with long-term use of natalizumab (Tysabri)

In all these cases, the sometimes lethal risks are accepted because the drug's benefits are thought to outweigh the risk. Clearly, however, no considered weighing of risks and benefits or modification of use to reflect risk is possible until risks are recognized. It is therefore worthwhile to consider how we detect serious risks.

2   How Do We Find Serious Risks?

There are four distinct patterns of serious risk and we detect these risks in different ways. The method depends on the frequency of the adverse effect and how often the event occurs spontaneously, i.e., without a drug cause.

2.1   Serious Adverse Effects That Are Not So Rare and Are Obviously Drug-Related

Serious adverse events that are relatively frequent can be detected in usual-size pre-marketing trial databases if these are large enough, e.g., in a large single study or in a pooled analysis of 1,000–3,000 patients, and if rates of the events are markedly higher than spontaneous rates. Thus:

1. Studies of anticoagulants for treatment of atrial fibrillation or platelet inhibitors in acute coronary syndrome show major bleeding rates of 3–5%, compared to background rates of well under 1%.
2. Studies of clozapine revealed a roughly 1.5% rate of agranulocytosis, compared to background rates of essentially zero.
3. The anti-inflammatory TNF blockers (infliximab, adalimumab, certolizumab, and others), used for rheumatoid arthritis, psoriasis, and inflammatory bowel disease, have been found to increase the rates of lymphomas and opportunistic infections compared to controls.
4. Oncologic drug studies reveal a wide range of effects on erythropoiesis, lymphocytes, platelets, and granulocytes, often with superinfections, again, events that only rarely occur spontaneously.

2.2 Rare Serious Adverse Effects That Are Obviously Drug-Related Because They Have Very Low Rates of Spontaneous Occurrence

Less common serious risks (e.g., events occurring at a rate of one per thousand) can sometimes be detected in clinical trials if they are interpretable as single cases, e.g., severe hepatic necrosis, acute renal failure, Stevens–Johnson syndrome, hematologic events (aplastic anemia, agranulocytosis, thrombocytopenia), although concomitant treatment and illness can render interpretation of single cases more difficult. In general, the probability is about 95% of seeing at least one case of an adverse effect occurring at a rate of one per thousand in a 3,000 patient sample, but pre-marketing databases often have fewer patients than this so that very rare events will often be missed.

Such events are readily detected post-marketing, however, usually as spontaneous reports, and they can generally be reliably attributed to the treatment (unless the drug-induced events are extremely rare, e.g., less than 1/50,000–100,000), because the events rarely occur spontaneously. This would mean, if cases of such an adverse event are seen, that the risk ratio for the event in relation to drug use is large, surely >10 and probably >100, and a causal relationship is highly credible, as the drug withdrawals (Table 1) and many warnings for hepatic necrosis, torsade de pointes arrhythmias, Stevens–Johnson syndrome, and agranulocytosis show.

In recent years it has become possible to anticipate the occurrence of two serious, rare, drug-related adverse effects by detecting a surrogate for these effects in clinical studies: (1) finding a specific hepatocellular injury that is not itself usually accompanied by severe hepatic failure, but that predicts the occurrence of cases of life-threatening hepatic necrosis, and (2) finding prolongation of the corrected electrocardiographic QT interval (QTc) that is not life-threatening but that predicts the occurrence of torsade de pointes arrhythmias (TdP) and sudden death.

Table 1 History of drug safety withdrawals

Drug	Year approved	Year withdrawn	Data source	Adverse effect
Azaribine (Triazure)	1975	1976	1	Arterial thrombosis
Phenformin		1978	2	Lactic acidosis
Ticrynafen (Selacryn)	1979	1980	1	DILI
Benoxaprofen (Oraflex)	1982	1982	1	DILI
Zomepirac (Zomax)	1980	1983	1	Anaphylaxis
Methaqualone (Qualude)	1960s	1984	1	Overdose very hard to treat
Nomifensine (Merital)	1984	1986	1	Hemolytic anemia
Suprofen (Suprol)	1985	1987	1	Acute renal failure
Encainide[a] (Enkaid)	1986	1991	3a	Mortality (HR=2)
Temafloxacin (Omniflox)	1992	1992	1	Hemolysis, renal failure
Flosequinan (Manoplax)	1992	1993	3a	Mortality (HR – 1.5)
Fenfluramine (Pondimin)	1973	1997	2	Valvulopathy
Terfenadine (Seldane)	1985	1998	1, 4	TdP
Mibefradil (Posicor)	1997	1998	1	Drug–drug interactions causing TdP and rhabdomyolysis
Bromfenac (Duract)	1997	1998	1	DILI
Trovafloxacin[b] (Trovan)	1997	1998	1	DILI
Astemizole (Hismanil)	1988	1999	1, 4	TdP
Grepafloxacin (Raxar)	1997	1999	1, 4	TdP
Troglitazone (Rezulin)	1997	2000	1	DILI
Cisapride (Propulsid)	1993	2000	1, 4	TdP
Alosetron[c] (Lotronex)	2000	2000	1	Ischemic colitis; constipation needing surgery
PPA (phenylpropanolamine)	<1962	2000	2	Hemorrhagic stroke
Rapacuronium (Raplon)	1999	2001	1	Bronchospasm
Cerivastatin (Baycol)	1997	2001	1, 2	Higher rate of rhabdomyolysis than other statins
Etretinate	1986	2002	1	Birth defects
Levacetyl methadol (Orlaam)	1993	2003	1, 4	TdP
Rofecoxib (VIOXX)	1999	2004	3a	AMI
Natalizumab[c] (Tysabri)	2000	2005	1	PML
Pemoline (Cylert)	1975	2005	1	DILI
Valdecoxib (Bextra)	2001	2005	1	Stevens–Johnson syndrome
Gatifloxacin (Tequin)	1999	2006	1	Hyperglycemia and hypoglycemia

Table 1 (continued)

Drug	Year approved	Year withdrawn	Data source	Adverse effect
Pergolide (Permax)	1998	2007	2	Valvulopathy
Tegaserod (Zelnorm)	2002	2007	3b	CV events
Aprotinin (Trasylol)	1993	2008	3a	Increased mortality
Sibutramine (Meridia)	1997	2010	3a	CV events
Propoxyphene	<1962	2010	2, 4	Mortality, esp in overdose

DILI drug-induced liver injury, *TdP* torsade de pointes, *PML* progressive multifocal leukoencephalopathy
Data sources:
1= individual cases
2 = epidemiologic data
3 = RCT's: 3a large trials; 3b MetaA
4 = Evidence of QT prolongation
[a]Important toxicity, but withdrawal not FDA encouraged
[b]NOT withdrawn, but limited
[c]Returned to market

It is now standard [2] to examine patients in drug development programs for hepatic aminotransferase elevations and for a pattern of abnormalities in individual cases referred to as meeting Hy's Law (named after hepatologist Hy Zimmerman): a substantial aminotransferase elevation and increase of serum bilirubin to above 2 mg/dL, with no evidence of hepatic obstruction (elevated alkaline phosphatase), and no evidence of other causes of liver injury (hepatitis viruses, acute heart failure, or other hepatic disease). Zimmerman found that 10% or more of patients who had hepatocellular injury sufficient to cause jaundice would go on to hepatic failure [3]. Observing even one or two Hy's Law cases in a New Drug Application (NDA) database has led to rejection of marketing applications for lumiracoxib, ximelagatran, dilevalol, and tasosartan (the first 3 of which were marketed in Europe and withdrawn because of hepatotoxicity), usually without any documented cases of life-threatening liver injury, and has represented an early signal of subsequent problems with bromfenac and troglitazone, which were withdrawn from the US market.

Virtually all drugs are now studied in a thorough QT study (TQT), as called for in ICH E-14 [Clinical Evaluation of QT/QTc Interval Prolongation and Proarrhythmic Potential for Non-Antiarrhythmic Drugs [4]]. A TQT study is a controlled observation of the QTc prolonging effects seen on an electrocardiogram (ECG) of a drug compared to placebo and (usually) to an active control with a modest QTc prolonging effect. QTc prolongation is a well-recognized predictor of TdP (torsade de pointes-type ventricular tachycardia), which can be fatal. QTc prolongation of more than a modest amount (above >10 msec) leads to close electrocardiographic observations in phase 3 studies, and larger effects (e.g., >20 msec, can lead to rejection of an application (e.g., sertindole) and to particular care and ECG monitoring in use if the drug is needed despite the risk (e.g., sotalol and dofetilide for maintaining sinus rhythm after conversion of atrial fibrillation, arsenic trioxide for promyelocytic leukemia).

2.3 A Serious Adverse Effect That Can Occur Spontaneously, with Reasonable Frequency, and That Is Therefore Not Obviously Drug-Related, but Whose Rate Is Greatly Increased by a Drug

Some serious adverse effects of drugs that would not have been interpretable from spontaneous reports, because the adverse events were often seen in the population receiving the drug, have been identified as drug-related in epidemiologic studies because the risk ratio was quite large, at least 4–5 (deep vein thrombosis and pulmonary embolism for oral contraceptives [5], endometrial cancer from unopposed postmenopausal estrogen [6], valvulopathy with fenfluramine or pergolide [7, 8], many teratogenic effects, vaginal cancer after exposure to diethylstilbestrol [9]). Of course, many epidemiologic studies report far smaller increases and there is debate as to when (at what risk ratio) these become credible [10]. In general, however, uncertainty grows as the risk estimate decreases and epidemiologists have suggested thresholds of two- to threefold [11, 12] Whatever the limit, however, it is clear that smaller increases in risk (i.e., below the credibility limit for epidemiologic studies) are also of clinical interest and methods of discovering them are critical.

2.4 Serious Events That Occur Spontaneously and Are Only Modestly (<1.5-Fold) Increased in Rate by the Drug

Typically, the adverse effects of interest in these cases are cardiovascular (CV) but they could also be tumors, or adverse outcomes of the disease, such as increased asthma deaths in people treated with long-acting beta-agonists [13]. As noted, views will differ on the size of risk increases that can be reliably detected or ruled out, but it is reasonably clear that although increases of 30–50% in serious CV events would be of major concern for widely used drugs, particularly when the goal of treatment is symptomatic (long-term pain relief) or risk reduction (oral hypoglycemics, cholesterol lowering drugs, anti-arrhythmics, antihypertensives, chemoprevention drugs), most observers would not find epidemiologic data definitive in such cases.

But large enough clinical trials, or pooled data from a number of smaller trials, can detect such effects and have been called for [14], and used [15, 16] both premarketing and post-marketing, to do so. There is growing interest in the conduct of such trials, an important change in focus on how to monitor safety (see Sect. 4).

3 How Have the Serious Risks Post-marketing That Led to Drug Withdrawal Been Detected?

Table 1 lists 35 drugs withdrawn from the market (in a few cases temporarily) since 1970 for safety reasons. The table shows both the adverse effect that led to withdrawal and the source of the data (types discussed in Sect. 2) documenting the adverse effect. The table does not address instances in which pre-marketing studies identified the risks (some of these are considered below), so that drugs were never marketed, or instances in which critical safety findings did not result in drug withdrawal but led to restrictive labeling. The large majority of withdrawals resulted from individual case reports to FDA (or reported in the literature) but some recent withdrawals were based on findings in controlled trials or meta-analyses.

4 Evolving Concerns

As Table 1 shows, the large majority of adverse effects leading to drug withdrawal were deadly, but rare, events, detected by FDA's spontaneous reporting system (AERS, the Adverse Reaction Reporting System), sometimes with cases reported in the literature. The vast improvement in the spontaneous adverse effect reporting system (AERS had <50,000 reports per year in the 1970s but has gradually grown to over 600,000 in recent years) can now detect these adverse effects very rapidly; the hepatotoxicity of bromfenac and troglitazone and adverse reactions arising from drug–drug interactions with mibefradil (TdP with several drugs and rhabdomyolysis with simvastatin) were detected within a few months.

Recent experiences showing modestly increased rates of common serious adverse outcomes of widely used drugs, however, have focused attention on the desirability of conducting longer and larger controlled trials, especially for chronically administered drugs. Such trials could undoubtedly have detected the large risks of thromboembolic disease with oral contraceptives, endometrial cancer with estrogen replacement therapy, and valvulopathy with fenfluramine, increases well above two- to threefold that were detected in epidemiologic studies, but it is also clear that they can detect much smaller increases in serious event rates, i.e., 30–50%, especially in high risk patients.

There is growing interest in being able to detect such modest increases in important adverse outcomes. Such adverse effects have been detected in the past, but several recent situations, both pre- and post-marketing, have greatly increased interest, generally involving drugs directed at cardiovascular endpoints, because of highly unexpected findings:

- COX-2 selective NSAIDs and NSAIDs more generally may increase CV risk.
- Rosiglitazone may increase CV risk, and it and other oral hypoglycemics are used in a high-risk population.
- Erythropoietin increased CV risk in dialysis and pre-dialysis patients, also a high risk population; it also promoted tumor growth in several groups of cancer patients.
- Studies of long-acting beta agonists showed an increase rate of asthma exacerbation.

- The Women's Health Initiative Trial (WHI) found adverse effects of estrogen/progesterone replacement on CV outcomes and carcinogenicity [17].
- Torcetrapib, a drug that raised HDL cholesterol and lowered LDL cholesterol, increased CV risk (pre-marketing) [15].
- Meta-analyses of antidepressants showed increased suicidality [18, 19] in children and young adults.

Before reflecting on where this new interest might lead, it is useful to consider the past history of randomized trials that have shown safety problems.

5   Past Outcome Trials Examining CV Events

Most of the randomized controlled trials (RCTs) that have shown or looked for adverse CV effects have been studies of CV diseases, or, less commonly, an examination of CV effects in non-CV disease, which were carried out for two principal reasons:

1. In most cases the trials sought to show a beneficial effect on an outcome because there was a known favorable effect on a surrogate endpoint. That is, there was no adverse hypothesis, and therefore no ethical issue involved in randomizing to drug or placebo.
2. In some cases there was an existing safety concern about a drug that seemed valuable (e.g., with clear short-term benefit and strong suspicion of longer term benefit, but no proof of this), so that the study was aimed at both confirming long-term benefit and assessing safety concerns. In some of the cases the CV concern that arose in long-term use was a complete surprise.

5.1   *Attempts to Show Benefit*

5.1.1   University Group Diabetes Program [20]

The University Group Diabetes Program (UGDP), a National Institutes of Health (NIH) trial conducted in the late 1960s, sought to show the value of improved glucose control with insulin, given as fixed or variable doses, and tolbutamide, a sulfonylurea oral hypoglycemic, compared to placebo. It showed an adverse effect of tolbutamide on cardiovascular deaths compared to the other treatments, a point made in labeling for all sulfonylureas since then, although the results have been challenged and are controversial.

5.1.2 Subsequent Trials in Diabetes Mellitus (DM)

Numerous studies in type 2 diabetes (recently stopped ACCORD [21], an NIH trial, and many other commercial, and government-sponsored European and U.S. trials) have failed to show the hoped-for benefit on CV outcomes. Indeed, ACCORD reported that very tight control in type 2 diabetes led to a roughly 25% increase in mortality.

5.1.3 CAST

The Cardiac Arrhythmia Suppression Trial (CAST), an NIH trial [22], was intended to show improved survival compared to placebo in post-infarction patients with ≥ 6 ventricular premature beats (VPBs) per hour (that rate was a known risk factor for sudden death) in patients given an effective (VPB-suppressing) antiarrhythmic. To be randomized patients had to respond to encainide or flecainide with substantial reduction of VPB's (mean response 70%; median response 100%). The expectation of benefit at the onset of the trial was so strong that it used a one-sided hypothesis and some questioned the ethics of the trial. CAST showed approximately 2.4-fold increase in mortality in the treated patients, a stunning surprise. CAST II [23] showed a similar result for ethmosin.

5.1.4 NSAIDs (Rofecoxib, Celecoxib)

The studies of COX-2 selective NSAIDs that were most suggestive of increased CV risk were designed to show

- Reduced risk of major GI bleeds (VIGOR [24], TARGET [25], EDGE [26]). This could be considered an attempt to validate the documented surrogate effect of decreased endoscopic ulcers.
- Reduced rate of colon polyp formation (APC and PreSAP [27] trials of cele-coxib); approve trial of rofecoxib) [28] or improvement in Alzheimer's disease (ADAPT trial of celecoxib) [29].

5.1.5 Erythropoietin

Three outcome studies were intended to confirm the common belief that titrating people to higher hemoglobin levels would be good for them (survival, quality of life), as epidemiologic data had suggested. Instead, there were unfavorable effects on stroke and survival, thus far not well explained [30–32].

5.1.6   Postmenopausal Estrogens

Epidemiological data led to the belief that estrogen/progestin postmenopausal treatment would have a favorable effect on CV outcome in older women. The Women's Health Initiative Trial [16] examined those effects in a randomized trial and found no benefit but an increased rate of adverse cardiovascular outcomes and breast cancer.

5.1.7   Torcetrapib

Torcetrapib was the first drug to have an important HDL-raising effect, an effect that overwhelming epidemiologic data predicted would be beneficial. Instead, the ILLUMINATE study [15] showed a 58% increase in mortality, perhaps the result of a BP-raising effect.

5.2   Attempts to Resolve a Safety Concern, Where Short-Term Clinical Benefit Had Been Demonstrated

Experience with two classes of CV drugs (inotropic drugs for congestive heart failure (CHF) and antiarrhythmics generally) raised concern about possible adverse effects on survival. The Division of Cardiorenal Products in FDA has therefore required, for more than 2 decades, that these drugs be studied, prior to approval, to assess CV risk. Such studies were practical because the CV event rate in CHF and most arrhythmias was high, making reasonably sized studies possible, and were considered ethical because an important benefit was expected.

5.2.1   CHF

Early experience with beta-agonists raised concern that inotropes (or at least some inotropes) might worsen outcome, leading to the requirement for outcome trials prior to approval for inotropic agents that improved exercise tolerance. Studies of various sympathomimetics, whether direct (beta agonists, such as dobutamine) or indirect (phosphodiesterase inhibitors, including milrinone, flosequinan, vesnarinone), all of which had shown clear favorable short-term effects on exercise tolerance, showed adverse effects on survival. The PROMISE Study [16], which randomized 1,088 patients with severe chronic heart failure to milrinone or placebo, each added to standard treatment, showed a 34% increase in cardiovascular mortality (p = 0.016). The PROFILE study (not published in full) comparing flosequinan to placebo showed a highly significant 48% increase in mortality in a 1,900 patient trial (p = 0.0004). A randomized placebo-controlled study of vesnarinone [33] showed a dose-related decrease in survival on the drug. In all of these cases the very high risk patients in the trials allowed studies of reasonable size to detect the adverse CV outcomes.

5.2.2 Antiarrhythmics

Since the CAST experience the FDA has sought assurance, in at least some setting, that any marketing application for an antiarrhythmic drug does not adversely affect CV outcome.

The application for sotalol for preventing recurrence of atrial fibrillation had the post-AMI Julien [34] trial (18% reduction of mortality, although not statistically significant), while the dofetilide application had 2 "Diamond" [35, 36] studies showing no adverse outcome in patients with CHF or post-infarction. Dronedarone, also for use in maintaining sinus rhythm, showed increased mortality in patients with recent CHF exacerbation, but the large effectiveness trial supporting approval (ATHENA) [37], which excluded such patients, showed numerically higher survival and a highly significant reduction in cardiovascular hospitalizations.

6 Recent Outcome Studies Raising New Issues

The studies described above have sobering implications because they showed that drugs with favorable effects on surrogate and even short-term clinical endpoints can have serious adverse effects, often unanticipated. Not surprisingly, there is particular concern when drug recipients are already at high risk, as is the case with patients with CHF and arrhythmias, diabetes, chronic kidney disease, and lipid abnormalities. Whether all drugs used long-term in high-risk patients need outcome data prior to, or even after, approval has not been determined and practice to date has depended on past experience and the specifics of the clinical studies needed to establish effectiveness. Thus, as noted, any antiarrhythmic agent or drug for CHF has needed outcome data prior to approval. Drugs that are used as anticoagulants to prevent embolic events in atrial fibrillation or used in various stages of CAD to inhibit platelet aggregation to prevent CV death, stroke, and myocardial infarction (clopidogrel, prasugrel, ticagrelor, iiB/iiiA inhibitors) have no credible surrogate measure and so have uniformly been studied in large outcome studies to demonstrate benefit; these studies, at the same time, are large enough to assess adverse outcomes.

Cardiovascular drugs have not uniformly been expected to be studied in outcome trials, in part because of what appeared to be reassuring past experience. Antihypertensives, for example, are approved based on evidence of sustained BP effects, with no requirement for outcome studies before or after approval. Depending on your view, ALLHAT [38] supports or challenges that position, finding at most modest differences between an angiotensin-converting enzyme inhibitor (ACEI), a calcium channel blocker (CCB), a diuretic, and an alpha blocker, although the last was clearly less effective in treating or preventing heart failure. A problem in designing such trials would be the great difficulty in defining a safety margin to rule out, as almost all patients will be on more than one drug and probably different drugs. In ALLHAT, for example, the groups randomized to the ACEI and CCB could not receive an added diuretic (a test drug in the study), a drug that greatly enhances effectiveness of ACEIs and that would help deal with CCB fluid retention. In any event, the lack of need for outcome studies does not mean the effect of treatments may not differ, as suggested by the LIFE Study [39], which showed a greater effect on stroke for losartan than atenolol, and the ACCOMPLISH Study [40], which showed a better effect of amlodipine than hydrochlorothiazide, each added to benazepril, on major adverse cardiovascular events (MACE) plus CV hospitalization.

LDL-lowering drugs have been approved based on the basis of effects on LDL, but all currently marketed HMGCoA reductase inhibitors (statins) have subsequently had at least one favorable outcome study conducted after approval. There seems little doubt that the torcetrapib experience will be strongly considered in deciding whether HDL-raising drugs will need pre-approval outcome studies.

Outcome studies with nonsteroidal anti-inflammatory drugs (NSAIDs), including rofecoxib, celecoxib, etoricoxib, and lumiracoxib, have affected the expectations for new NSAIDs; although FDA has prepared no formal guidance on the class, the database for lumiracoxib had well over 10,000 patients. There is reason to hope the ongoing >20,000 patient PRECISION study comparing ibuprofen, naproxen, and celecoxib, which is designed to rule out a >30% increased CV risk for celecoxib, compared to naproxen, will shed light on this class. Also of interest is the mechanism of the adverse CV effects seen with, for example, rofecoxib. Elevated BP is generally considered the leading candidate cause, but that might have been expected to lead to excess strokes, not the increase in acute myocardial infarction actually seen.

Finally, the still somewhat controversial results of individual and pooled studies of rosiglitazone have focused attention on the long-term effects of oral hypo-glycemic agents, a class of drugs used in a high CV risk population. The meta-analysis receiving most [41] attention included over 40 relatively short-term placebo and active controlled trials of rosiglitazone and added 2 larger longer-term trials, ADOPT [42] and DREAM [43], whose results were of course known before the analysis. The combined data supported (p = 0.03) an effect on nonfatal MI and leaned toward an adverse effect on survival (p = 0.06). Interestingly, the short-term studies supported the adverse mortality effect while ADOPT, DREAM, and a later, longer study, RECORD [44] did not suggest an adverse effect on survival. However one interprets these results, they powerfully raised the question of what data we should be available at the time of marketing an oral hypoglycemic drug and afterward.

The recent SCOUT [45] trial of sibutramine, an effective weight loss drug, has raised similar issues related to this class of drugs, which are also used in high-risk population. The SCOUT trial showed a 16% increase in the rate of the primary endpoint (CV death, nonfatal MI and non-fatal stroke) in the sibutramine-treated patients, although there was no effect on CV death. Sibutramine had a modest effect on BP and heart rate and more generally, has sympathomimetic properties, possibly a problem in high-risk patients.

7 Outcome Data at the Time of Approval and Afterward

Where there is documented reason for concern about cardiovascular outcomes with a particular drug intended for long-term use, especially a drug intended for high-risk patients, or concern about a drug class, as FDA concluded there was for antiarrhythmics and drugs for CHF, and, more recently, for NSAIDs, an outcome study would generally be expected pre-marketing (perhaps unless there was strong effectiveness in an untreated or hard-to-treat population). But suppose there is no documented reason for concern. Are there some conditions in which reassurance about long-term effects should be sought nonetheless?

There was a fair consensus in the literature, and many specific suggestions [46] that oral hypoglycemics should in fact be studied in a way that could rule out an excessive CV risk. Risk was sometimes linked to use of a surrogate marker, HbA1c, as the effectiveness endpoint for these drugs, but that seems something of a distraction, as improved glucose control is well accepted as a surrogate that predicts improved microvascular outcomes. A far more forceful argument is that in drugs intended for people at high risk, it is appropriate to expect, as a condition of approval, that an applicant should rule out an unacceptable cardiovascular risk of the drug [47]. Following a July 2008 meeting of the Endocrinologic and Metabolic Drugs Advisory Committee, FDA published in December 2008 a final guidance [14] calling for:

- Pre-marketing demonstration, generally based on pooled data from controlled trials, that there is not an unacceptable increase in CV risk, indicated by an upper bound of the 95% CI for risk of less than 1.8 for test drug (but a point estimate much above 1 would also be a concern).
- Post-approval demonstration, obviously in a larger database, that the 95% CI upper bound for CV risk is less than 1.3.

These studies are plainly demanding but not unreasonably daunting if the trials include patients at higher risk (with many events). For a class of drugs directed at a population with high CV risk, this requirement seems hard to dispute. The 1.8 and 1.3 upper bounds are arbitrary (but reasonable, and similar to the goal in the large PRECISION trial of celecoxib, ibuprofen, and naproxen).

FDA has not applied the oral hypoglycemic policy to additional areas and remains conscious of the tension between the desirability of expanded efforts to assure pre-market safety and potential effects of increased cost and duration of study on the drug development process. These issues have arisen with respect to weight loss drugs and drugs for asthma (following the outcome results with long-acting beta-agonists), [13] but could be raised for many other chronically used drugs.

The problems of design and analysis posed by such trials are quite formidable:

- Unless the population is at high risk, CV studies will have little chance of showing an adverse effect unless they are enormous (or unless a very high upper bound for the risk is used).
- In many cases, studies will need to be quite long, acceptable for outcome studies, but very hard to achieve in symptomatic conditions, where even in active control trials, dropouts are very common.
- In symptomatic settings, long-term placebo control is unrealistic and the risk of potential active controls is often unevaluated.
- If a study represents a follow-up of even a weak suggestion of harm, ethical concerns have been raised, at least for drugs without unusual benefits. That has not stopped the PRECISION study, but TIDE, a planned controlled comparative study of rosiglitazone and pioglitazone, has been suspended for this reason.
- The large outcome trials are taking years, even decades, to be conducted. Perhaps a higher upper bound would be an acceptable trade-off for a quicker answer?

We all know that results from epidemiologic studies can vary, but recent experience shows that RCT results can vary too when effects are small. How sure of the results will we be able to be?

- ASA secondary prevention: the largest trial (AMIS) [48] showed no significant overall effect and survival was actually leaning adversely; iib/iiia inhibitor trials in ACS vary from 0 to 50% reduction in death plus AMI at 30 days.
- Of 3 placebo-controlled celecoxib trials of similar size, one (APC) showed more than a doubling of risk, one showed no risk at all (PreSAP), and the third showed a small increase in risk that was numerically smaller than the risk of naproxen in that trial, a drug thought by many to have lowest risk of the NSAIDS (ADAPT).
- A fairly strong mortality effect in the short-term studies in the Nissen meta-analysis of rosiglitazone was not seen at all in ADOPT, DREAM, and RECORD. For AMI's in that meta-analysis, in contrast, short-term studies did not show a significant effect (there was numerical increase in AMIs, however) and only by adding in the larger studies (ADOPT and DREAM) did a significant effect emerge. None of this is to suggest what answer is correct in this case or to suggest poor analytic process, but it does show the problem of selection in meta-analyses as well as the problem of variable results.

In addition, there are other considerations related to value and cost–benefit

- Requiring outcome data might affect drug development. The antiarrhythmic policy is "associated with" with minimal antiarrhythmic development for ventricular arrhythmias (implanted defibrillators may have influenced this also) and new pharmacologically novel CHF treatments are very scarce. On the other hand, many trials with 10–20,000 patients are needed and carried out in development programs for antiplatelet drugs and anticoagulants. That is, the need for large outcome trials in those areas has not prevented active drug development.

- How likely, absent an animal or human signal, is a bad outcome for a drug with a beneficial effect on symptoms. If such outcomes are very hard to detect, and detection is uncertain, how worthwhile is it to study this compared to other important questions?
- Expanded ability to conduct large trials (e.g., in HMO-type environments) would greatly enhance our ability to do such trials.

8 Conclusion

There is clearly a new interest in possible modest increases in serious adverse effects of chronic-use drugs and a growing desire to assess the potential for such effects before and after a drug is marketed. Interest has spread from cardiovascular drugs (where it has long been present because of experience with antiarrhythmics and various inotropes) to other chronic-use drugs, including antidiabetics, NSAIDs, and chronic-use asthma drugs. As noted above, adverse long-term effects will already have been detected for drugs that have their effectiveness evaluated in long-term studies (e.g., antiplatelet drugs, bisphosphonates and other bone-preserving agents, adjuvant chemotherapy) that are of substantial size and measure important outcomes, at least if the right population is studied. But there are many other long-term treatments whose usual controlled studies are relatively short term, and for these we need to examine our expectations.

References

1. US Food and Drug Administration (2005) Guidance for industry: pre-marketing risk assessment
2. US Food and Drug Administration (2009) Guidance for industry: drug-induced liver injury: premarketing clinical evaluation
3. Zimmerman HJ (1978) Drug-induced liver disease. In: Hepatotoxicity, the adverse effects of drugs and other chemicals on the liver, 1st edn. Appleton-Century-Crofts, New York, pp 351–353
4. US Food and Drug Administration Guidance for Industry: E14 clinical evaluation of QT/QTc interval prolongation and proarrhythmic potential for non-antiarrhythmic drugs (2005)
5. Vessey MP, Doll R (1968) Investigation of relation between use of oral contraceptives and thromboembolic disease. A further report. Br Med J 2:651–657
6. Weiss NS, Szekely DR, English DR (1975) Endometrial cancer in relation to patterns of menopausal estrogen use. JAMA 242:261–264
7. Connolly HM, Crary JL, McGoon MD (1997) Valvular heart disease associated with fenfluramine – phentermine. N Engl J Med 337:581–588
8. Zachikoff C, Rochon P, Lang A (2007) Cardiac valvulopathy associated with pergolide use. Can J Neurol Sci 33:27–33
9. Herbst AL, Ulefelder H, Poskanzer DC (1971) Adenocarcenoma of the vagina. Association of maternal stilbesterol therapy with tumor appearance in young women. N Engl J Med 284: 878–881

10. Temple R (1999) Meta-analysis and epidemiologic studies in drug development and post-marketing surveillance. JAMA 281:841–844
11. Taubes G (1995) Epidemiology faces its limits. Science 269:164–169
12. Shapiro S (2000) Bias in the evaluation of low-magnitude associations: an empirical perspective. Am J Epidemiol 151:939–945
13. Nelson HS, Weiss ST, Bleecker ER et al (2006) The Salmeterol Multicenter Asthma Research Trial: a comparison of usual pharmacotherapy for asthma or usual pharmacotherapy plus salmeterol. Chest 129:15–26 [Erratum, Chest 2006; 129:1393]
14. US Food and Drug Administration Guidance for Industry: Diabetes mellitus – evaluating cardiovascular risk in new antidiabetic therapies to treat type 2 diabetes (2008)
15. Barter PJ, Caulfield M, Eriksson M et al (2007) Effects of torcetrapib in patients at high risk for coronary events. N Engl J Med 357:2109–2122
16. Packer M, Carver J, Rodeheffer R et al (1991) Effect of oral milrinone on mortality in severe chronic heart failure. The PROMISE Study Research Group. N Engl J Med 325:1468–1475
17. Writing group for the Women's Health Initiative Investigators (2002) Risks and benefits of estrogen plus progestin in healthy postmenopausal women. JAMA 288:321–333
18. Hammad TA, Laughren T, Racoosin J (2006) Suicidality in pediatric patients treated with antidepressants. Arch Gen Psychiatry 63:332–339
19. Stone M, Laughren T, Jones ML et al (2009) Risk of suicidality in clinical trials of antidepressants in adults: analysis of proprietary data submitted to US Food and Drug Administration. BMJ 339:2880
20. Meinart CL, Knatterud GL, Prout TE et al (1970) A study of the effects of hypoglycemic agents on vascular complications in patients with adult-onset diabetes. II. Mortality results. Diabetes 19(Suppl 1):789–830
21. The Action to Control Cardiovascular Risk in Diabetes Study Group (2008) Effects of intensive glucose lowering in type 2 diabetes. N Engl J Med 358:2545–2559
22. The Cardiac Arrhythmia Suppression Trial (CAST) Investigators (1989) Preliminary report: effect of encainide and flecainide on mortality in a randomized trial of arrhythmia suppression after myocardial infarction. N Engl J Med 321:406–412
23. The Cardiac Arrhythmia Suppression Trial II Investigators (1992) Effect of the antiarrhythmic agent moricizine on survival after myocardial infarction. N Engl J Med 327:227–233
24. Bombardier C, Laine L, Reicin A et al (2000) Comparison of upper gastrointestinal toxicity of rofecoxib and naproxen in patients with rheumatoid arthritis. VIGOR Study Group. N Engl J Med 343:1520–1528
25. Farkouh ME, Kirshner H, Harrington RA et al (2004) Comparison of lumiracoxib with naproxen and ibuprofen in the Therapeutic Arthritis Research and Gastrointestinal Event Trial (TARGET), cardiovascular outcomes: randomized controlled trial. Lancet 364:675–684
26. Baraf HSB, Fuentealba C, Greenwald M et al (2007) Gastrointestinal side effects of etoricoxib in patients with osteoarthritis: results of the Etoricoxib versus Diclofenac Sodium Gastrointestinal Tolerability and Effectiveness (EDGE) trial. J Rheumatol 34(2):408–420
27. Solomon SD, Pfeffer MA, McMurray JJV et al (2006) Effect of celecoxib on cardiovascular events and blood pressure in two trials for the prevention of colorectal adenomas. Circulation 114:1028–1035
28. Bresalier RS, Sandler RS, Quan H et al (2005) Cardiovascular events associated with rofecoxib in a colorectal adenoma chemoprevention trial. N Engl J Med 352:1092–1102
29. ADAPT Research Group (2006) Cardiovascular and cerebrovascular events in the randomized, controlled Alzheimer's Disease anti-inflammatory prevention trial (ADAPT). PLOS Clin Trials e33. doi: 10.1371
30. Besarab A, Bolton WK, Browne JK et al (1998) The effects of normal as compared with low hematocrit values in patients with cardiac disease who are receiving hemodialysis and epoetin. N Engl J Med 339:584–590
31. Singh AK, Szczech L, Tang KL et al (2006) Correction of anemia with epoetin alfa in chronic kidney disease. N Engl J Med 355:2085–2098

32. Pfeffer MA, Burdmann EA, Chen CY et al (2009) A trial of darbepoetin alfa in type 2 diabetes and chronic kidney disease. N Engl J Med 361:2019–2032
33. Cohn JN, Goldstein SO, Greenberg BH et al (1998) A dose-dependent increase in mortality with vesnarinone among patients with severe heart failure. Vesnarinone Trial Investigators. N Engl J Med 339:1810–1816
34. Julian DG, Prescott RJ, Jackson FS et al (1982) Controlled trial of sotalol for one year after myocardial infarction. Lancet 1:1142–1147
35. Torp-Pederson C, Moller M, Block-Thompson PE et al (1999) Dofetilide in patients with congestive heart failure and left ventricular dysfunction. N Engl J Med 341:857–865
36. Kober L, Thomson PEB, Motter M et al (2000) Effect of dofetilide in patients with recent myocardial infarction and left-ventricular dysfunction: a randomized trial. Lancet 356: 2052–2058
37. Hohnloser SH, Crigns HJGM, van Eickels M et al (2009) Effect of dronedarone on cardiovascular events in atrial fibrillation. N Engl J Med 360:668–678
38. The ALLHAT Officers and Coordinators for the ALLHAT Collaborative Research Group (2002) Major outcomes in high-risk hypertensive patients randomized to angiotensin-converting enzyme inhibitor or calcium channel blocker vs diuretic: The Antihypertensive and Lipid-Lowering Treatment to Prevent Heart Attack Trial (ALLHAT). JAMA 288:2981–2997
39. Dahlof B, Devereaux R, Kieldson SE et al (2002) Cardiovascular morbidity and mortality in the Losartan Intervention For Endpoint reduction in hypertension study (LIFE): a randomized trial against atenolol. Lancet 359:995–1003
40. Jamerson K, Weber MA, Bakris GL et al (2008) Benazepril plus amlodipine or hydrochlorothiazide for hypertension in high-risk patients. N Engl J Med 359:2417–2428
41. Nissen SE, Wolski K (2007) Effect of rosiglitazone on the risk of myocardial infarction and death from cardiovascular causes. N Engl J Med 356:2457–2471
42. Kahn SE, Haffner SM, Heise MA et al (2006) Glycemic durability of rosiglitazone, metformin, or glyburide monotherapy. N Engl J Med 355:2427–2443
43. The DREAM Trial Investigators (2006) Effect of ramipril on the incidence of diabetes. N Engl J Med 355:1551–1562
44. Home PD, Pocock SJ, Beck-Neilsen H et al (2009) Rosiglitazone evaluated for cardiovascular outcomes in oral agent combination therapy for type 2 diabetes (RECORD): a multicentre, randomized, open-label trial. Lancet 373:2125–2135
45. James WP, Caterson ID, Coutinho W et al (2010) Effect of sibutramine on cardiovascular outcomes in overweight and obese subjects. N Engl J Med 363:905–917
46. Psaty BM, Furburg CD (2007) The record on rosiglitazone and the risk of myocardial infarction. N Engl J Med 357:67–69
47. Joffe HV, Parks MH, Temple R (2010) Impact of cardiovascular outcomes on the development and approval of medications for the treatment of diabetes mellitus. Rev Endocr Metab Disord 11:21–30
48. The Aspirin Myocardial Infarction Research Group (1980) The aspirin myocardial infarction study: final results. Circulation 62:79–84

Part V
Special Topics

Designing, Monitoring, and Analyzing Group Sequential Clinical Trials Using the `RCTdesign` Package for R

Daniel L. Gillen and Scott S. Emerson

Abstract The use of group sequential methodology has become widespread in the conduct of clinic trials. As each clinical trial presents unique scientific, statistical, and logistical constraints, it is important to carefully evaluate candidate group sequential designs to ensure desirable operating characteristics. At the implementation stage of a clinical trial design it is also essential to account for deviations from original design specifications in order to control operating characteristics such as type I and II error rates. These changes might include the number and/or timing of analyses as well as deviations from the originally assumed variability of outcome measures. Due to the computational complexity involved in evaluating, monitoring, and analyzing a group sequential procedure, specialized software is required. In this manuscript we demonstrate how the `RCTdesign` package (www.rctdesign. org) in R can be used to select, implement, and analyze a group sequential stopping rule. Throughout, we illustrate trial design and monitoring in the context of a group sequential survival trial of an experimental monoclonal antibody in patients with relapsed chronic lymphocytic leukemia (CLL).

1 Introduction

The use of group sequential methodology has become widespread in the conduct of clinic trials. Many authors have addressed the design [6, 22, 25, 32, 36], implementation [3, 18], and analysis [7, 34] of group sequential trials.

D.L. Gillen (✉)
Department of Statistics, 2226 Donald Bren Hall, University of California,
Irvine, CA 92697-1250, USA
e-mail: dgillen@uci.edu

S.S. Emerson
Department of Biostatistics, University of Washington, Seattle, WA, USA

T.R. Fleming and B.S. Weir (eds.), *Proceedings of the Fourth Seattle Symposium in Biostatistics: Clinical Trials*, Lecture Notes in Statistics 1205,
DOI 10.1007/978-1-4614-5245-4_11, © Springer Science+Business Media New York 2013

In the general case, a stopping rule is defined for a schedule of analysis occurring at times $t_1, t_2, \ldots, t_J$, which may be random. Often, the analysis times are in turn defined according to the statistical information available at each analysis. In the case of a statistical model that has statistical information proportional to the sample size accrued to the study, such an approach is equivalent to defining the sample sizes $N_1, N_2, \ldots, N_J$ at which the analysis will be performed. For $j = 1, \ldots, J$, we calculate a specified test statistic T_j based on observations available at time t_j. The outcome space for T_j is then partitioned into stopping set $\mathcal{S}_j$ and continuation set $\mathcal{C}_j$. Starting with $j = 1$, the clinical trial proceeds by computing T_j, and if $T_j \in \mathcal{S}_j$, the trial is stopped. Otherwise, T_j is in the continuation set $\mathcal{C}_j$, and the trial gathers additional observations until time t_{j+1}. By choosing $\mathcal{C}_J = \emptyset$, the empty set, the trial must stop at or before the J-th analysis.

All of the most commonly used group sequential stopping rules are included if we consider continuation sets of the form $\mathcal{C}_j = (a_j, b_j] \cup [c_j, d_j)$ such that $-\infty \leq a_j \leq b_j \leq c_j \leq d_j \leq \infty$. Quite often, these boundaries are interpreted as the critical values for a decision rule. For instance, in a clinical trial comparing two active treatments A and B, test statistics less than a_j might correspond to decisions for the superiority of treatment A, test statistics exceeding d_j might correspond to decisions for the inferiority of treatment A, and test statistics between b_j and c_j might correspond to decisions for approximate equivalence between the two treatments.

As each clinical trial presents unique scientific, statistical, and logistical constraints, it is important to carefully evaluate candidate group sequential designs to ensure desirable operating characteristics. [9] describe a variety of frequentist design characteristics which might be examined in the most commonly encountered statistical problems. Among them are

1. The scientific measures of treatment effect which will correspond to early termination for futility and/or efficacy.
2. The sample size requirements as described by the maximal sample size and summary measures of the sample size distribution (e.g., mean, 75th percentile) as a function of the hypothesized treatment effect.
3. The probability that the trial would continue to each analysis as a function of the hypothesized treatment effect.
4. The frequentist power to reject the null hypothesis as a function of the hypothesized treatment effect, with the type I error corresponding to the power under the null hypothesis.
5. The frequentist inference (adjusted point estimates, confidence intervals, and P values), which would be reported were the trial to stop with results corresponding exactly to a boundary.

At the implementation stage of a clinical trial design it is also essential to account for deviations from original design specifications in order to control operating characteristics such as type I and II error rates [3, 18]. These changes might include the number and/or timing of analysis as well as deviations from the originally assumed variability of outcome measures. Finally, at the completion of a group sequential test it is important that point and interval estimates be adjusted to account for bias that arises through repeated testing, particularly when the implemented stopping boundaries allow for early stopping under more modest effect sizes [7, 34].

Due to the computational complexity involved in evaluating, monitoring, and analyzing a group sequential procedure, specialized software is required. Multiple software packages can be used for the design and/or analysis of group sequential trials [4, 24, 27]. The RCTdesign package (www.rctdesign.org) for R statistical software is an extension of the SeqTrial module for SPlus [28]. RCTdesign is a comprehensive package that allows users to choose from a full array of previously proposed group sequential stopping rules, monitor an ongoing trial using standard constrained boundaries techniques, and report bias-adjusted results at the conclusion of a clinical trial.

In this manuscript we demonstrate how the RCTdesign package can be used to select, implement, and analyze a group sequential stopping rule. Throughout, we illustrate trial design and monitoring in the context of a clinical trial of an experimental monoclonal antibody in patients with relapsed chronic lymphocytic leukemia (CLL). Section 2 provides an evaluation of candidate clinical trial designs based upon commonly considered frequentist operating characteristics. Section 3 describes previously proposed methods for flexibly monitoring a group sequential test. An example implementing the constrained boundaries algorithm [3] is presented, and adjusted inference is discussed. In Sect. 4, we present additional issues that should be considered when designing and monitoring a clinical trial to investigate an intervention for which the effect may be hypothesized to vary with the duration of time since initiation. Section 5 concludes with a discussion of the importance of thorough evaluation in the selection of a group sequential stopping rule along with areas of current and future research.

2 Evaluation of a Group Sequential Trial for a Censored Time-to-Event Endpoint

In this section we illustrate the evaluation of statistical operating statistics in the context of a randomized, double-blind, placebo-controlled clinical trial of an experimental monoclonal antibody in patients with relapsed CLL. Treatment of CLL tends to focus on controlling disease symptoms through the use of chemotherapy, radiation therapy, biological therapy, or bone marrow transplantation. Recently there have been multiple trials to assess the efficacy of treating CLL via monoclonal antibodies that target markers which are heavily expressed by CLL cells. In one of these trials, patients with relapsed CLL were randomly assigned to receive an experimental antibody or placebo, in addition to a standard chemotherapeutic regime. The intervention was administered intravenously once a week for four weeks and patients were followed for the primary endpoint of overall survival. It was anticipated that the median survival time among patients treated with placebo would be approximately 16 months and that the distribution of survival times among this group would be approximately exponentially distributed. It was hoped that patients receiving the antibody would experience a 33% reduction in the hazard for death and that the effect of treatment on the hazard would remain roughly constant over time.

In the discussion of the operating characteristics which follows, we will use comparisons similar to (but not exactly the same as) those explored by the collaborators in the CLL study. In all cases, we consider level 0.025 one-sided hypothesis tests appropriate for testing a null hypothesis $H_0 : \theta \geq 1$ versus the lesser alternative $H_1 : \theta \leq 0.67$, where θ represents the hazard ratio comparing treatment to control. Throughout, a one-to-one randomization scheme is assumed.

To illustrate the evaluation process, we consider candidate designs as derived from the unified family of group sequential stopping rules [17]. As noted in Sect. 1, all of the most commonly used group sequential stopping rules are included if we consider continuation sets of the form $C_j = (a_j, b_j] \cup [c_j, d_j)$ such that $-\infty \leq a_j \leq b_j \leq c_j \leq d_j \leq \infty$. Particular families of group sequential designs correspond to parameterized boundary functions which relate the stopping boundaries at successive analysis according to the proportion of statistical information accrued and the hypothesis rejected by the boundary. For instance, letting Π_j represent the proportion of the maximal statistical information available at the j-th analysis (e.g., $\Pi_j = N_j/N_J$ for the most commonly used analytic models), then for some specified parametric function $f_d()$, the boundary function for the upper boundary might be given by $d_j = f_d(\theta_d, \Pi_j)$, where θ_d is the hypothesis rejected when $T_j > d_j$. Furthermore, many of the group sequential design families previously described can be expressed in a parameterization which has $d_j = f(\theta_d, g(\Pi_j; A_d, P_d, R_d, G_d))$ with boundary shape function

$$g(\Pi; A, P, R, G) = (A + \Pi^{-P}(1 - \Pi)^R)G$$

where parameters A, P, and R are typically specified by the user to attain some desired level of conservative behavior at the earliest analyses, and critical value G might be found in an iterative search to attain some specified operating characteristics (e.g., frequentist type I error and power) when the stopping rule is to be used as the basis of a decision rule. In this parameterization, taking $A = R = 0$ yields a one-parameter family of stopping boundaries where larger values of P result in increased conservatism of the stopping rule meaning that it is more difficult to stop at early analyses for a given treatment effect. In the unified family [17], the boundaries are expressed on the treatment effect scale and the boundary hypothesis is merely a shift of the boundary shape function so that

$$d_j = \theta_d + g(\Pi_j; A_d, P_d, R_d, G_d)$$
$$a_j = \theta_a + g(\Pi_j; A_a, P_a, R_a, G_a).$$

For the remainder of the manuscript we will focus on the following candidate designs. RCTdesign code to compute each of the above stopping rules is provided in Appendix A.

1. *Fixed.Sample*: A fixed sample study with 263 events providing 90.1% power to detect the alternative H_1.
2. *SymmOBF.2, SymmOBF.3, SymmOBF.4*: One-sided symmetric stopping rules that treat the null and alternative hypotheses symmetrically [6] and utilize O'Brien–Fleming boundary relationships having a total of 2, 3, and 4 equally spaced analyses, respectively, and a maximal sample size of 263 events.
3. *SymmOBF.Power*: One-sided symmetric stopping rule with O'Brien–Fleming boundary relationships, a total of 4 equally spaced analysis and the total sample size selected to provide 90.1% power to detect the alternative H_1.
4. *Futility.5, Futility.8, Futility.9*: One-sided stopping rules from the unified family [17] with a total of four equally spaced analyses, with a maximal sample size of 263 events, and having O'Brien–Fleming lower (efficacy) boundary relationships and upper (futility) boundary relationships corresponding to boundary shape parameters $P = 0.5$, 0.8, and 0.9, respectively. In this parameterization of the boundary shape function, parameter P is a measure of conservatism at the earliest analysis. $P = 0.5$ corresponds to Pocock boundary shape functions, and $P = 1.0$ corresponds to the more conservative O'Brien–Fleming boundary relationships.
5. *Eff11.Fut8, Eff11.Fut9*: One-sided stopping rules from the unified family [17] with a total of 4 equally spaced analysis, with a maximal sample size of 263 events, and having lower (efficacy) boundary relationships corresponding to boundary shape parameter $P = 1.1$ and upper (futility) boundary relationships corresponding to boundary shape parameters $P = 0.8$ and 0.9, respectively.
6. *Fixed.Power*: A fixed sample study which provides the same power to detect H_1 as the *Eff11.Fut8* trial design.

2.1 Evaluation of Stopping Boundaries

It is important that clinical trialists not be surprised by the conditions under which a particular stopping rule suggests that a trial might continue or stop early. As such, we believe that it is of paramount importance that the stopping boundary at each analysis be considered as the stopping rule is selected. [9] note that there are a number of scales on which the boundaries can be examined. While there exists a one-to-one relationship between these scales, the statistical and scientific utility of the scales varies depending upon one's background. In the context of the CLL trial, we may consider any of the following test statistics as the basis for the definition of the stopping rule at interim analysis j:

1. *Partial sum statistic*: S_j, the partial likelihood based score function for $\log(\theta)$ in a proportional hazards regression model.
2. *Crude estimate of treatment effect*: $\hat{\theta}_j$, the estimated hazard ratio from a proportional hazards model.
3. *Normalized Z statistic*: Z_j, the score statistic for testing H_0.

4. *Fixed sample P value statistic*: $P_j = \Phi(Z_j)$, where $\Phi(\cdot)$ represents the cumulative distribution function corresponding to the standard normal distribution.
5. *Error spending statistic*: An error spending statistic can be defined for any of the four boundaries based on an arbitrary hypothesized value for the true treatment effect. For instance, if a group sequential stopping rule were defined for the partial sum statistic and the observed value of the test statistic at the j-th analysis were $S_j = s_j$, a lower type I error spending statistic defined for the null hypothesis $H_0 : \theta = \theta_0$ would have

$$
E_{aj} = \frac{1}{\alpha_L} \left(Pr\left[S_j \leq s_j, \bigcap_{k=1}^{j-1} S_k \in C_k \mid \theta = \theta_0 \right] \right.
$$
$$
\left. + \sum_{\ell=1}^{j-1} Pr\left[S_\ell \leq a_\ell, \bigcap_{k=1}^{\ell-1} S_k \in C_k \mid \theta = \theta_0 \right] \right),
$$

where α_L is the lower type I error of the stopping rule defined by

$$
\alpha_L = \sum_{\ell=1}^{J} Pr\left[S_\ell \leq a_\ell, \bigcap_{k=1}^{\ell-1} S_k \in C_k \mid \theta = \theta_0 \right].
$$

6. *Bayesian posterior probabilities*: $B_j(\theta_0) = Pr(\theta \leq \theta_0 \mid S_j = s_j)$, the posterior probability that the null hypothesis $H_0 : \theta \geq \theta_0$ is false under a specified prior distribution.
7. *Conditional power statistics*: The conditional probability that the test statistic at the final (J-th) analysis would exceed the threshold for declaring statistical significance, where we condition on the observed statistic $S_j = s_j$ at the j-th analysis and assume some particular value for the true treatment effect θ. For instance, we might define a conditional power statistic using a threshold a_J defined for the partial sum statistic. Such a threshold would represent the critical value for declaring statistical significance at the J-th analysis. Using an alternative hypothesis $H_1 : \theta = \theta_1$ conditional power would be computed as

$$
C_j(a_J, \theta_1) = Pr(S_J < a_J \mid S_j = s_j; \theta = \theta_1)
$$

Alternatively, a conditional power statistic might use the current best estimate of the treatment effect $\hat{\theta}_j$ in place of θ_1.
8. *Predictive probability statistics*: The Bayesian predictive probability that the test statistic would exceed some specified threshold at the final analysis. In the case of a threshold a_J defined for the partial sum statistic, a predictive probability statistic may be computed as

$$
H_j(a_J, \zeta, \tau^2) = \int Pr(S_J < a_J \mid S_j = s_j, \theta)\, p(\theta \mid S_j = s_j)\, d\theta
$$

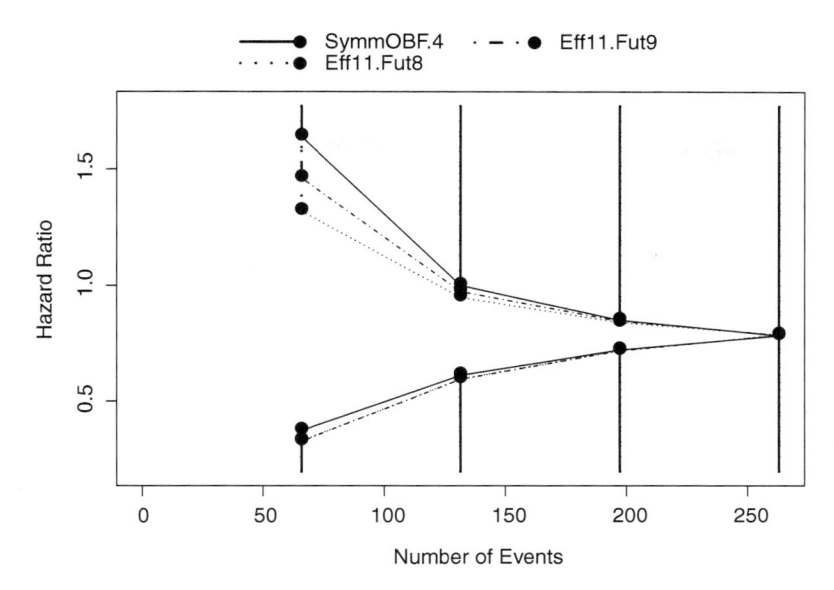

Fig. 1 Stopping boundaries on the scale of the crude estimate of treatment effect (estimated hazard ratio). In the case of the CLL trial, stopping boundaries for level 0.025 one-sided stopping rules for a maximum of 263 events and various levels of conservatism for the efficacy (*lower*) and futility (*upper*) boundary relationships

Returning to the CLL trial, we find it most useful to consider stopping boundaries on the scientifically relevant scale of the estimated treatment effect. By graphing the stopping boundaries versus the number of events (or statistical information) available at each analysis, we can see both the degree of conservatism employed at the earliest analysis and the worst case sample size requirements for the study. In Fig. 1 we display the stopping boundaries for the *SymmOBF.4*, *Eff11.Fut9*, and *Eff11.Fut8* stopping rules, all of which use the same level of significance. These three designs all have a maximal sample size of 263 events but differ in the boundary shape function used for the efficacy (lower) and futility (upper) boundary, ranging in conservatism (higher values of P yield a more conservative stopping rule). By comparing *Eff11.Fut9* and *Eff11.Fut8*, it can be seen that altering the futility boundary has only minimal effects on the efficacy boundary. We can also see from Fig. 1 that at the planned first analysis ($N = 66$ events) the O'Brien–Fleming boundary shape function would suggest early termination for futility only if the estimated hazard ratio were 1.639 or larger—a difference that may be deemed too large. The futility boundary shape function for the *Eff11.Fut8* stopping rule, on the other hand, would allow early termination for futility when the observed hazard ratio is 1.319. Similar comparisons may be made with respect to the efficacy bound. It is worth noting that in many cases the extreme conservatism of the *Eff11.Fut9* and *Eff11.Fut8* efficacy bounds may be desired at early analyses because stopping a trial early for efficacy would preclude the collection of longer-term safety data in a controlled setting. `RCTdesign` code to generate the resulting boundary plot and to create a table of the stopping boundaries on different scales is provided in Appendix A.

2.2   Frequentist Type I Error and Power

The most commonly used definition for statistical evidence against a null hypothesis is to consider the probability of falsely rejecting the null hypothesis. In fact, regulatory agencies often use this criterion as a de facto standard for strength of evidence that will be attained in a clinical trial design. Thus, when specifying a group sequential stopping rule, clinical trialists most often constrain the type I error associated with a decision boundary to some prescribed level, typically 0.05 for a two-sided test and 0.025 for a one-sided test.

Similarly, it is often the case that the sample size to be used in a clinical trial is determined by computing the sample size that will allow estimation of the treatment effect with specified precision (often according to the width of a 95% confidence interval) or that will allow a decision to reject the null hypothesis to be made with high probability (e.g., 80%, 90%, 95%, or 97.5% statistical power) when a specific alternative hypothesis is true. This criterion of statistical power is of particular interest from a scientific standpoint: It describes the probability that the clinical trial will discriminate between the two viable scientific hypotheses represented by the null and alternative hypotheses. Hence, basic scientists, clinical researchers, epidemiologists, and biostatisticians often focus on the statistical power of the study to detect a hypothesis representing the minimal treatment effect which is of clinical importance.

Figure 2 displays power curves for some stopping rules considered in the design of the CLL trial. In this figure we compare the effect of increasing the number of interim analysis on the statistical power when the maximal sample size is maintained at 263 events. Rather than displaying the absolute power curve as in Fig. 2a, we often find it most convenient to display the power relative to some reference design. In Fig. 2b, we examine the loss of power relative to a fixed sample clinical trial for several stopping rules which vary in the number of interim analyses. With the O'Brien–Fleming boundary relationships considered in this figure, we see relatively little loss of power: A one-sided symmetric design with O'Brien–Fleming relationships and a total of four equally spaced analyses [6] loses at most 0.019 power (from 68.5 to 66.6%) relative to a fixed sample analysis with the same maximal sample size.

Table 1 compares the power of the *Fixed.Sample*, *Eff11.Fut9*, and *Eff11.Fut8* stopping rules under specific hypotheses and provides the alternative hypotheses for which the various designs have prescribed statistical power. From this table it is apparent that the introduction of either of these stopping rules has relatively minimal impact on the statistical power of the study. This in turn means that the introduction of either of these stopping rules has relatively little effect on the scientific interpretation of a failure to reject the null hypothesis. More specifically,

a

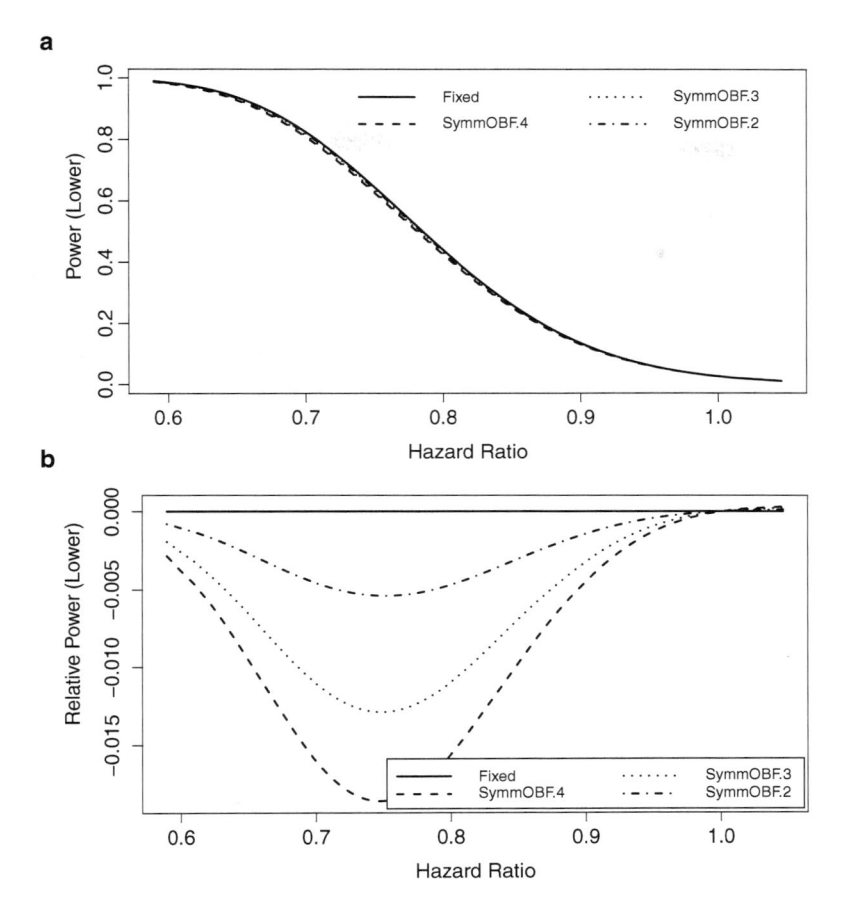

b

Fig. 2 Power curves and difference in power relative to a fixed sample design for a fixed sample design and one-sided symmetric tests with O'Brien–Fleming ($SymmOBF.J$) boundary relationships with $J = 2, 3$, or 4 analysis. All designs have type I error of 0.025 under the null hypothesis $H_0 : \theta \geq 1$ and a maximal sample size of 263 events

using a confidence level of 95% as the statistical criterion for evidence, a failure to reject the null can be interpreted as a rejection of a hazard ratio corresponding to the alternative for which the design attains a power of 0.975: equal to 0.617 using the *Fixed.Sample* design, 0.610 using the *Eff11.Fut9* design, and 0.607 using the *Eff11.Fut8* design. We note that this difference in rejected alternatives is due to the fact that the maximal sample size was not increased when a stopping rule was introduced. With an increase in the maximal sample size, we can maintain the magnitude of the alternative rejected by a failure to reject the null hypothesis.

Table 1 Comparison of operating characteristics of three candidate stopping rules: (*upper panel*) detectable alternatives and mean sample size for fixed power; (*lower panel*) power and mean sample size for fixed alternative

	Fixed.Sample Stopping rule		Eff11.Fut9 Stopping rule		Eff11.Fut8 Stopping rule	
Power	Hazard ratio	Average samp size	Hazard ratio	Average samp size	Hazard ratio	Average samp size
0.800	0.708	263	0.703	207	0.702	204
0.900	0.670	263	0.665	196	0.663	194
0.950	0.641	263	0.635	185	0.633	184
0.975	0.617	263	0.610	176	0.607	174
Hazard ratio	Power	Average samp size	Power	Average samp size	Power	Average samp size
1.00	0.025	263	0.025	163	0.025	154
0.75	0.645	263	0.628	214	0.624	211
0.67	0.901	263	0.889	198	0.885	196
0.60	0.985	263	0.981	172	0.980	172

2.3 Sample Size Distribution

In a fixed sample clinical trial, if the sample size is chosen to attain some prespecified statistical power, one of the first operating characteristics considered is whether obtaining that sample size is feasible logistically and financially. Clinical trial collaborators also have to consider whether the sample size would provide credible scientific evidence. In the presence of data collected using a stopping rule, the actual sample size obtained during the conduct of a clinical trial is a random variable with a distribution that depends on the magnitude of the true treatment effect—a dependence that is, of course, behind the ethical motivation for interim analyses: We want to use fewer patients when one treatment is markedly inferior to another or not sufficiently superior to warrant further investigation. Thus, when examining the sample size requirements of a particular clinical trial design, we will be interested in summary measures of the probability distribution for the sample size. The maximal sample size will be of interest for the feasibility of accrual, just as it is in a fixed sample trial. Examination of the curves for the average sample size (ASN = average sample number) and various quantiles of the sample size distribution provides some indication of the values that might reasonably be attained under various hypotheses. In the case of a survival endpoint, statistical information is (at least partially) dictated by the number of observed events. In this case it is natural to consider summary measures of the distribution of the required number of events.

In Fig. 3 we compare the average and 75th percentile of the distributions of required events for the group sequential stopping rules considered for the futility boundary in the CLL trial. From this figure it can be seen that substantially

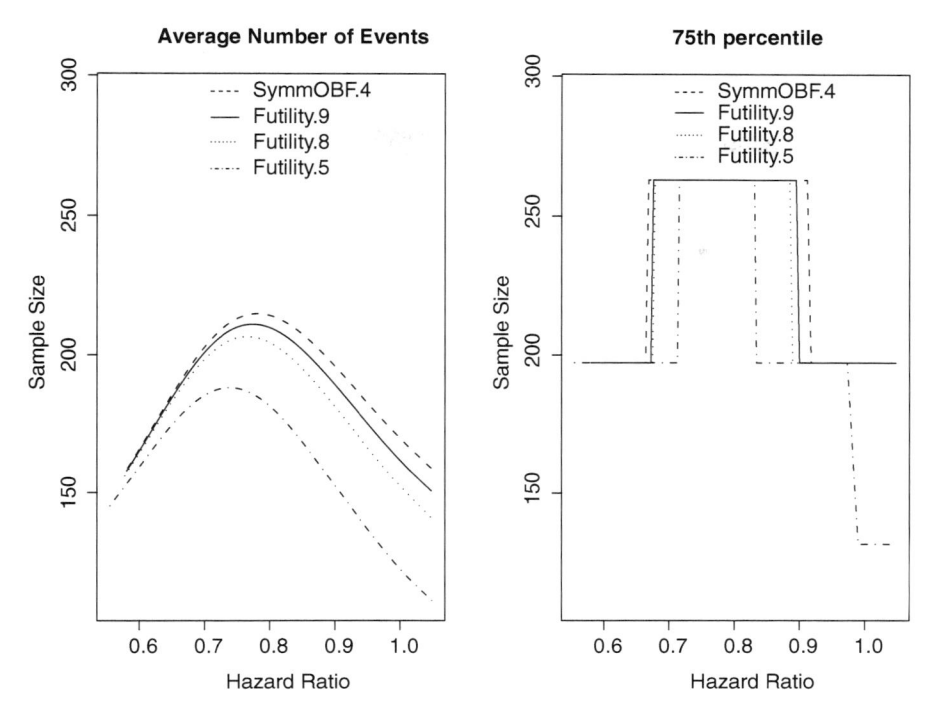

Fig. 3 Average and 75th percentile of the distribution of required events as a function of the hypothesized treatment effect. In the case of the CLL trial, stopping boundaries for level 0.025 one-sided stopping rules for a maximum of 263 events and having O'Brien–Fleming efficacy (*lower*) boundary relationships and various levels of conservatism for the futility (*upper*) boundary relationships

smaller numbers of events would be accrued on average as the futility (upper) boundary becomes successively less conservative. Of course, because the maximal number of events does not differ among these stopping rules, the power curves will vary. Therefore, the ultimate selection of a stopping rule involved simultaneous graphical comparisons of the average event curves and the respective power curves (not shown here, but analogous to those shown in Fig. 2) in order to judge the acceptability of trade-offs between the loss of power and gains in average number of events.

2.4 Stopping Probabilities

When more detail about the stopping behavior of the group sequential trial design is desired, the probability of stopping at each analysis time can be examined as a function of the hypothesized true treatment effect. Figure 4 displays the cumulative

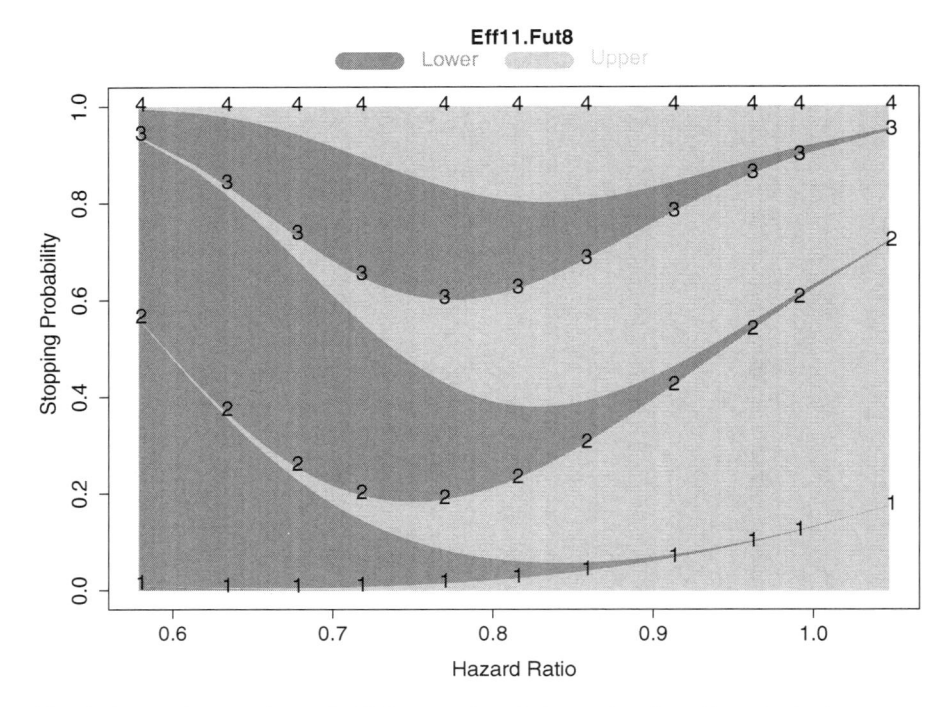

Fig. 4 Cumulative stopping probabilities at each analysis as a function of hypothesized treatment effect. The one-sided level 0.025 stopping rule to test the null hypothesis $H_0 : \theta \geq 0$ has a maximum of four equally spaced analysis with an efficacy (*lower*) boundary shape function corresponding to $P = 1.1$ and a futility (*upper*) boundary shape function corresponding to $P = 0.8$ in the unified family of group sequential designs

stopping probability at each analysis versus the true treatment effect. For any given hypothesized hazard ratio (x-axis) the vertical distance up to each contour line represents the cumulative probability that the trial will stop at or before the corresponding analysis time (as depicted by the number of the contour). In this figure, the shading indicates the probability with which a decision at stopping will be made for the alternative hypothesis (i.e., when the test statistic is less than the lower boundary) or the null hypothesis (i.e., when the test statistic is greater than the upper boundary). Thus from this figure we can see that under the *Eff11.Fut8* stopping rule, when the true treatment effect corresponds to a hazard ratio of $\theta = 0.70$, the probability of stopping at or before the third analysis is approximately 0.67, and as the shading below that curve is generally the darker color, the predominant decision will be one to reject the null hypothesis. Furthermore, by examining the stopping boundaries on the scale of the crude estimate of treatment effect (Fig. 1), it can be seen that the stopping rule would only recommend continuing past the third analysis if the observed hazard ratio comparing treatment to placebo was between 0.717 and 0.838, a situation that may look promising enough to invest in the larger sample size.

2.5 *Frequentist Inference at the Stopping Boundaries*

In order to ensure the scientific and statistical credibility of the study results, it is important to examine the statistical inference that would be reported if the study were to be terminated early. Of particular interest is whether estimates of treatment effect would indeed be extreme enough to convince the scientific community that action should be taken with less precision in the estimates. When using frequentist inference, we typically consider point estimates of treatment effect with small bias and mean squared error, and we consider the precision of such estimates using 95% confidence intervals. Strength of evidence against a null hypothesis is often quantified by the P value—the probability that results as or more extreme than those actually obtained would be observed when the null hypothesis is true. These same frequentist measures are possible in the setting of group sequential stopping rules, though the calculation of the estimates, confidence intervals, and P values must use the correct sampling distribution. Further discussion of inferential procedures that account for group sequential testing is presented in Sect. 3.2.

In the process of evaluating group sequential designs, it is useful to consider the inference associated with outcomes which correspond exactly to the stopping boundaries. Clearly, if such outcomes are scientifically and statistically convincing, more extreme results would also be acceptable. Figure 5 displays such hypothetical inference for the stopping boundaries of the *Eff11.Fut8* stopping rule. The top and bottom panels display the adjusted point estimates (bias adjusted mean, BAM, as described by Whitehead [33]) and the sample mean ordering based 95% confidence intervals and P values for hypothetical results which correspond to the futility (upper) and efficacy (lower) boundaries, respectively. Also displayed for reference are horizontal lines corresponding to the null hypothesis $\theta = 1$ and the alternative hypothesis $\theta = 0.67$. From this plot we see the extreme conservatism of the efficacy boundary. At the first analysis, we would stop the study early with a decision for efficacy only if we could with high confidence rule out that the treatment effect was less extreme than an alternative far beyond that which we considered in the design of the trial (i.e., the 95% confidence interval not only excludes the null hypothesis but also excludes an alternative corresponding to a hazard ratio of 0.54). On the other hand, the futility boundary is less conservative as evidenced by the fact that although results which would cause termination have ruled out a markedly beneficial effect of treatment, they have not established with high confidence that the treatment might have some small beneficial effect (i.e., the 95% confidence interval corresponding to results at the futility stopping boundary includes the null hypothesis of $\theta = 1$) (Fig. 5).

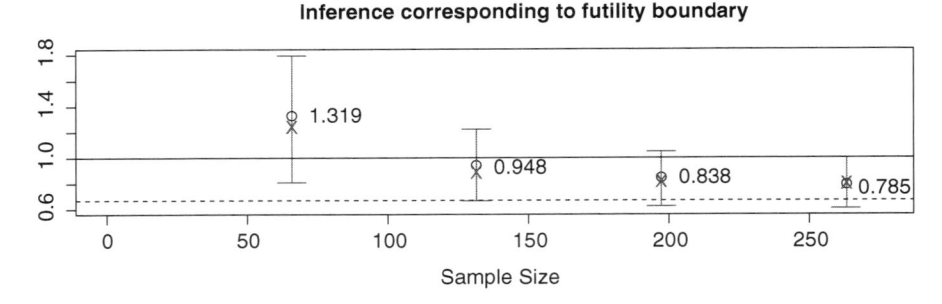

Fig. 5 Display of estimates and confidence intervals for observed trial results which correspond exactly to the stopping boundaries of a one-sided level 0.025 stopping rule to test the null hypothesis $H_0 : \theta \geq 1$ and having a maximum of four equally spaced analysis, an efficacy (*lower*) boundary shape function corresponding to $P = 1.1$ and a futility (*upper*) boundary shape function corresponding to $P = 0.8$ in the unified family of group sequential designs. Inference for the futility (*upper*) boundary is displayed in the *upper panel*, and inference for the efficacy (*lower*) boundary is displayed in the *lower panel*. All estimates, confidence intervals, and P values are adjusted for the stopping rule. Horizontal lines correspond to the null hypothesis $\theta = 1$ and the alternative hypothesis $\theta = 0.67$

2.6 Assessing the Implications of Varying Patient Accrual Patterns

The rate at which patients accrue will directly impact the observed censoring distribution in the trial when testing a time-to-event endpoint. For example, if accrual to the study were heavy at early times and slowed as the study progressed, then a majority of patients would tend to have high censoring times relative to the maximal follow-up of the trial. On the one hand, if the rate of accrual were low at the initial stages of the trial but increased towards the end of trial, then a majority of patients would tend to have low censoring times relative to the maximal follow-up. More rigorously, if T_L denotes the total follow-up for the trial and T_A denotes the duration of accrual, the probability that a subject is observed for an event over the course of the study is given by

$$1 - \int_0^{T_A} S_T(T_L - u) f_A(u) du,$$

where S_T denotes the survival function of the subject and f_A denotes the probability density function of the accrual distribution of the subject. Because of this, changes to the accrual distribution can have economic (the duration of the study), statistical (the rate of statistical information growth), and scientific (the length of time treatments are to be compared) implications on a clinical trial.

Under a proportional hazards treatment effect, the statistical information as derived from the partial likelihood is directly proportional to the number of events observed on the trial. This reduces the complexity of planning interim analyses but one must still translate between the number of observed events and when those events are to be expected in calendar time so that a Data Monitoring Committee can be convened for interim analyses. The translation from events to calendar time requires specification of the accrual rate of patients, the duration of accrual, the duration of continued follow-up after accrual is closed, the baseline survival distribution, and the treatment effect. Most, if not all, of these parameters are unknown to investigators at the design stage of a trial and must be assumed. Therefore we find it useful to explore the potential impact of varying assumptions on the timing of analysis and the overall duration of the trial. In RCTdesign patient accrual patterns can be explored at the time of design specification. To provide flexibility in the exploration process, accrual rates may be parameterized via a Beta(a, b) distribution or simulated from existing pilot data. Similarly, baseline survival may be parameterized via a Weibull distribution, a piece-wise constant hazard function, or simulated from existing pilot data.

In the context of the CLL trial, Fig. 6 depicts the event accrual rates and expected analysis times under fast (a) and slow (b) patient accrual patterns. In both cases, a total of 400 subjects were assumed to enroll over a period of 3 years and baseline survival in the placebo group was assumed to follow an exponential distribution with a median survival of 16 months. In Fig. 6a, a Beta$(1,10)$ accrual distribution was assumed while in Fig. 6b, a Beta$(10,1)$ distribution was assumed. In each figure, the solid line represents the cumulative number of subjects accrued to the trial as a function of calendar time, the small dashed line represents the number of subjects still at risk in the trial, and the large dashed line represents the cumulative number of events observed in the trial. Lighter dashed lines depict estimates under the null hypothesis ($\theta = 1$) and darker dashed lines depict estimates under the full design alternative ($\theta = 0.67$). Entry distributions have been chosen to be extreme to highlight the impact of the patient accrual patterns. Specifically, under fast accrual the first interim analysis is estimated to take place between 7 and 8 months after study start. From a clinical perspective, this may be too soon to begin assessing efficacy because long-term survival effects are generally of primary interest. Conversely, under slow early accrual the first interim analysis is expected to take place more than 3 years after recruitment into the trial began. In the context of the trial, this may be too long of a wait to assess futility, particularly in light of the fact that by this time all 400 patients will have been recruited to the trial

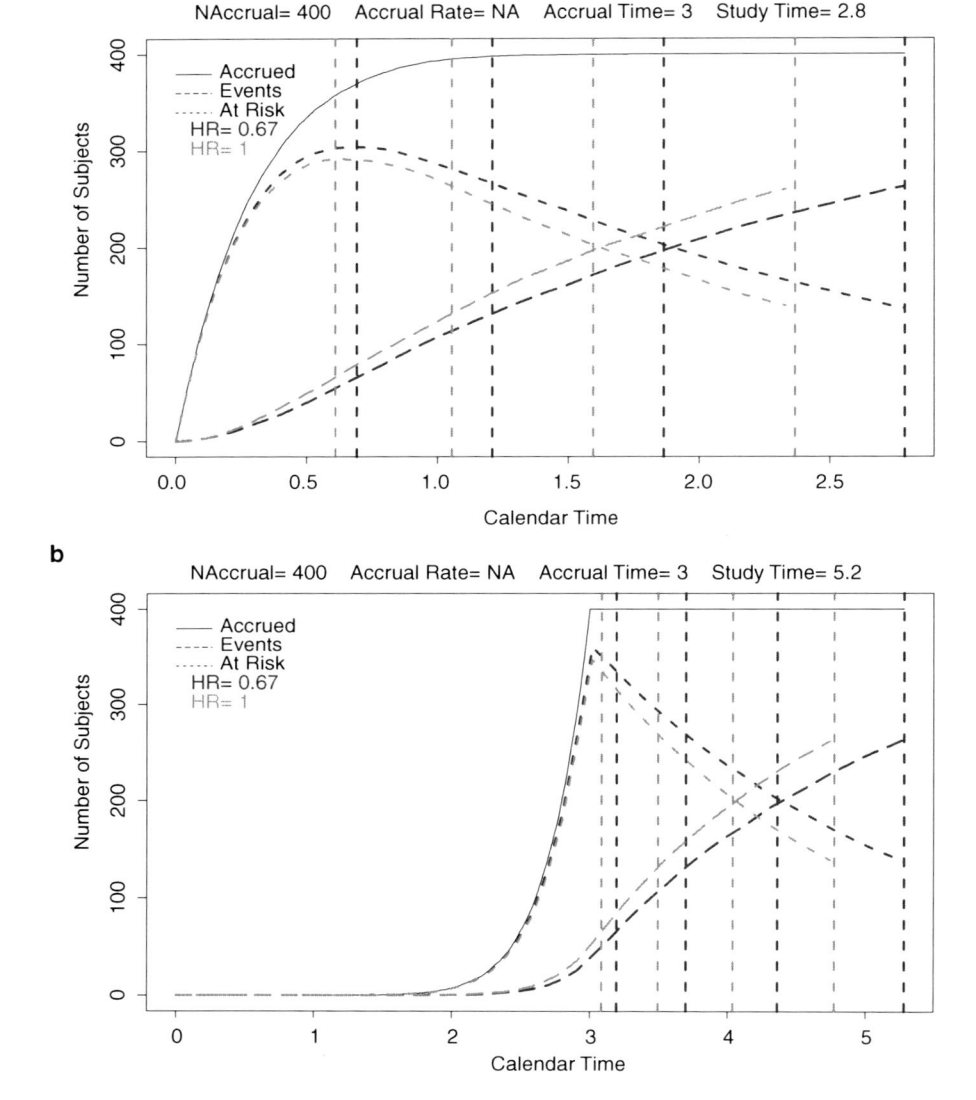

Fig. 6 Expected event accrual rates and analysis times under fast (**a**) and slow (**b**) patient accrual patterns. Analysis times are for one-sided level 0.025 stopping rule to test the null hypothesis $H_0 : \theta \geq 1$ and having a maximum of four equally spaced analysis, an efficacy (*lower*) boundary shape function corresponding to $P = 1.1$ and a futility (*upper*) boundary shape function corresponding to $P = 0.8$ in the unified family of group sequential designs. In each figure, the *solid line* represents the cumulative number of subjects accrued to the trial as a function of calendar time, the *small dashed line* represents the number of subjects still at risk in the trial, and the *large dashed line* represents the cumulative number of events observed in the trial

and treated. Also of note is the total expected duration of the study under each scenario. Under the full alternative, the total study time could be as little as 2.8 years if early accrual is fast and as long as 5.2 years if early accrual is slow. Beyond the obvious clinical implications of estimating the treatment effect in a controlled setting for these different periods of time, the cost of running a trial for longer periods of time may not be feasible for a sponsor.

3 Implementing a Group Sequential Design

3.1 Flexible Implementation of Stopping Rules Based on Constrained Boundaries

The stopping rule chosen in the design of a clinical trial serves as a guideline to a Data Monitoring Committee as it makes the decision to recommend continuing or stopping a clinical trial. If all aspects of the conduct of the clinical trial adhered exactly to the conditions stipulated during the design, the stopping rule obtained during the design phase could be used directly. However there are usually at least two complicating factors that must be dealt with during the conduct of the clinical trial. First, the schedule of interim analysis does not follow that used in the design of the trial. Often, meetings of the Data Monitoring Committee are scheduled according to calendar time, and thus the sample sizes available for analysis at any given meeting is a random variable. Similarly, accrual may be slower or faster than planned, thereby resulting in a different number of interim analyses than was originally planned. Either of these eventualities will necessitate modifications of the stopping rule, because the exact stopping boundaries are dependent upon the number and timing of analysis. Second, the estimate for response variability that was used at the design phase is typically incorrect. Often very crude estimates of response variability or baseline event rates are used at the design phase. As the trial progresses, more accurate estimates are to be used. Clearly the operating characteristics of particular stopping rules are heavily dependent on the variability of response measurement. In order to address these issues, flexible methods of implementing stopping rules have been developed which allow the clinical trialist to maintain at least some of the operating characteristics of the stopping rule. Typically such flexible methods always maintain the size (type I error) at the prescribed level. A choice must then be made as to whether the maximal sample size or the power to detect the design alternative should be maintained.

The flexible methods of implementing stopping rules in RCTdesign are based on the idea of computing a stopping boundary for the current interim analysis in such a way that the desired operating characteristics are satisfied and that the stopping rule is constrained to agree with the stopping boundaries used at all previously conducted interim analysis. Algorithmically, the monitoring strategy proceeds as follows:

1. At the first analysis, the stopping boundaries are derived by using the parametric boundary shape family specified in the design. The exact stopping boundary is computed by considering the proportion Π_1 of statistical information available at that first analysis. The value of Π_1 depends on which operating characteristics of the stopping rule the trial designer chooses to preserve:

   (a) If the maximal sample size (or number of events), N, is to be maintained, $\Pi_1 = N_1/N$. Here N_1 represents the number of subjects (or events) accrued at the first analysis.

   (b) If the power of the test to detect the design alternative is to be maintained, a schedule of future analysis is assumed and a stopping rule using the design parametric family (possibly constrained) is found which has the desired power. This consists of searching for the value of N which has the correct type I error and power to detect the alternative for the parametric design family for the assumed schedule of interim analysis. In either case, interpolation of the exact, minimum, or maximum constraints specified at the design stage is used to derive any constraints for the interim analysis specified by the assumed schedule of future analysis (which may differ from the schedule specified at the design stage). In cases where statistical information is dependent upon a variance parameter, the current best estimate of the statistical information contributed by a single sampling unit is used instead of the estimate supplied at the design stage.

2. At later interim analysis, the exact stopping boundaries used at previously conducted interim analysis are used as exact constraints at those analysis times, and the stopping boundaries at the current analysis, and all future analyses specified by an assumed schedule of future analysis are computed using the parametric family of designs specified at the design stage. The basic approach is that described for the first analysis, in which the proportion of statistical information at the j-th analysis is computed based either on the planned maximal sample size N if that operating characteristic is to be maintained, or it is computed based on a recomputation of a sample size which takes into account the new schedule of interim analysis and the current best estimate of the statistical information contributed by a single sampling unit. In either case, $\Pi_j = Nj/N$ is used as the proportion of statistical information available at the j-th analysis.

It should be noted that when a variance parameter is reestimated at each analysis, the stopping boundaries at previously conducted interim analysis depend upon which boundary scale is used when constraining the stopping rules at those analyses. That is, if the value of the variance parameter used in computing the stopping rule is constant over the course of the study, it is irrelevant which boundary scale is used for the constraints at previously conducted analyses. If, as is usually the case, the estimate of the variance parameter varies over the study, there will be some difference between the boundaries obtained. There is no clear advantage for one such scale over another.

This approach based on constrained boundaries is a generalization of the error spending approach of [18, 23]: That approach corresponds to boundary constraints specified on the error spending scale. More recently, [3] suggested the above constrained boundaries algorithm to allow a clinical trialist to constrain the stopping rule on any scale (e.g. the sample mean scale) and for any parametric family of designs (e.g. the unified family of group sequential designs).

To illustrate the use of the constrained boundaries approach in RCTdesign, Fig. 7 depicts data simulated in the context of the CLL trial. To demonstrate the method, suppose that the *Eff11.Fut8* design (boundaries depicted in Fig. 1) was the chosen stopping rule for the trial. Data were simulated under uniform patient accrual over 3 years assuming exponential survival times, with a median survival of 16 months in the placebo arm and a median survival of 22.9 months in the antibody arm (corresponding to a hazard ratio of 0.70). Figures (a)–(c) depict the observed survival curves and estimates of treatment effect at three interim analyses taking place at 1.5, 2.75, and 3.5 years after the start of trial enrollment. For reference, subfigure (d) depicts the data that would have been observed if a fixed sample design were performed after a total of 263 events were observed (occurring at 4.11 years after the start of trial enrollment).

Table 2 depicts the observed statistics at each of the three interim analyses, including the total number of observed events, the estimated hazard ratio (not adjusted for the stopping rule), and the normalized Z statistic (also not adjusted or the stopping rule). In addition to the observed statistics at each analysis, Table 2 yields the modified stopping rule obtained from the constrained boundaries algorithm. Of note, the first analysis took place after 49 events were observed in the study and not the originally planned 66 events. This earlier analysis time results in a much wider continuation interval at the first analysis when compared to the original *Eff11.Fut8* stopping boundaries depicted in Fig. 1. Given the observed hazard ratio of 0.46, the stopping rule suggested continuation of the trial and new stopping thresholds were derived using the original parametric family under a specified timing for the future analyses while maintaining an overall type I error rate of 0.025. The algorithm was again implemented at the second analysis occurring after 146 events were observed (differing from the previously assumed 132 events). We note that the stopping thresholds at the first analysis remained unchanged, while future stopping boundaries are recomputed. Again, the stopping rule suggested continuation of the study. The process was repeated at the third interim analysis, where a hazard ratio of 0.70 was computed (not adjusted for the stopping rule) after observing 208 events. At this analysis, the stopping rule suggested stopping the trial in favor of efficacy. Figure 8 provides a visual comparison of the original *Eff11.Fut8* (solid lines), having a maximum of four equally spaced analyses, an efficacy (lower) boundary shape function corresponding to $P = 1.1$ and a futility (upper) boundary shape function corresponding to $P = 0.8$ in the unified family of group sequential designs, and the final implemented design (dashed lines) using constrained boundaries to account for variation in the originally planned timing of analysis. In the figure, "X" denotes the observed point estimate (hazard ratio) at the three interim analysis.

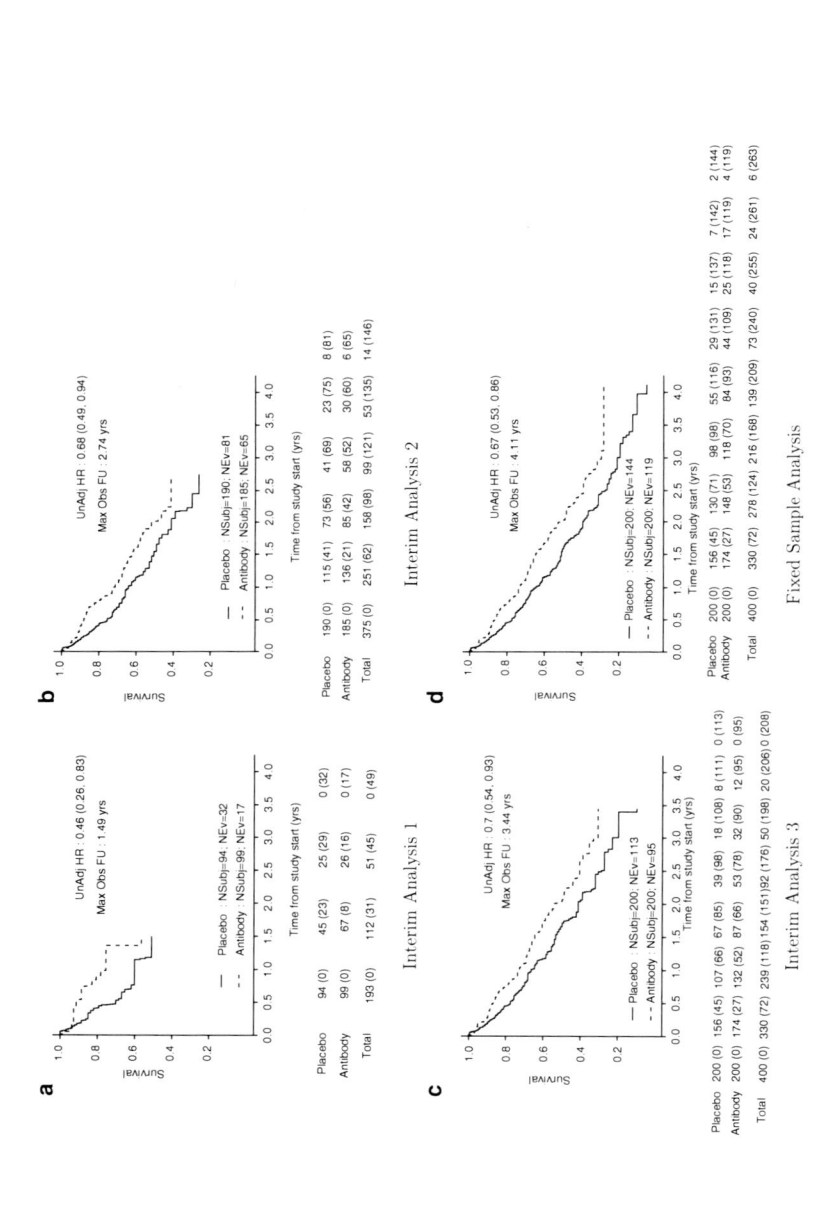

Fig. 7 Data simulated in the context of the CLL trial. Figures (**a**)–(**c**) depict the observed survival curves and estimates of treatment effect at the three interim analysis times taking place at 1.5, 2.75, and 3.5 years after the start of trial enrollment. Figure (**d**) depicts the data that would have been observed if a fixed sample design were performed after a total of 263 events were observed (occurring at 4.11 years after the start of trial enrollment). In each plot, numbers under the *x*-axis indicate the number of patients at risk and (the cumulative number of events) observed at 6-month intervals

Table 2 Implementation of the original *Eff11.Fut8* using constrained boundaries to account for variation in the originally planned analysis times. Original analysis times were planned at 66, 132, 198, and 263 events Data were simulated in the context of the CLL trial and are depicted in Fig. 7. Due to deviations from patient and event accrual rates, the first three interim analysis actually took place at 49, 146, and 208 events

	Observed statistics			Modified stopping boundaries[a,b]			Stopping rule
Analysis	No. events	Crude HR	Normalized Z statistic	Time	Efficacy	Futility	recommendation
1	49	0.462	−2.628	NEv= 49	0.214	1.619	Continue
	–	–	–	NEv=132	0.595	0.947	
	–	–	–	NEv=198	0.718	0.837	
	–	–	–	NEv=263	0.784	0.784	
2	49	0.462	−2.628	NEv= 49	0.214	1.619	Continue
	146	0.678	−2.342	NEv=146	0.629	0.915	Continue
	–	–	–	NEv=198	0.717	0.837	
	–	–	–	NEv=263	0.784	0.784	
3	49	0.462	−2.628	NEv= 49	0.214	1.619	Continue
	146	0.678	−2.342	NEv=146	0.629	0.915	Continue
	208	0.704	−2.522	NEv=208	0.730	0.826	Stop (efficacy)
	–	–	–	NEv=263	0.784	0.784	

[a]NEv denotes the observed number of events
[b]Stopping boundaries are displayed on the scale of the estimated hazard ratio

3.2 Adjusted Inference

As previously stated, the use of a group sequential stopping rule generally alters the sampling distribution of usual fixed sample statistics. Therefore special techniques must be used to compute point estimates, interval estimates and P values. Commonly reported point estimates include the usual maximum likelihood estimate (MLE), the median unbiased estimator (MUE; see [35]), the BAM [33], and the Rao–Blackwell adjusted unbiased estimate (RBUE; [19]).

In order to compute a MUE, P value, or confidence interval which adjusts for the stopping rule used in a group sequential trial, an ordering of possible clinical trial outcomes must be chosen. There is no uniformly optimal choice for such an ordering. In group sequential testing, the issue is how to treat outcomes observed at different analyses (see [7]). RCTdesign offers two approaches: the sample mean ordering [7] and the analysis time ordering [31].

The sample mean ordering judges one result more extreme than another according to whether the estimate of the treatment effect is more extreme. Thus, a treatment effect measured by a hazard ratio of 0.6 is lower than a treatment effect measured by a hazard ratio of 0.7, regardless of the analysis time. In the analysis time ordering, results that led to earlier termination of the study are judged to be more extreme than those observed at later analyses. Results that exceed an upper

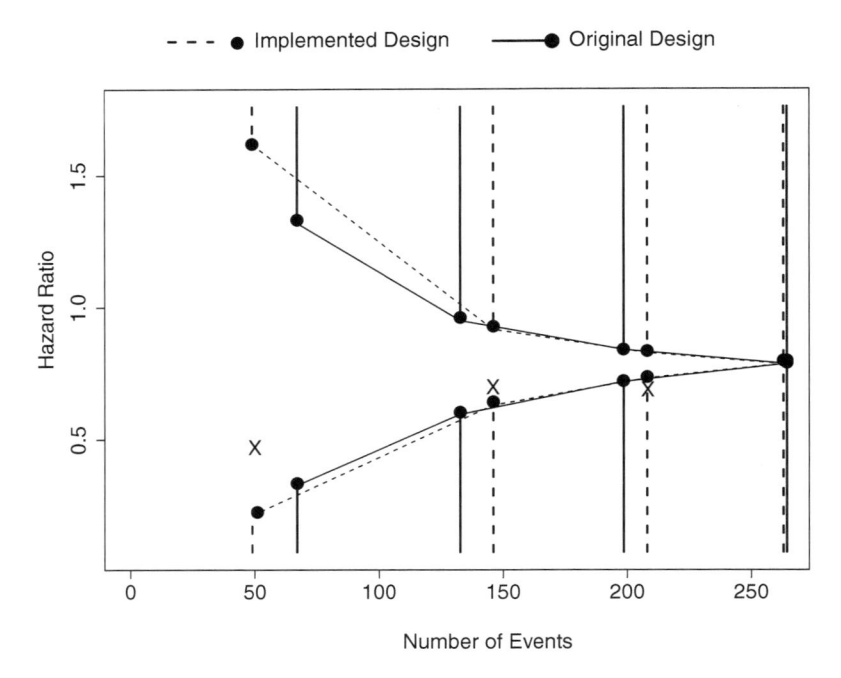

Fig. 8 Comparison of the original *Eff11.Fut8* (*solid lines*), having a maximum of four equally spaced analysis, an efficacy (*lower*) boundary shape function corresponding to $P = 1.1$ and a futility (*upper*) boundary shape function corresponding to $P = 0.8$ in the unified family of group sequential designs, and the final implemented design (*dashed lines*) using constrained boundaries to account for variation in the originally planned timing of analysis. "X" denotes the observed point estimate (hazard ratio) at the first three analysis. As indicated in the plot, the stopping rule recommended stopping at the third analysis so that no observed estimate is provided at the final analysis

boundary for the treatment effect at a specific analysis are higher than all results exceeding the upper boundary at later analyses, and also higher than all results less than the lower boundary at any analysis. Thus, a treatment effect measured by a hazard ratio of 0.6, which was judged so high as to warrant early termination of the study, is less extreme than a hazard ratio of 0.7 which was similarly judged high enough to warrant termination of the study at an earlier analysis.

Emerson and Fleming [7] investigated the relative behavior of the sample mean and analysis time orderings with respect to the average width of confidence intervals. The sample mean ordering tends to average shorter confidence interval lengths for the same coverage probabilities. Gillen and Emerson [14] more recently showed that under a time-varying treatment effect, the sample mean ordering tends to attain higher power relative to the analysis time ordering in the sense that the probability of attaining a small P value is higher with the sample mean ordering when compared to the analysis time ordering. Finally, the analysis time ordering is not defined for two-sided group sequential tests that allow early stopping under both the null and

Table 3 Inference adjusted for the *Eff11.Fut8* stopping rule. Data were simulated in the context of the CLL trial and are depicted in Fig. 7. Due to variability in patient and event accrual rates, the first three interim analysis actually took place at 49, 146, and 208 events. Based upon the sequential boundaries the trial was stopping at the third interim analysis

Result	Analysis time ordering		Sample mean ordering
Unadjusted estimate		0.7044	
Adjusted estimates			
BAM		0.7127	
RBadj		0.7167	
MUE	0.7074		0.7153
Adjusted inference			
95% CI	(0.5382, 0.9313)		(0.5469, 0.9347)
P value	0.006906		0.007238

alternative analysis. For these reasons, the sample mean ordering is the recommended method of computing ordering-dependent inference in RCTdesign. However, the sample mean ordering does depend on the number and timing of future analysis, but such dependence was found to be fairly slight by Emerson and Fleming [7].

Table 3 depicts the resulting inference at the conclusion of the simulated CLL trial. Based upon the implemented *Eff11.Fut8* design the trial was stopped at the third analysis. The observed hazard ratio (unadjusted for the stopping rule) was 0.7044. As can be seen from Table 3, each of the adjusted estimates are attenuated towards the null hypothesis. This adjustment for bias is slight in the example due to the conservativeness of the *Eff11.Fut8* stopping rule. Had a less conservative design been chosen, a larger difference between the unadjusted and adjusted estimates would have been observed. Also reported in Table 3 are the corrected 95% confidence intervals and *P* values based upon the analysis time and sample mean orderings. Again the two orderings produce similar results. This is because the trial continued to the penultimate analysis before stopping. Had the trial stopped earlier, at the first analysis for example, the difference in the inference obtained from the two orderings would have been more extreme.

4 Consideration of Potential Time-Varying Treatment Effects

The methods discussed in this manuscript have focused on settings in which the measure of treatment effect does not vary with time. However, it is often the case that a given treatment might have a delayed effect within individuals or that the effect of treatment might dissipate over time. Special issues arise in such settings. For instance, when using nonparametric statistics to analyze survival data exhibiting nonproportional hazards one must consider (among other things):

1. The formulation of alternatives at which operating characteristics are to be evaluated.
2. The rate of information growth of the test statistic for appropriately timing interim analysis.
3. The changing censoring distribution across interim analysis and its impact on the asymptotic distribution of the test statistic under alternatives.

In a further extension to the evaluation paradigm demonstrated here, [16] describe one general approach to the evaluation of clinical trial designs in the setting of nonproportional hazards. Gillen and Emerson [16] note that in the presence of nonproportional hazards survival data, nonparametric methods such as the $G^{\rho,\gamma}$ family of weighted logrank statistics [11] are often used and the evaluation of stopping rules is no longer a trivial task. Specifically, nonparametric test statistics do not necessarily correspond to a parameter of clinical interest, thus making it difficult to characterize alternatives at which operating characteristics are to be computed. It is shown that this sometimes leads to contradictions when reporting clinically meaningful measures of treatment effect in the event that they do not correspond to the nonparametric statistic on which testing is based. Gillen and Emerson [16] go on to describe re-sampling approaches which might be used to construct alternatives under nonproportional hazards when preexisting pilot data are available. Those methods can be implemented using the RCTdesign package as a foundation for generating stopping boundaries.

It was noted in Sect. 2.6 that under a proportional hazards treatment effect, statistical information is directly proportional to the number of events observed on the trial. In this case one only needs to estimate the calendar time that a specified number of events is likely to occur in order to schedule interim analyses. However, when testing is based upon a weighted statistic, such as the $G^{\rho,\gamma}$ family of weighted logrank statistics (perhaps to emphasize particular time intervals where treatment effects are of greatest clinical importance), the growth of statistical information is nonlinear with respect to the cumulative number of observed events (see [13]). Specifically, the amount of information contributed by each event is dependent upon when the event occurred as well as the accrual distribution. Building on the work of [2, 3, 13] describe a general constrained boundaries algorithm that can be used to flexibly monitor a group sequential survival trial under nonlinear information growth patterns. This procedure modifies the usual constrained boundaries algorithm described in Sect. 3.1 by using observed survival and accrual data at each interim analysis to predict the information growth curve, then mapping information accrual to calendar time. Because the method is an extension of the constrained boundaries approach implemented in RCTdesign it can easily be implemented in the current software.

Finally, multiple authors have noted that the parameter consistently estimated by the Cox proportional hazards model and the logrank statistic are dependent upon the observed censoring distribution when the proportional hazards assumption does not hold (cf. [15, 29]). This dependence is not only on the total length of follow-up observed in the trial, but also on the shape of the underlying censoring distribution.

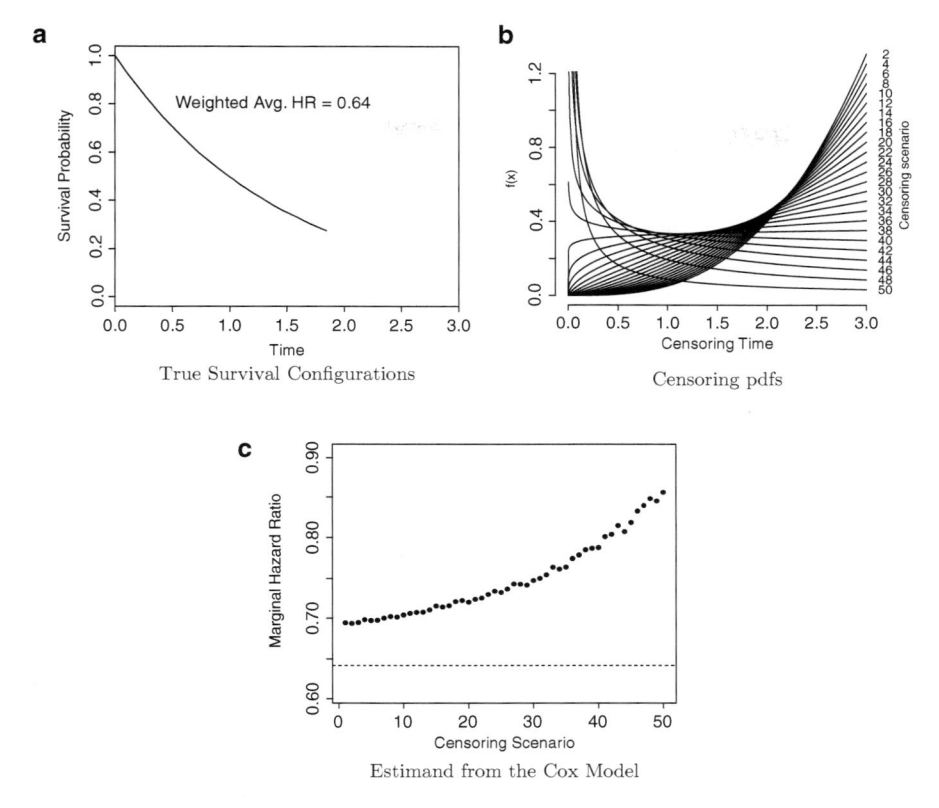

Fig. 9 Example illustrating the effect of the censoring distribution on the parameter consistently estimated by the Cox proportional hazards model under 50 different censoring distributions (shown in subfigure (**b**)). Data were generated under the survival configurations presented in subfigure (**a**) and the resulting estimand from each censoring scenario is plotted in subfigure (**c**)

As an illustration, Fig. 9 depicts the effect of the censoring distribution on the parameter consistently estimated by the Cox proportional hazards model under 50 different censoring distributions (shown in Fig. 9b). In this simulation study, survival curves were generated under the piecewise constant hazard ratio alternative depicted in Fig. 9a. With no censoring over 3 years the Cox model consistently estimates a "marginal" or "weighted" hazard ratio of 0.64. However, as censoring is introduced Fig. 9c illustrates that the parameter consistently estimated by the Cox model can vary from 0.67 (no censoring) to 0.87 (heavy early censoring as depicted in scenario 50). To remove this dependence, [37] suggested an inverse probability of censoring estimator that assumes a common censoring pattern across all comparison groups. Boyd et al. [1] later extended the weighted estimator to allow for group-dependent censoring in the case of a two-sample comparison and derived a consistent variance estimator in this case. Most recently Nguyen and Gillen developed a censoring robust reweighted estimator for discrete survival outcomes in the two sample setting

[21] and proposed a method to provide robust estimation of survival effects under covariate-dependent censoring in observational studies [20]. Because it is necessary to a priori specify the estimation and testing procedure to be used in a clinical trial, the above estimators are attractive in that they limit the influence of study accrual/dropout patterns on trial results under a misspecified model. In addition, although these estimators are not directly implemented in RCTdesign at the present time, the ability to monitor a normalized Z statistic using RCTdesign provides clinical trialists with a software tool that can be adapted to monitor any statistic that can be suitably normalized.

5 Discussion

In this manuscript we have demonstrated how the RCTdesign package can be used to select, implement, and analyze a group sequential stopping rule. The RCTdesign package aids in the complete evaluation of a clinical trial design by easily allowing clinical trialists to compare a broad range of candidate designs with respect to:

1. The scientific measures of treatment effect which will correspond to early termination for futility and/or efficacy.
2. The sample size requirements as described by the maximal sample size and summary measures of the sample size distribution (e.g., mean, 75th percentile) as a function of the hypothesized treatment effect.
3. The probability that the trial would continue to each analysis as a function of the hypothesized treatment effect.
4. The frequentist power to reject the null hypothesis as a function of the hypothesized treatment effect, with the type I error corresponding to the power under the null hypothesis.
5. The frequentist inference (adjusted point estimates, confidence intervals, and P values) which would be reported were the trial to stop with results corresponding exactly to a boundary.
6. The frequentist power to obtain a point estimate above some relevant threshold.
7. The expected timing of interim analysis as a function of patient accrual patterns.

After the selection of a group sequential stopping rule, flexible implementation of the sequential boundaries using a constrained boundaries approach was demonstrated. This method easily accounts for deviations in planned variance, timing, and number of analysis in order to maintain some of those operating characteristics specified at the design stage. With careful evaluation of stopping rules and methods for flexibly implementing those rules under changing circumstances, there seems little reason to resort to less efficient adaptive designs such as those based on using conditional power to re-design a study [26] or Fisher's "self-designing clinical trial" [10]. The most frequently cited motivation for using such adaptive designs include the possibility that at an interim analysis a clinical trialist might observe treatment effects that were promising, but not statistically significant, and thus want to continue the clinical trial to obtain a larger sample size. Of course, as noted in this manuscript, by examining the stopping boundary on the scale of the estimated treatment effect, all such possibilities can truly be considered at the design stage, and there is no real need to accommodate adaptive designs based solely on the estimate of the primary measure of treatment effect. Additionally, if conditions external to the trial suggest a change in the clinical or economic importance of particular alternative hypotheses or estimates of treatment effect, redesign of the clinical trial can proceed without materially affecting the type I error, because in that setting the factors affecting the redesign of the trial are not based on the trial results. This then argues that there is no real need for using adaptive designs. Furthermore, there are distinct disadvantages to the adaptive methods, most notably those related to the loss of statistical efficiency [5, 30].

The CLL case study used throughout this manuscript considered a survival endpoint and the design approach relied on a semi-parametric (proportional hazards) model. Robust methods for the analysis of survival data under a time-varying treatment effect remain an active area of research. Section 4 discusses multiple approaches to modify common survival statistics in order to limit the impact the censoring distribution in these settings. While these methods are effective for removing the dependence of the resulting estimand on the censoring distribution under fixed support, they do not address the dependence of these estimators on the underlying length of trial follow-up. This is a particular problem in the case of sequential testing where interim analysis inherently truncate the observed support of the survival distribution. Gillen [12] proposes one method for quantifying uncertainty in future treatment effects by utilizing a random walk approach to generate future alternatives which might reasonably be observed conditional upon data collected up to the time of an interim analysis. Similar methods could also be used in the design, evaluation, and monitoring of longitudinal studies, since the potential for time-varying treatment effects in these settings forces one to consider future alternative which might arise following an interim analysis.

Finally, the current manuscript has focused on the evaluation of frequentist operating characteristics. Increasingly, however, there has been much interest in the design and analysis of clinical trials under a Bayesian paradigm. While not demonstrated here, the RCTdesign package also allows for the Bayesian evaluation of group sequential designs. For further reading on this topic, the reader should see [8].

Appendix A RCTdesign Code to Recreate the CLL Examples in Sects. 2 and 3 Using R

```
##
#####   Definition of candidate designs for the CLL trial
##
```

```
Fixed.Sample <- seqDesign( prob.model = "hazard", arms = 2,
                           null.hypothesis = 1.,
                           alt.hypothesis = 0.67,
                           ratio = c(1., 1.),
                           nbr.analysis = 1,
                           test.type = "less",
                           sample.size=263,
                           power = "calculate",
                           alpha = 0.025 )
SymmOBF.2 <- update( Fixed.Sample, nbr.analysis=2, P=c(1,1),
                           sample.size=263,
                           power="calculate" )
SymmOBF.3 <- update( SymmOBF.2, nbr.analysis = 3 )
SymmOBF.4 <- update( SymmOBF.2, nbr.analysis = 4 )
SymmOBF.Power <- update( SymmOBF.4, power = 0.901 )
Futility.5 <- update( SymmOBF.4, P=c(1,.5) )
Futility.8 <- update( SymmOBF.4, P=c(1,.8) )
Futility.9 <- update( SymmOBF.4, P=c(1,.9) )
Eff11.Fut8 <- update( SymmOBF.4, P=c(1.1,.8) )
Eff11.Fut9 <- update( SymmOBF.4, P=c(1.1,.9) )
Fixed.Power <- update( Fixed.Sample, nbr.analysis=1,
                           power=0.8853 )


##
#####   Figure 1 : Comparison of stopping boundaries on crude
                             estimate of treatment effect
                             scale
##
seqPlotBoundary(    SymmOBF.4, Eff11.Fut8, Eff11.Fut9,
                           lty=c(1,3,4), col=1,
                           stagger=0, fixed=FALSE )
seqBoundary( Eff11.Fut8, scale="X" )
seqBoundary( Eff11.Fut8, scale="Z" )
1-seqBoundary( Eff11.Fut8, scale="P" )


##
#####   Figure 2 : Comparison of statistical power curves
##
seqPlotPower(SymmOBF.4,SymmOBF.3,SymmOBF.2, lty=1:4, col=1,
                           lwd=2 )
seqPlotPower(SymmOBF.4,SymmOBF.3,SymmOBF.2, reference=TRUE,
                           lty=1:4, col=1, lwd=2 )


##
#####   Table 1 : Computation of power and alternative tables
                             for the Eff11.Fut8 design
##
seqOC( Eff11.Fut8, power=c(.8,.9,.95,.975) )
seqOC( Eff11.Fut8, theta=c(1,.75,.67,.60) )


##
#####   Figure 3 : Comparison of sample size distributions
##
```

```
seqPlotASN(SymmOBF.4,Futility.9,Futility.8,Futility.5,
                         fixed=FALSE, lty=c(2,1,3,4),
                         col=1, lwd=2)

##
#####   Figure 4 : Depiction of stopping probabilities
##
seqPlotStopProb(Eff11.Fut8)

##
#####   Figure 5 : Statistical inference on the boundaries
##
plot(seqInference(Eff11.Fut8))

##
#####   Figure 6a : Patient accrual patterns (early accrual)
##
Eff11.Fut8Extd.early <- seqDesignExtd(prob.model = "hazard",
                         arms = 2, null.hypothesis
                         = 1., alt.hypothesis = 0.67,
                         ratio = c(1., 1.),
                         nbr.analysis = 4,
                         test.type = "less",
                         alpha = 0.025,
                         sample.size=263,
                         power="calculate",
                         P=c(1.1,.8),
                         accrualSize=400,
                         accrualTime=3, bShapeAccr=10,
                         eventQuantiles=16/12,
                         nPtsSim=10000, seed=0)
seqPlotPHNSubjects(Eff11.Fut8Extd.early)

##
#####   Figure 6b : Patient accrual patterns (late accrual)
##
Eff11.Fut8Extd.late <- seqDesignExtd(prob.model = "hazard",
                         arms = 2,
                         null.hypothesis
                         = 1., alt.hypothesis = 0.67,
                         ratio = c(1., 1.),
                         nbr.analysis = 4,
                         test.type = "less",
                         alpha = 0.025,
                         sample.size=263,
                         power="calculate",
                         P=c(1.1,.8),
                         accrualSize=400,
                         accrualTime=3, aShapeAccr=10,
                         eventQuantiles=16/12,
                         nPtsSim=10000, seed=0)
seqPlotPHNSubjects(Eff11.Fut8Extd.late)
```

```
##
#####    Simulation of CLL data
##
set.seed( 123456 )
n <- 200
grp1 <- rexp( n, rate=.75*log(2) )
grp2 <- rexp( n, rate=(.75*log(2))*.70 )
trueSurv <- c( grp1, grp2 )
entry <- runif( 2*n, 0, 3 )
grp <- rep( 0:1, each=n )

##  First analysis at 1.5 years after study start
analysisTime <- 1.5
obsSurv <- ifelse( trueSurv + entry <= analysisTime, trueSurv,
                                 analysisTime-entry )
event <- ifelse( obsSurv == trueSurv, 1, 0 )
cllData <- as.data.frame( cbind( grp, entry, obsSurv, event ) )
cllData <- cllData[ cllData$obsSurv > 0, ]
resp <- Surv( cllData$obsSurv, cllData$event )
interim1 <- seqMonitor( Eff11.Fut8, response=resp,
                                 treatment=cllData$grp,
                                 future.analysis=c(132,198,263) )

##  Second analysis at 2.75 years after study start
analysisTime <- 2.75
obsSurv <- ifelse( trueSurv + entry <= analysisTime, trueSurv,
                                 analysisTime-entry )
event <- ifelse( obsSurv == trueSurv, 1, 0 )
cllData <- as.data.frame( cbind( grp, entry, obsSurv, event ) )
cllData <- cllData[ cllData$obsSurv > 0, ]
resp <- Surv( cllData$obsSurv, cllData$event )
interim2 <- seqMonitor( interim1, response=resp,
                                 treatment=cllData$grp,
                                 future.analysis=c(198,263) )

##  Third analysis at 3.5 years after study start
analysisTime <- 3.5
obsSurv <- ifelse( trueSurv + entry <= analysisTime, trueSurv,
                                 analysisTime-entry )
event <- ifelse( obsSurv == trueSurv, 1, 0 )
cllData <- as.data.frame( cbind( grp, entry, obsSurv, event ) )
cllData <- cllData[ cllData$obsSurv > 0, ]
resp <- Surv( cllData$obsSurv, cllData$event )
interim3 <- seqMonitor( interim2, response=resp,
                                 treatment=cllData$grp,
                                 future.analysis=c(263) )

##
#####    Figure 8 : Comparison of implemented and original
                                 design
##
plot( interim3, dsnLbls=c("Implemented Design", "Original
                                 Design") )
```

```
##
#####    Table 3 : Inference adjusted for the stopping rule
##
print( interim3 )
```

References

1. Boyd A, Kittelson J, Gillen D (2012) Estimation of treatment effect under nonproportional hazards and covariate dependent censoring. Stat Med [Epub ahead of print]
2. Brummel S, Gillen D (2012) Flexibly monitoring group sequential survival trials using constrained boundaries. Revised for Journal of Biopharmaceutical Statistics
3. Burington BE, Emerson SS (2003) Flexible implementations of group sequential stopping rules using constrained boundaries. Biometrics 59:770–777
4. Cytel Software Corporation (2000) EaSt. A software package for the design and interim monitoring of group-sequential clinical trials. Cambridge, Mass
5. Emerson SS (2006) Issues in the use of adaptive clinical trial designs. Stat Med 25:3270–3296
6. Emerson SS, Fleming TR (1989) Symmetric group sequential test designs. Biometrics 45: 905–923
7. Emerson SS, Fleming TR (1990) Parameter estimation following group sequential hypothesis testing. Biometrika 77:875–892
8. Emerson SS, Kittelson JM, Gillen DL (2007) Bayesian evaluation of group sequential designs. Stat Med 26:1431–1449
9. Emerson SS, Kittelson JM, Gillen DL (2007) Frequentist evaluation of group sequential designs. Stat Med 26:5047–5080
10. Fisher LD (1998) Self-designing clinical trials. Stat Med 17:1551–1562
11. Fleming TR, Harrington DP (1991) Counting processes and survival analysis. Wiley, New York
12. Gillen DL (2009) A random walk approach for quantifying uncertainty in group sequential survival trials. Comput Stat Data Anal 53(3):603–620
13. Gillen DL, Emerson SS (2005) Information growth in a family of weighted logrank statistics under repeated analysis. Seq Anal 24(1):1–22
14. Gillen DL, Emerson SS (2005) A note on P-values under group sequential testing and nonproportional hazards. Biometrics 61(2):546–551
15. Gillen DL, Emerson SS (2007) Non-transitivity in a class of weighted logrank statistics under non-proportional hazards. Stat Probab Lett 77(2):123–130
16. Gillen DL, Emerson SS (2011) Evaluating a group sequential design in the setting of non-proportional hazards UW Biostatistics Working Paper Series. Working Paper 307. http://biostats.bepress.com/uwbiostat/paper307
17. Kittelson JM, Emerson SS (1999) A unifying family of group sequential test designs. Biometrics 55:874–882
18. Lan KKG, DeMets DL (1983) Discrete sequential boundaries for clinical trials. Biometrika 70:659–663
19. Liu A, Hall WJ (1999) Unbiased estimation following a group sequential test. Biometrika 86:71–78
20. Nguyen V, Gillen D (2012) Robust inference in semiparametric discrete hazard models for observational studies. Revised for Journal of the American Statistical Association
21. Nguyen V, Gillen D (2012) Robust inference in semiparametric discrete hazard models for randomized clinical trials. Lifetime Data Anal 18:446–69
22. O'Brien PC, Fleming TR (1979) A multiple testing procedure for clinical trials. Biometrics 35:549–556
23. Pampallona S, Tsiatis A, Kim K (1995) Spending functions for the type i and type ii error probabilities of group sequential tests. Technical report. http://76.12.5.166/papers/usefun.pdf

24. PEST (2000) Planning and evaluation of sequential trials. The MPS Research Unit, The University of Reading, Reading
25. Pocock SJ (1977) Group sequential methods in the design and analysis of clinical trials. Biometrika 64:191–200
26. Proschan MA, Hunsberger SA (1995) Designed extension of studies based on conditional power. Biometrics 51:1315–1324
27. SAS Institute Inc (2005) SAS OnlineDoc 9.1.3, SAS/SEQDESIGN, Cary, NC
28. TIBCO Software Inc (2000) S-Plus SeqTrial. Palo Alto, Ca
29. Struthers CA, Kalbfleisch JD (1986) Misspecified proportional hazard models. Biometrika 73:363–369
30. Tsiatis AA, Mehta CR (2003) On the inefficiency of the adaptive design for monitoring clinical trials. Biometrika 90:367–378
31. Tsiatis AA, Rosner GL, Mehta CR (1984) Exact confidence intervals following a group sequential test. Biometrics 40:797–803
32. Wang SK, Tsiatis AA (1987) Approximately optimal one-parameter boundaries for group sequential trials. Biometrics 43:193–199
33. Whitehead J (1986) On the bias of maximum likelihood estimation following a sequential test. Biometrika 73:573–581
34. Whitehead J (1986) Supplementary analysis at the conclusion of a sequential clinical trial. Biometrics 42:461–471
35. Whitehead J (1997) The design and analysis of sequential clinical trials. Wiley, New York
36. Whitehead J, Stratton I (1983) Group sequential clinical trials with triangular continuation regions. Biometrics 39:227–236 (corr: V39 p1137)
37. Xu R, O'Quigley J (2000) Estimating average regression effect under non-proportional hazards. Biostatistics (Oxford) 1(4):423–439

Genetic Markers in Clinical Trials

B.S. Weir and P.J. Heagerty

Abstract The current availability of dense sets of marker SNPs for the human genome is having a large impact on genetic studies and offers new possibilities for clinical trials. This chapter offers a unified basis for the analysis of marker and response data, emphasizing the central importance of the correlation, or linkage disequilibrium, between SNP markers and the genes that affect response. It is convenient to phrase the development of association mapping in the language of quantitative genetics, using additive and non-additive components of variance. A novel feature of dense SNP data is that good estimates can be made of actual inbreeding and relatedness. These estimates are more relevant than values predicted from family pedigree, and are all that are available in the absence of family data.

The dimensionality of SNP marker datasets has required the development of new methods that are appropriate for a large number of statistical comparisons, and the development of computational methods that allow high-dimensional regression. These methods are reviewed here, as is the use of biological annotation for both viewing the relevance of empirical associations, and to structure analysis in order to focus on those markers with the highest expectation for association with the outcomes under study.

1 Introduction

This chapter explores the statistical issues surrounding the use of SNPs in clinical trials and genome-wide association studies, and it contains the material presented in a short course by the authors. It is based, in part, on their experience with two NHGRI-funded consortia: GENEVA [3, 12], a collection of genome-wide

B.S. Weir (✉) • P.J. Heagerty
Department of Biostatistics, University of Washington, Box 357232, Seattle,
WA 98195-7232, USA
e-mail: bsweir@uw.edu

T.R. Fleming and B.S. Weir (eds.), *Proceedings of the Fourth Seattle Symposium in Biostatistics: Clinical Trials*, Lecture Notes in Statistics 1205, DOI 10.1007/978-1-4614-5245-4_12, © Springer Science+Business Media New York 2013

association studies, and GARNET, a collection of randomized clinical trials. It also reflects our work as a data coordinating center for a number of randomized clinical trials including evaluation of vertebroplasty for osteoporotic fractures [11] and surgery for carpal tunnel syndrome [10], performed through the Center for Biomedical Statistics at the University of Washington.

At the time of the Fourth Seattle Symposium on Biostatistics there were 199 clinical trials listed at www.clinicaltrials.gov that were collecting genetic information on participants. The entry for trial NCT01106144, for example, states:

> The main component in the treatment of acute myeloid leukemia (AML) is consist of anthracycline (such as daunorubicin or idarubicin) and cytarabine. Inter-individual variability of transport/ metabolism of the chemotherapeutic agent and several genetic pathways involved in the drug action might be associated with different response following the treatment for AML usually consisted of chemotherapy and/or transplantation. One of potential pathways involved in the drug action is DNA repair pathway, accordingly single nucleotide polymorphisms (SNPs) in the DNA repair machinery pathway might be a predictive marker for therapy outcomes in AML.

This chapter focusses on the use of SNPs for clinical trials.

2 Single Nucleotide Polymorphisms

Information about the genetic constitution of an individual in a study is often provided by technologies that reveal SNP profiles. Each of us receives one genome, including 23 chromosomes, from each of our parents and the genome can be described by the base type (A,C,G, or T) at each of the three billion nucleotides in the genomic DNA sequence. There can be constraints on which bases can be present at each nucleotide position but there is now documentation of 25 million or so positions at which there is variation among people (http://www.1000genomes.org). The low rate of change with which one base may be replaced by another means that most SNPs have only two possible states in a population, such as A and C. If the frequency of type A in a population is $p_A = 0.8$, then C is termed the minor allele and the minor allele frequency (MAF) is 0.2.

Individuals may be typed at specific target regions of the genome but it is generally cost-effective to type many SNPs with platforms that give whole-genome data. The OMNI5 chip produced by the Illumina company allows five million SNPs to be typed (http://www.illumina.com/products), most of them with MAF values over 0.01 in publicly available data sets such as HapMap or 1000 Genomes (www.hapmap.org, or www.1000genomes.org). In a recent review, [5] listed sets of studies where associations of SNPs with drug response had been sought, often resulting in highly significant results.

3 Associations

The use of genetic markers for mapping disease genes or as biomarkers in clinical trials depends on associations between genetic variants and observed or measured traits. We first examine associations between genetic variants before taking up the association of markers with traits or outcomes.

It is convenient to describe associations between pairs of alleles in terms of correlations. At one locus, the correlation coefficient is an *inbreeding coefficient* and at two loci, the correlation depends upon *linkage disequilibrium*. For marker and trait locus pairs, the squared correlation coefficient is the key parameter.

3.1 *Allelic Association at One Locus*

For a set of n individuals in a sample from one population, it is convenient to replace every allele by an indicator variable for, say, allele A at locus **A**. For allele k ($k = 1, 2$) in individual j ($j = 1, 2, \ldots, n$), these indicator variables x_{jk} are defined as

$$x_{jk} = \begin{cases} 1 & \text{allele is of type } A \\ 0 & \text{otherwise} \end{cases}$$

Taking averages over all samples from the population of these Bernoulli variables is straightforward:

$$\mathcal{E}(x_{jk}) = p_A$$
$$\mathcal{E}(x_{jk}^2) = p_A$$
$$\mathrm{Var}(x_{jk}) = p_A(1 - p_A)$$

where p_A is the allele frequency for A.

Now the product of the two x's for one individual is nonzero only if the individual is homozygous AA, and this leads to the covariance of indicator variables within individuals:

$$\mathcal{E}(x_{jk}x_{jk'}) = P_{AA}, \quad k \neq k'$$
$$\mathrm{Cov}(x_{jk}, x_{jk'}) = P_{AA} - p_A^2$$

where P_{AA} is the genotype frequency for AA.

The (within-population) inbreeding coefficient f_A at locus **A** is defined to allow the reparameterization of genotype frequencies in terms of allele frequencies:

$$P_{AA} = p_A^2 + p_A(1 - p_A)f_A$$

$$P_{Aa} = 2p_A(1 - p_A) - 2p_A(1 - p_A)f_A$$
$$P_{aa} = (1 - p_A)^2 + p_A(1 - p_A)f_A$$

This imposes no constraints on genotypic proportions and it preserves the usual reduction of genotypic frequencies to allele frequencies:

$$p_A = P_{AA} + \frac{1}{2}P_{Aa}, \quad p_a = P_{aa} + \frac{1}{2}P_{As}$$

The inbreeding coefficient can be seen to be the correlation coefficient of the indicator variables for the two alleles carried by an individual at a locus. This follows because

$$\text{Var}(x_{jk}) = p_A(1 - p_A)$$
$$\text{Cov}(x_{jk}, x_{jk'}) = p_A(1 - p_A)f_A, \quad k \neq k'$$
$$\text{Corr}(x_{jk}, x_{jk'}) = f_A$$

Because genotypic frequencies are bounded by allele frequencies above and zero below,

$$0 \leq P_{AA} = p_A^2 + p_A p_a f_A \leq p_A$$

there are bounds on the inbreeding coefficient

$$\max\left(-\frac{p_A}{p_a}, -\frac{p_a}{p_A}\right) \leq f_A \leq 1$$

Sample Values If a sample of n individuals is found to have counts n_{AA}, n_{Aa}, n_{aa} for genotypes AA, Aa, aa, the sample allele frequencies, denoted by tildes, are

$$\tilde{p}_A = \frac{1}{2n}(2n_{AA} + n_{Aa}) = \tilde{P}_{AA} + \frac{1}{2}\tilde{P}_{Aa}$$

and these have means and variances over all samples from the same population of

$$\mathcal{E}(\tilde{p}_A) = p_A$$
$$\text{Var}(\tilde{p}_A) = \frac{1}{2n}p_A(1 - p_A)(1 + f_A).$$

A structured population is shown in Fig. 1, where the subpopulations have distinct allele frequencies p^*. Among samples from the ith subpopulation the allele counts are binomially distributed : $(2n\tilde{p}_i) \sim \text{Binomial}(2n, p_i^*)$ providing there is Hardy–Weinberg equilibrium ($f = 0$) in that subpopulation. We will return to variation among subpopulations later.

Population

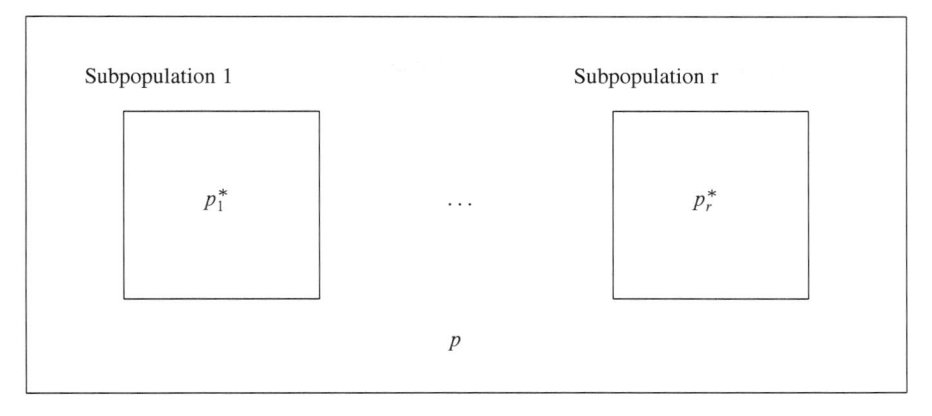

Fig. 1 Allele frequencies in a substructured population

3.2 *Allelic Association at Two Loci*

A *gamete* is the set of genetic material, in the egg or sperm, passed from parent to child and a *haplotype* is a relatively small region on one chromosome. For the present purposes the terms are essentially interchangeable, but "gamete" will be used as it has greater generality.

If data are available for a set of n gametes, indicator variables x_A and x_B can be defined for loci **A** and **B** in the same way as that above for one locus. For gamete j:

$$x_{j_A} = \begin{cases} 1 & \text{if gamete carries } A \\ 0 & \text{otherwise} \end{cases}$$

$$x_{j_B} = \begin{cases} 1 & \text{if gamete carries } B \\ 0 & \text{otherwise} \end{cases}$$

As the product $x_{j_A} x_{j_B}$ is nonzero only if the gamete is of type AB it has expectation $\mathcal{E}(x_{j_A} x_{j_B}) = P_{AB}$, where P_{AB} is frequency of that gamete type. Therefore

$$\mathcal{E}(x_{j_A}) = p_A, \text{Var}(x_{j_A}) = p_A(1 - p_A)$$

$$\mathcal{E}(x_{j_B}) = p_B, \text{Var}(x_{j_B}) = p_B(1 - p_B)$$

$$\mathcal{E}(x_{j_A} x_{j_B}) = P_{AB}, \text{Cov}(x_{j_A}, x_{j_B}) = D_{AB} = P_{AB} - p_A p_B$$

The quantity D_{AB} is defined to be the (gametic) linkage disequilibrium between alleles A and B.

The correlation of indicator variables at two loci is

$$\rho_{AB} = \mathrm{Corr}(x_{j_A}, x_{j_B}) = \frac{D_{AB}}{\sqrt{p_A(1 - p_A)p_B(1 - p_B)}}$$

and this is the two-locus analog of the inbreeding coefficient f. It is the parameter that determines the behavior of all genetic association tests. In practice, use is made of the squared sample value

$$r_{AB}^2 = \frac{\tilde{D}_{AB}^2}{\tilde{p}_A(1 - \tilde{p}_A)\tilde{p}_B(1 - \tilde{p}_B)}$$

Because gamete frequencies are bounded above by allele frequencies and below by zero it can be seen that

$$0 \le D_{AB} + p_A p_B \le p_A \, , \, 0 \le -D_{AB} + p_A p_b \le p_A$$

$$0 \le \rho^2 \le \min\left(\frac{p_A p_b}{p_a p_B}, \frac{p_a p_B}{p_A p_b}\right) \le 1$$

The two loci need equal allele frequencies ($p_A = p_B$) for ρ_{AB}^2 to attain the value 1.

Allelic Association at Two Unphased Loci It is generally the case that only genotypic data, rather than gametic data, are available and this suggests another measure of linkage disequilibrium. The indicator variables now need two subscripts: j ($j = 1, 2, \ldots, n$) for individual and k for gamete ($k = 1, 2$) within individual. Summing the indicator values at each locus:

$$X_{j_A} = x_{j1_A} + x_{j2_A}$$

$$X_{j_B} = x_{j1_B} + x_{j2_B}$$

provides indicators X_{j_A} having values $2, 1, 0$ with probabilities P_{AA}, P_{Aa}, P_{aa} and indicators X_{j_B} having values $2, 1, 0$ with probabilities P_{BB}, P_{Bb}, P_{bb}.

The means, variances, and covariances of the genotypic indicators are

$$\mathcal{E}(X_{j_A}) = 2p_A, \mathrm{Var}(X_{j_A}) = 2p_A(1 - p_A)(1 + f_A)$$

$$\mathcal{E}(X_{j_B}) = 2p_B, \mathrm{Var}(X_{J_B}) = 2p_B(1 - p_B)(1 + f_B)$$

$$\mathcal{E}(X_{j_A} X_{j_B}) = 4P_{AABB} + 2P_{AABb} + 2P_{AaBB} + P_{AaBb}$$

$$\mathrm{Cov}(X_{j_A}, X_{j_B}) = 2D_{AB}^c$$

These equations introduce the "composite" linkage disequilibrium D_{AB}^c and

$$\text{Corr}(X_{jA}, X_{jB}) = \frac{D_{AB}^c}{\sqrt{p_A p_a (1 + f_A) p_B p_b (1 + f_B)}}$$

With Hardy–Weinberg equilibrium, $f_A = f_B = 0$ and $D_{AB}^c = D_{AB}$. In this special case it is straightforward, although computationally challenging, to recover gamete frequencies from genotypic frequencies and it is possible to work only with gametic disequilibria.

3.3 Subgroup Analysis

Before considering association mapping methods that depend on linkage disequilibrium between marker and trait loci, we consider evaluating treatment effects in genotype subgroups. In a small modification of previous notation, the genotype indicator X_{lj} is the number of copies of the minor allele for the lth SNP in the jth individual, and we could consider a binary grouping: marker l is positive if $X_{lj} \geq 1$ and it is negative if $X_{lj} = 0$. Subjects can be placed into marker-positive and marker-negative subgroups.

Subgroup treatment effects Δ_{lg} are the differences in responses Y between the two treatment groups $Tx = 1$ and $Tx = 0$, for that subgroup:

$$\Delta_{lg} = \mathcal{E}(Y_j | X_{lj} = g, Tx = 1) - \mathcal{E}(Y_j | X_{lj} = g, Tx = 0) \tag{1}$$

The first question of interest is whether or not there are subgroups that have strong treatment effects, or evidence for harm: $H_0 : \Delta_{lg} = 0$. Within a subgroup, a test statistic for treatment effect is $z = \hat{\Delta}_{lg} / \sqrt{V_{lg}}$, where $\hat{\Delta}_{lg}$ is the observed effect for SNP l in that subgroup and V_{jg} is an estimate of the variance of the effect.

As an example of a study with which we have had experience, we refer to an evaluation of compound "X" by GlaxoSmithKline in which the main objective of the analysis is to identify genetic markers that influence the clinical efficacy of the compound for the treatment of disease "D."

A second question is whether or not there are subgroups that have treatment effects that are larger (or smaller) than the overall treatment effect. In other words, are there "enhanced" treatment effects? If $\bar{\Delta}$ is the treatment effect averaged over subgroups, or simply the overall marginal treatment effect:

$$\bar{\Delta} = \mathcal{E}(Y_j | Tx = 1) - \mathcal{E}(Y_j | Tx = 0)$$

this question is $H_0 : \Delta_{lg} = \bar{\Delta}$. This is equivalent to $H_0 : \Delta_{lg} = \bar{\Delta}_{lg^c}$ where g, g^C are the subgroups $X_{lj} = g, X_{lj} \neq g$.

4   Association Mapping

Association methods use random samples from a population and are alternatives to linkage methods based on pedigrees. The associations depend on linkage disequilibrium between marker and trait loci instead of depending on linkage between those loci as in pedigree methods.

Suppose that a quantitative trait locus **T** contributes to a trait of interest. The QTL genotype cannot be observed but maybe it can be inferred, and the location of the QTL estimated, from observations on the trait and the genotype at a genetic marker **M**. Individuals have observable marker genotypes and unobservable trait or response genotypes.

Each marker genotypic class $M_u M_v$ is composed of a mixture of elements from each of the QTL classes, $T_r T_s$, where the proportion of QTL class $T_r T_s$ contained within marker class $M_u M_v$ is $Pr(T_r T_s | M_u M_v) = \Pr(T_r T_s M_u M_v)/ \Pr(M_u M_v)$. With random mating, joint **TM** genotype frequencies are products of gamete frequencies as shown in Table 1, and gamete frequencies differ from products of allele frequencies because of linkage disequilibrium as shown in Table 2.

Trait Variables   A treatment of association mapping also requires genetic variables Z and G for loci **M** and **T**. The values of Z are assigned for the marker, whereas the values G represent the genetic contributions to measured trait variables, disease status, or treatment response. The G's are not under control of the investigator. In either case, the Hardy–Weinberg assumption provides the following expressions for the means and variances:

$$\mathcal{E}(Z) = \mu_Z = p_M^2 Z_{MM} + 2 p_M p_m Z_{Mm} + p_m^2 Z_{mm}$$

$$\mathcal{E}(G) = \mu_G = p_T^2 G_{TT} + 2 p_T p_t G_{Tt} + p_t^2 G_{tt}$$

$$\mathrm{Var}(Z) = \sigma_{A_M}^2 + \sigma_{D_M}^2$$

$$\mathrm{Var}(G) = \sigma_{A_T}^2 + \sigma_{D_T}^2$$

Table 1 Two-allele genotypic frequencies

	TT	Tt	tt
MM	P_{MT}^2	$2 P_{MT} P_{Mt}$	P_{Mt}^2
Mm	$2 P_{MT} P_{mT}$	$2 P_{MT} P_{mt} + 2 P_{Mt} P_{mT}$	$2 P_{Mt} P_{mt}$
mm	P_{mT}^2	$2 P_{mT} P_{mt}$	P_{mt}^2

Table 2 Two-allele gametic frequencies

	T	t
M	$P_{MT} = p_M p_T + D_{MT}$	$P_{Mt} = p_M p_t - D_{MT}$
m	$P_{mT} = p_m p_T - D_{MT}$	$P_{mt} = p_m p_t + D_{MT}$

The "additive" and "dominance" components of variance are

$$\sigma_{A_M}^2 = 2p_M p_m [p_M(Z_{MM} - Z_{Mm}) + p_m(Z_{Mm} - Z_{mm})]^2$$
$$\sigma_{A_T}^2 = 2p_T p_t [p_T(G_{TT} - G_{Tt}) + p_t(G_{Tt} - G_{tt})]^2$$

$$\sigma_{D_M}^2 = p_M^2 p_m^2 (Z_{MM} - 2Z_{Mm} + Z_{mm})^2$$
$$\sigma_{D_T}^2 = p_T^2 p_t^2 (G_{TT} - 2G_{Tt} + G_{tt})^2$$

and the covariance of Z and G depends on the linkage disequilibrium ρ_{MT} between **M** and **T**:

$$\text{Cov}(G, Z) = \rho_{MT}\sigma_{A_T}\sigma_{A_M} + \rho_{MT}^2\sigma_{D_T}\sigma_{D_M}$$

If either Z or G are purely additive, then

$$\text{Cov}(G, Z) = \rho_{MT}\sigma_{A_T}\sigma_{A_M}$$

whereas if either is purely nonadditive

$$\text{Cov}(G, Z) = \rho_{MT}^2\sigma_{D_T}\sigma_{D_M}$$

The choice of marker coding, i.e. whether Z has only additive variance, only nonadditive variance, or a combination of the two, will determine the nature of trait genetic effects that can be detected by association mapping.

Suppose the measured trait or response variable has value Y where $Y = G + E$, the sum of the genetic effect G of locus **T** and all other effects E. These other effects may be supposed to have mean zero and to be independent of both G and the marker variable Z. Then

$$\mathcal{E}(Y) = \mathcal{E}(G)$$
$$\text{Cov}(Y, Z) = \text{Cov}(G, Z)$$
$$\text{Var}(Y) = \sigma_{A_T}^2 + \sigma_{D_T}^2 + V_E$$

4.1 Continuous Traits

Regression Trait values Y may be regressed on marker variables Z. The regression coefficient has parametric value

$$\beta_{YZ} = \frac{\text{Cov}(Y, Z)}{\text{Var}(Z)} = \frac{\rho_{MT}\sigma_{A_T}\sigma_{A_M} + \rho_{MT}^2\sigma_{D_T}\sigma_{D_M}}{\sigma_{A_M}^2 + \sigma_{D_M}^2}$$

Marker variable Z is often chosen to be additive, e.g $Z_{MM} = 2, Z_{Mm} = 1, Z_{mm} = 0, \sigma^2_{D_M} = 0$, and then

$$\beta_{YZ} = \rho_{MT} \frac{\sigma_{A_T}}{\sigma_{A_M}}$$

Evidence for a nonzero regression slope is therefore evidence for linkage disequilibrium between trait and marker loci. This, in turn, is generally regarded as evidence for genomic proximity of these loci. A cluster of SNPs with nonzero regression coefficients is likely to delineate the region of a chromosome containing a trait locus.

The marker variable could also be made to have zero additive variance, e.g. $Z_{MM} = p_m, Z_{Mn} = 0, Z_{mm} = p_M$, and then

$$\beta_{YZ} = \rho^2_{MT} \frac{\sigma_{D_T}}{\sigma_{D_M}}$$

The size of the regression coefficient is lower than in the additive case, partly because $\rho^2_{AB} \leq \rho_{AB}$ and partly because it is generally the case that $\sigma^2_{D_T} \leq \sigma^2_{A_T}$.

For any scoring of the marker genotypes, a significant regression coefficient implies a significant linkage disequilibrium measure ρ_{MT} between marker and disease loci.

Correlation It may be more convenient to work with the correlation of Y and Z. For an additive marker variable

$$\text{Corr}(Y, Z) = \rho_{YZ} = \rho_{MT} h_Y^{(T)}$$

where $(h_Y^{(T)})^2 = \sigma^2_{A_T} / (\sigma^2_{A_T} + \sigma^2_{D_T} + V_E)$ is the (narrow sense) *heritability* of trait Y due to locus **T**. Sample values r_{YZ} for the correlation ρ_{YZ} can be transformed to normal variables with Fisher's transformation

$$z = \frac{1}{2} \ln \left(\frac{1 + r_{YZ}}{1 - r_{YZ}} \right)$$

and then standard theory for correlation coefficients provides that, for $\alpha\%$ significance level and $(1 - \beta)\%$ power, the necessary sample size n is (approximately)

$$n = \left[\frac{2(z_{\alpha/2} + z_\beta)}{\ln \left(\frac{1 + \rho_{YZ}}{1 - \rho_{YZ}} \right)} \right]^2 + 3$$

For 90 % power, $z_\beta = 1.28$. For 90 % power and 1 % or 0.001 % significance level and for an SNP with $\rho^2_{MT} = 0.8$ to the disease gene and a trait with per-locus heritability $(h_Y^{(T)})^2 = 0.2$ these sizes are about 85 or 185. Although heritabilities of

0.2 are not uncommon, these are values over all causal loci and the per-locus values are much smaller.

Analysis of Variance Instead of regressing trait values on marker scores, the trait means could be compared among marker classes. The expected trait means follow as

$$\mathcal{E}(Y|M_u M_v) = \sum_{r,s} G_{rs} \Pr(T_r T_s | M_u M_v)$$

$$= \sum_{r,s} Grs \Pr(T_r M_u, T_s M_v)/\Pr(M_u M_v)$$

in general. For a trait locus with only two alleles, T, t, for marker homozygote MM and still assuming Hardy–Weinberg equilibrium

$$\mathcal{E}(Y|MM) = (G_{TT} P_{MT}^2 + 2G_{Tt} P_{MT} P_{Mt} + G_{tt} P_{Mt}^2)/p_M^2$$

The trait means among the three marker genotype classes are

$$\mathcal{E}(Y|MM) = \mu_G + 2\rho_{MT} A/p_M + \rho_{MT}^2 D/p_M^2$$

$$\mathcal{E}(Y|Mm) = \mu_G + \rho_{MT} A(1/p_M - 1/p_m) - \rho_{MT}^2 D/(p_M p_m)$$

$$\mathcal{E}(Y|mm) = \mu_G - 2\rho_{MT} A/p_m + \rho_{MT}^2 D/p_m^2$$

where $A = \sigma_{AT}\sqrt{(p_M p_m)}$, $D = \sigma_{DT}(p_M p_m)$, so that an analysis of variance will also test that $\rho_{MT} = 0$ and the test will be affected by both additive and dominance effects at the trait locus.

4.2 Dichotomous Traits

Case Only The case–control approach starts with independent samples of individuals who are either affected or not affected with a disease and compares marker frequencies between the two groups. The following development also applies to two arms of a clinical trial. The MM marker frequency among cases is

$$\Pr(MM|\text{Case}) = p_M^2 + \frac{1}{\mu_G}\left[p_M \rho_{MT} A + \rho_{MT}^2 \sigma_{D_T} D\right]$$

$$\Pr(Mm|\text{Case}) = 2p_M p_m + \frac{1}{\mu_G}\left[(p_m - p_M)\rho_{MT} A - 2\rho_{MT}^2 D\right]$$

$$\Pr(mm|\text{Case}) = p_m^2 + \frac{1}{\mu_G}\left[-p_m \rho_{MT} A + \rho_{MT}^2 D\right]$$

Combining the genotypic frequencies to give allele frequencies:

$$\Pr(M|\text{Case}) = p_M + \frac{\rho_{MT}\sigma_{A_T}}{2\mu_G}\sqrt{2p_M p_m}$$

$$\Pr(m|\text{Case}) = p_m - \frac{\rho_{MT}\sigma_{A_T}}{2\mu_G}\sqrt{2p_M p_m}$$

Case-only HWE Testing The inbreeding coefficient at the marker locus in the case population, from the earlier definition of f, now written as $f = [\Pr(MM|\text{Case}) - \Pr(M|\text{Case})^2]/\{\Pr(M|\text{Case})[1 - \Pr(M|\text{Case})]\}$, is

$$f = \frac{\rho_{MT}^2(2\mu_G\sigma_{D_T} - \sigma_{A_T}^2)}{(\mu_G\sqrt{2p_M/p_m} + \rho_{MT}\sigma_{A_T})(\mu_G\sqrt{2p_m/p_M} - \rho_{MT}\sigma_{A_T})}$$

so that a test for Hardy–Weinberg equilibrium ($f = 0$) at the marker among cases is actually a test for linkage disequilibrium between marker and trait loci in the whole population. The power of this test depends on nf^2 which is proportional to ρ_{MT}^4 so the power will decrease quickly as ρ_{MT} decreases.

It is common for investigators to assume a multiplicative trait model (i.e., additive on a log scale), but that leads to Hardy–Weinberg equilibrium at marker loci among cases since then $2\mu_G\sigma_{D_T} = \sigma_{A_T}^2$.

Case–Control An argument similar to that above provides the marker genotype frequencies among controls:

$$\Pr(MM|\text{Control}) = p_M^2 - \frac{1}{1-\mu_G}\left[p_M\rho_{MT}A + \rho_{MT}^2 D\right]$$

$$\Pr(Mm|\text{Control}) = 2p_M p_m - \frac{1}{1-\mu_G}\left[(p_m - p_M)\rho_{MT}A - 2\rho_{MT}^2 D\right]$$

$$\Pr(mm|\text{Control}) = p_m^2 - \frac{1}{1-\mu_G}\left[-p_m\rho_{MT}A + \rho_{MT}^2 D\right]$$

Adding these to give allele frequencies:

$$\Pr(M|\text{Control}) = p_M - \frac{\rho_{MT}A}{2(1-\mu_G)}$$

$$\Pr(m|\text{Control}) = p_m + \frac{\rho_{MT}A}{2(1-\mu_G)}$$

The simplest case–control test compares marker allele frequencies between the two samples and it is clearly equivalent to testing that $\rho_{MT} = 0$ since

$$\Pr(M|\text{Case}) - \Pr(M|\text{Control}) \propto \rho_{MT}\sigma_{A_T}\sqrt{2p_M p_m}$$

The test is not affected by nonadditivity at the trait locus.

Table 3 Notation for trend test

	$i = 0$	$i = 1$	$i = 2$	
Marker genotype	MM	Mm	mm	Total
Marker variable	Z_0	Z_1	Z_2	
Case counts	r_0	r_1	r_2	R
Control counts	s_0	s_1	s_2	S
Total counts	n_0	n_1	n_2	N

If the allelic counts for M, m in cases and controls are laid out in a 2×2 table, the contingency-table chi-square test statistic has 1 df. An alternative is to work with the 3×2 table of marker genotype counts in cases and controls and calculate a 2 df chi-square test statistic. This test is affected by both additivity and nonadditivity at the trait locus but it is sensitive to errors in genotype calls for rare alleles. The main problem with the allelic case–control test is its sensitivity to departures from Hardy–Weinberg equilibrium, and for this reason there is preference for trend tests.

Trend Test The Armitage trend test is based on a score statistic U. Using the notation in Table 3:

$$U = \sum_{i=0}^{2} Z_i \left(\frac{S}{N} r_i - \frac{R}{N} s_i \right)$$

This is also the sample covariance between marker variable Z and disease status scored as 0 or 1 for case or control.

With random sampling, the case and control counts are multinomially distributed and the expected value of U is

$$\mathcal{E}(U) = \frac{SR}{N} \sum_i Z_i (R_i - S_i)$$

where R_i, S_i are the expected values of r_i, s_i. This expected value can be written as

$$\mathcal{E}(U) = \frac{1}{\mu_G(1 - \mu_G)} \left[\rho_{MT} \sigma_{A_T} \sigma_{A_M} + \rho_{MT}^2 \sigma_{D_T} \sigma_{D_M} \right]$$

showing that it is zero when there is linkage equilibrium $\rho_{MT} = 0$.

The variance of U is

$$\text{Var}(U) = \frac{S^2 R}{N^2} \left(\sum_i Z_i^2 R_i - \left(\sum_i Z_i R_i \right)^2 \right) + \frac{SR^2}{N^2} \left(\sum_i Z_i^2 S_i - \left(\sum_i Z_i S_i \right)^2 \right)$$

Under the hypothesis of no association, $R_i = S_i$, $\mathcal{E}(U) = 0$ and

$$\text{Var}(U) = \frac{SR}{N} \left(\sum_i Z_i^2 R_i - \left(\sum_i Z_i R_i \right)^2 \right) = \frac{SR}{N} \left(\sigma_{A_M}^2 + \sigma_{D_M}^2 \right)$$

Assuming normality for U, the score test statistic is

$$X^2 = \frac{U^2}{\widehat{\text{Var}}(U)} = \frac{N(N \sum_i r_i Z_i - R \sum_i n_i Z_i)^2}{SR[N \sum_i n_i Z_i^2 - (\sum_i n_i Z_i)^2]}$$

and this is distributed as $\chi^2_{(1)}$ under the hypothesis $H_0 : \rho_{MT} = 0$.

It is usual to consider a linear trend test, say $Z_0 = 0, Z_1 = 1, Z_2 = 2$, so that $\sigma^2_{D_M} = 0$ and

$$X^2 = \frac{N[N(r_1 + 2r_2) - R(n_1 + 2n_2)]^2}{SR[N(n_1 + 4n_2) - (n_1 + 2n_2)^2]}$$

This will provide a test for additive effects at the disease locus. Setting $X_0 = p_m, X_1 = 0, X_2 = p_M$ gives $\sigma^2_{A_M} = 0$ and a test for nonadditive effects.

Effects of Inbreeding From the form of the allelic case–control test statistic

$$X_A^2 = \frac{2N[N(r_1 + 2r_2) - R(n_1 + 2n_2)]^2}{SR[2N(n_1 + 2n_2) - (n_1 + 2n_2)^2]}$$

and the previous form of the genotypic linear trend test statistic it can be shown that

$$\mathcal{E}(X_A^2) \approx (1 + f)$$

$$\mathcal{E}(X_T^2) \approx 1$$

when there is inbreeding to extent f in the population. The trend test is therefore robust to departures from Hardy–Weinberg equilibrium. The other general concern about association tests are that they are sensitive to population structure.

Effect of Population Structure The effect of population structure on association tests can be phrased in terms of the variation in allele frequencies over subpopulations (Fig. 1). This variation reflects the dependence among individuals imposed by the history of the population. If x_{jk} indicates the allelic state of allele k in individual j, it is now necessary to consider that these states are dependent among individuals, as indicated by joint probability $P_{A,A}$ for two individuals each carrying A:

$$\mathcal{E}(x_{jk} x_{j'k'}) = P_{A,A}, \quad j \neq j', k \neq k'$$

This is no longer p_A^2 as it was for the analyses within populations.

The expected value of squared sample allele frequency for a single subpopulation is changed to:

$$\mathcal{E}(\tilde{p}_A^2) = P_{A,A} + \frac{1}{2n}(p_A + P_{AA} - 2P_{A,A})$$

Population

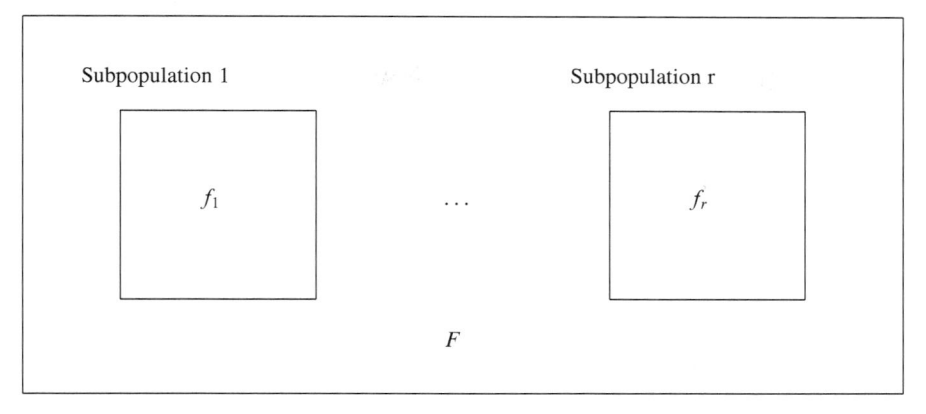

Fig. 2 Inbreeding coefficients in a structured population. Within a subpopulation: $P_{AA}^* = (p_A^*)^2 + f p_A^*(1 - p_A^*)$. Over all subpopulations: $P_{AA} = p_A^2 + F p_A (1 - p_A)$

so that the (total) variance is

$$\mathrm{Var}(\tilde{p}_A) = (P_{A,A} - p_A^2) + \frac{1}{n}(P_{AA} - P_{A,A}) + \frac{1}{2n}(p_A - P_{AA})$$

With this evolutionary perspective there is need for a new parameterization for joint allele frequencies to reflect the variation over subpopulations as well as over samples from one subpopulation:

$$P_{AA} = p_A^2 + p_A(1 - p_A)F$$

$$P_{A,A} = p_A^2 + p_A(1 - p_A)\theta$$

The total inbreeding coefficient F still refers to alleles within individuals but is for all individuals in the collection of subpopulations (see Fig. 2). The coancestry coefficient θ_i is for alleles in two individuals in the ith subpopulation. A common value θ is assumed here for all subpopulations and the subpopulations are assumed to be independent ($\theta_i = \theta, \theta_{ii'} = 0$ in Fig. 3). The frequency p_A is now the average over all subpopulations, and the total variance is

$$\mathrm{Var}(\tilde{p}_A) = p_A(1 - p_A)\left[\theta + \frac{1}{n}(F - \theta) + \frac{1}{2n}(1 - F)\right]$$

There are three components of variance: among populations $p_A(1 - p_A)\theta$, among individuals within populations $p_A(1 - p_A)(F - \theta)$, and among alleles within individuals $p_A(1 - p_A)(1 - F)$, with a total variance of $p_A(1 - p_A)$.

Population

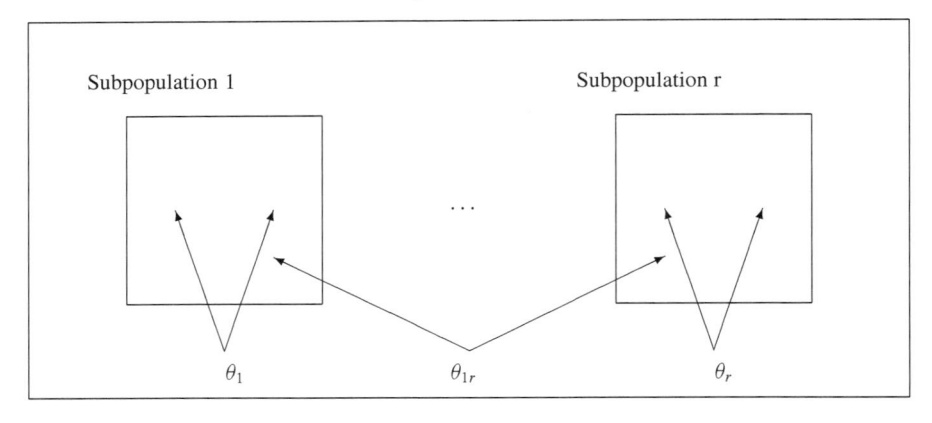

Fig. 3 Coancestry coefficients in a structured population. Within the ith subpopulation: $P_{A.A} = p_A^2 + \theta_i p_A(1 - p_A)$. Between the i, i'th subpopulations: $P_{A.A} = p_A^2 + \theta_{ii'} p_A(1 - p_A)$

Within a subpopulation it is still the case that

$$P_{AA}^* = (p_A^*)^2 + f p_A^*(1 - p_A^*)$$

Taking expectation values over populations, and using $f = (F - \theta)(1 - \theta)$:

$$\mathcal{E}(p_A^*) = p_A$$

$$\mathcal{E}[(p_A^*)^2] = p_A^2 + \theta p_A(1 - p_A)$$

$$\mathcal{E}(P_{AA}^*) = [p_A^2 + \theta p_A(1 - p_A)] + f[p_A - p_A^2 - \theta p_A(1 - p_A)]$$

$$= p_A^2 + F p_A(1 - p_A)$$

If x_i, y_i, z_i are the proportions of cases, controls and all samples from the ith subpopulation, the case–control and trend test statistics have expectations

$$\mathcal{E}(X_A^2) \approx \frac{2RS\theta \sum_i (x_i - y_i)^2 + N(F - \theta) + N(1 - \theta)}{N(1 - \theta \sum_i z_i^2) - (F - \theta)/2 - (1 - \theta)/2}$$

$$\mathcal{E}(X_T^2) \approx \frac{2RS\theta \sum_i (x_i - y_i)^2 + N(F - \theta) + N(1 - \theta)}{N[(1 + F) - 2\theta \sum_i z_i^2]}$$

The behavior of these test statistics is therefore affected by both inbreeding (within subpopulations) and population structure (the existence of subpopulations).

If there is random mating within each subpopulation, $F = \theta$, and if there are equal numbers of cases and controls $R = S = N/2$. If there are many subpopulations, it is possible to ignore the term $F \sum_i z_i^2$ in the denominator and then

$$\mathcal{E}(X_A^2) = \mathcal{E}(X_T^2) \approx 1 + \frac{RF \sum_i (x_i - y_i)^2 - 2F}{1 + F}$$

as was given by Pritchard and Donnelly [14].

If there is only one subpopulation ($x_1 = y_1 = z_1 = 1$):

$$\mathcal{E}(X_A^2) \approx 1 + f$$

$$\mathcal{E}(X_T^2) \approx 1$$

as before.

5 Treatment Effects

In the previous section we considered individuals categorized by case/control status or by either of two treatment arms in a clinical trial. We now generalize this to allow for continuous treatments and we consider the joint effects of treatment and genotype on response. We preserve the notation of Y for response and X for genotype, and introduce S for treatment. For the jth subject and lth SNP we let μ_{lj} be the conditional mean response, recognizing that this depends on both genotype and treatment:

$$\mu_{lj} = \mathcal{E}(Y_j | X_{lj}, S_j)$$

with link function

$$g(\mu_{lj}) = \beta_0 + \beta_1 X_{lj} + \gamma_0 S_j + \gamma_1 X_{lj} S_j$$

For linear regression, $g(\mu) = \mu$ and for logistic regression $g(\mu) = \ln[\mu/(1 - \mu)]$.

In the previous section we accommodated a range of genetic models with the marker variable Z. We now express these models in terms of subgroup treatment effects as in Eq. (1). For an additive model, such as the genotype variable being the number of minor alleles, and for linear regression

$$\Delta_{l0} = \gamma_0$$

$$\Delta_{l1} = \gamma_0 + \gamma_1$$

$$\Delta_{l2} = \gamma_0 + 2\gamma_1$$

whereas for logistic regression the Δ's are treatment log-odds ratios specific for each genotype subgroup.

A dominant model regards the effects of one or two major alleles being the same and X_{lj} is replaced by 1 if there are one or no minor alleles and 0 if there are two minor alleles:

$$g(\mu_{lj}) = \beta_0 + \beta_1 \mathbf{1}(X_{lj} \geq 1) + \gamma_0 S_j + \gamma_1 \mathbf{1}(X_{lj} \geq 1)S_j$$

where the variable $\mathbf{1}(a)$ is 1 if a is true. This implies

$$\Delta_{l0} = \gamma_0$$

$$\Delta_{l1} = \gamma_0 + \gamma_1$$

$$\Delta_{l2} = \gamma_0 + \gamma_1$$

Conversely, a recessive model regards the effects of one or two minor alleles being the same and X_{lj} is replaced by 1 if there are no minor alleles and 0 if there are one or two minor alleles:

$$g(\mu_{lj}) = \beta_0 + \beta_1 \mathbf{1}(X_{lj} = 2) + \gamma_0 S_j + \gamma_1 \mathbf{1}(X_{lj} = 2)S_j$$

This implies

$$\Delta_{l0} = \gamma_0$$

$$\Delta_{l1} = \gamma_0$$

$$\Delta_{l2} = \gamma_0 + \gamma_1$$

A general, or nominal, model assigns different effect levels to each marker genotype:

$$g(\mu_{lj}) = \beta_0 + \beta_1 \mathbf{1}(X_{lj} = 1) + \beta_2 \mathbf{1}(X_{lj} = 2)$$

$$+ \gamma_0 S_i + \gamma_1 \mathbf{1}(X_{lj} = 1)S_j + \gamma_2 \mathbf{1}(X_{lj} = 2)S_j$$

This implies

$$\Delta_{l0} = \gamma_0$$

$$\Delta_{l1} = \gamma_0 + \gamma_1$$

$$\Delta_{l2} = \gamma_0 + \gamma_2$$

Table 4 Likelihoods for testing gene by treatment interaction

Model	Likelihood	Number of parameters	Maximum $\ln(L)$
Full	$X + S + X \times S$	$p + q$	$\ln(L_1)$
Null	$X + S$	p	$\ln(L_0)$

Table 5 Likelihood ratio tests for specific models

Model	Null parameters	LR test
Additive	γ_1	$\chi^2_{(1)}$
Dominant	γ_1	$\chi^2_{(1)}$
Recessive	γ_1	$\chi^2_{(1)}$
Nominal	γ_1, γ_2	$\chi^2_{(2)}$

Table 6 Power for gene by treatment interaction

Truth	Test assumes Additive	Nominal	Dominant
Additive	0.882	0.800	0.746
Dominant	0.607	0.611	0.746

5.1 Testing for Gene by Treatment Interaction

A general testing procedure uses the likelihood ratio test based on alternative pairs of models for treatment and genetic effects. To test for no gene by treatment interaction, the likelihoods are displayed in Table 4. Under the null hypothesis of no interaction

$$2[\ln(L_1) - \ln(L_0)] \sim \chi^2_{(q)}$$

In Table 5 we display the interaction test parameters and distributions for each of the genetic models.

Designing a study to test for gene by treatment interaction is made complicated by the true genetic model being unknown. There is a body of literature to suggest that complex traits are additive, reflecting the independent and additive effects of alleles at the trait loci [8] but also a suggestion that at least some genes act in a nonadditive fashion [1,20]. In Table 6 we show powers of likelihood ratio tests under different model assumptions when the true model is either additive or dominant. For simulations we used data sets consisting of 780 cases and 780 controls. For an additive structure we assumed additivity on the probability scale with a prevalence of 0.4 when $X_l = 0$ and 0.3, 0.2 for $X_l = 1, 2$, respectively. For a dominant model we used a prevalence of 0.4 when $X_l = 0$ and 0.28 when X_l is either 1 or 2. Use of logistic regression with an additive genetic effect on the log odds scale is only an approximation to the true data-generating model (e.g., additive on probability scale).

5.2   Multiple Comparisons

With millions of SNPs being scored or imputed for each study participant, the issue of multiple testing needs to be considered. If α^* is the per-test (per-SNP) false-positive error rate, then a set of L tests under the null is expected to produce $\alpha^* L$ false positives. For $L \sim 10^6$ this number can be large. The family-wise error rate (FWER) α is the probability of at least one false positive in a set of tests where all the null hypotheses are true. The Bonferroni approach sets the per-test error to $\alpha^* = \alpha/L$, or 5×10^{-8} for an FWER of 0.05 and one million tests. The Sidak approach uses $\alpha^* = 1 - (1 - \alpha)^{1/L}$, with the very similar value of 5.13×10^{-8} in this case.

These simple multiple comparison corrections are conservative and they may assume independent tests even though linkage disequilibrium prevents whole-genome sets of SNPs being independent. Permutation procedures can yield correct FWER values for dependent tests, at the expense of being computationally intensive and dataset dependent. These procedures keep the genetic profiles intact and permute the outcomes Y among individuals: in essence destroying any genotype-trait association and producing data for which the null hypotheses at each SNP are true. Repeated permutations lead to reference distributions for the single-SNP test statistics. Approximations were proposed by Nyholt [13].

5.3   Bayes' Factors

Genetics research is embracing "evidence" criteria such as likelihood ratios. In linkage studies, where the transmission of trait values and genotypes are traced down pedigrees, LOD scores based on likelihood ratios have long been used. The appeal of an alternative that does not rely on p-values, the probabilities of data assuming the null hypothesis to be true, is that power (probabilities when the null is not true) and sample size can be considered when choosing criteria for evaluating tests.

The Bayes Factor is the ratio of the probability of the data under the null to the probability under the alternative hypothesis. Wakefield [17] showed that an Approximate Bayes Factor (ABF) is given by

$$\text{ABF} = \sqrt{\frac{V + W}{V}} \exp\left(-\frac{Z^2}{2} \frac{W}{V + W} \right)$$

where the maximum likelihood estimate $\hat{\theta}$ of a parameter of interest is normally distributed with mean θ and variance V. The test statistic Z for the hypothesis $H_0 : \theta = 0$ is $Z = \hat{\theta}/\sqrt{V}$. The Bayesian aspect of the analysis is to assign a prior distribution for parameter θ, such as normal with mean 0 and variance W, and to decide in favor of the alternative hypothesis if

$$\text{ABF} \times \text{PO} < R \tag{2}$$

The prior odds PO is the ratio of the probabilities of the hypotheses before the data are collected, $PO = Pr(H_0)/Pr(H_1)$ and R is the ratio of costs: the cost of a false non-discovery divided by the cost of a false discovery. For example, R is the cost of a Type II error divided by that of a Type I error.

In practice, values are assigned to (PO/R) and then the ABF threshold is determined. It may be that PO is 10,000 and $R = 1$, so that the threshold is 10^{-4}. The ABF threshold is translated into a threshold for the test statistic from Eq. (2).

5.4 Bioinformatics Tools

The biological significance of an association found between an SNP and an outcome can be phrased in terms of the biological function of an SNP or the biological pathway to which it belongs. There are a variety of tools available to help this activity:

- UCSC Genome Bioinformatics (http://ucsc.genome.edu).
- Fast SNP (http://fastsnp.ibm.sinica.edu.tw).
- Gene Ontology (GO) (http://www.geneontology.org).

These and other tools were reviewed by Bansal et al. [1].

6 Analyses with Multiple Markers

For a set of individuals j there is information Y_j on the outcome of interest, on the treatment or dose S_j, and on the genetic profile $\mathbf{X}_j = \{X_{lj}, l = 1, 2, \ldots L\}$. A series of questions can be posed:

- How can the genetic markers be used to predict outcome?
- How can the genetic markers be used to score the individuals with respect to treatment benefit?
- How can the genetic markers be used to create a treatment decision function?

We address these questions in a generalized linear model framework:

$$\mathcal{E}(Y_j | \mathbf{X}_j, S_j) = \mu_j$$
$$g(\mu_j) = \beta(\mathbf{X}_j) + \gamma(\mathbf{X}_j) \times S_j$$

Hastie and Tibshirani [7] introduced a "varying coefficient model." As a simple example

$$g(\mu_j) = (\beta_0 + \beta_1 X_{1j} + \ldots + \beta_L X_{Lj}) + (\gamma_0 + \gamma_1 X_{1j} + \ldots + \gamma_L X_{Lj}) \times S_j$$

Major challenges to this work include

- How do we select SNPs to include in $\beta(\mathbf{X}_j)$ and $\gamma(\mathbf{X}_j)$?
- Should we also consider epistasis: gene by gene interactions, $X_{lj} \times X_{l'j}, l \neq l'$ or higher-order interaction?
- How can we fit a model when L, the number of SNPs, is much greater than n, the number of individuals?
- How do the model choice criteria reflect the ultimate clinical goal of the model (for example, prediction versus treatment selection)?

6.1 Regularization Methods

Tibshirani [16] introduced "lasso" for regression shrinkage and selection. He discussed maximizing an objective function, such as a likelihood, subject to constraints or a penalty. More generally, a set of parameters ` is estimated as

$$\hat{\boldsymbol{\theta}} = \underset{\theta}{\operatorname{argmax}} \left(\sum_j \ln \Pr(Y_j | \mathbf{X}_j, S_j, \grave{}) - \lambda \sum_j |\theta_j|^p \right)$$

There are three special cases:

- $p = 1$: Lasso [16] with penalty $\lambda \sum_j |\theta_j|$.
- $p = 2$: Ridge Regression [9] with penalty $\lambda \sum_j |\theta_j|^2$.
- $p = 1, 2$: Elastic Net [19] with penalty $\lambda_1 \sum_j |\theta_j| + \lambda_2 \sum_j |\theta_j|^2$.

Some comments about regularization methods are:

- Lasso tends to "select" variables by keeping $\hat{\beta}_l = 0$.
- Ridge regression tends to include all variables, but with small coefficients. This is essentially no selection.
- Lasso will not estimate a model with more nonzero coefficients than there are individuals.
- Fast algorithms exist for calculating regularization paths.
- Lasso tends to select only one variable from a set of highly correlated predictors.

6.2 Example

Wu et al. [18] presented an analysis of SNP data in a case–control setting, and conducted simulations to demonstrate the feasibility of allowing for interactions among SNPs. In their example they analyzed $n = 2,200$ subjects with 778 having Coeliac Disease and 1,422 as controls. Using LASSO Wu et al. [18] constructed

Table 7 Treatment selection example

Genotype	$\bar{Y}_j(0)$	$\bar{Y}_j(1)$	A_0	A_1	A^*
0 (30%)	10	20	0	1	1
1 (50%)	10	10	0	1	0
2 (20%)	15	5	0	1	0
Population mean			11	12	14

a multi-marker predictive model using $L = 310,637$ SNPs. In order to explore models of increasing dimension the authors chose the L_1 penalty parameter λ to obtain a fixed number (e.g., 5, 10, 20, 50) of predictors with nonzero coefficients, and used cross-validation to evaluate the accuracy of models with increasing dimension. Using a sequence of models has the attractive property that subsets of markers can be ordered in terms of their inclusion in the regression models. Rather than focusing on a specific model selection criterion such as the area under the ROC curve, or a statistical loss function, Wu et al. [18] evaluate a sequence of models of a specified dimensionality (such as using 50 SNPs). These authors clearly demonstrate the ability of modern penalized regression methods to consider development and evaluation of multi-marker models, and provide guidance for model development and the potential evaluation of interactions.

6.3 Treatment Selection

How can genetic marker analysis provide a scoring for treatment selection? To answer this question it is necessary to state the goals in statistical terms. Gunter et al. [6] formulated an action function and then defined the resulting population mean outcome that would result when using the specified action function:

$$\text{Action function: } A(\mathbf{X}_j) = a$$

$$\text{Population result: } \mathcal{E}_a \mathcal{E}_Y [Y_j(a) | A(\mathbf{X}_j) = a] = \mu_A$$

Here $Y_j(a)$ is the potential outcome for subject j if treated with choice a. For example, $a = 1$ may be "treat" and $a = 0$ may be "do not treat." Alternatively, a may be a dose level.

As a small example, consider the values shown in Table 7 for a single marker. There are three genetic marker values (0,1,2) and two treatment values (0,1). The function A_0 always assigns $A = 0$, while A_1 always assigns $A = 1$. However, the action function A^* is optimal in the sense it maximizes μ_A over all possible functions A.

With a vector $\mathbf{X}_j$ of genetic values the optimal action rule is

$$A^*(\mathbf{X}_j) : \text{argmax}_A \mu_A = \text{argmax}_A \mathcal{E}_a \mathcal{E}_Y [Y_j(a) | A(\mathbf{X}_j) = a]$$

The goal is to determine which components of $\mathbf{X}_j$ are prescriptive markers, i.e. those with qualitative interactions rather than simply having quantitative interactions with treatment.

The space of functions $\{A(x)\}$ has high dimension: with each genotype taking three values, and with L total genotypes there are 3^L possible genotypes that the function $A(x)$ can evaluate. In addition, there are two possible outcomes for each genotype evaluated (e.g., treat, or not treat) leading to $(3^L)^2$ binary actions a. Therefore, computation methods are needed to define model search strategies that can maximize the intended performance metric such as μ_A in order to identify an optimal allocation rule, A^*.

Gunter et al. [6] suggested that the following marginal characteristics of a marker are important for that marker to have prescriptive potential:

- Fraction with benefit:

$$p_{l1} = \mathcal{E}\left\{\mathbf{1}\left(\operatorname{argmax}_a \mathcal{E}[Y_j(a)|X_{lj}, A(X_{lj}) = a] = 1\right)\right\}$$

- Interaction magnitude:

$$D_l = \max_j \left\{\mathcal{E}[Y_j(a)|X_{lj}, a = 1] - \mathcal{E}[Y_j(a)|X_{lj}, a = 0]\right\}$$
$$- \min_j \left\{\mathcal{E}[Y_j(a)|X_{lj}, a = 1] - \mathcal{E}[Y_j(a)|X_{lj}, a = 0]\right\}$$

Since p_{l1} doesn't capture the number of subjects who have their treatment changed because of their genetic profile, Gunter et al. [6] suggest using $P_l = p_{l1}(1 - p_{l1})$. The motivation for considering marginal measures for X_{lj} is to provide an algorithm that can search among candidate functions $A(\mathbf{X}_j)$ using an attractive subset of $\mathbf{X}_j$.

Gunter et al. [6] then suggest two criteria for ranking markers:

$$U_l = \text{Scale}(P_l) \times \text{Scale}(D_l)$$
$$\text{Scale}(x_l) = (x_l) - \min_k x_k)/(\max_k x_k - \min_k x_k)$$

The second criterion measures the impact on the mean outcome using X_{lj} optimally to direct treatment:

$$T_l = \mathcal{E}_X\left\{\max_a \mathcal{E}[Y_j(a)|X_{lj}, A = a]\right\} - \max(\mu_{A_0}, \mu_{A_1})$$
$$= \mu_{A^*} - \max(\mu_{A_0}, \mu_{A_1})$$

With all these quantities defined, we can state the selection algorithm of Gunter et al. [6]:

1. Use lasso with K-fold cross-validation to obtain an additive model estimate of $\mathcal{E}[Y_j | \mathbf{X}_j, S_l]$.
2. Estimate U_l and/or T_l, then rank $\mathbf{X}_l$.
3. For $h = 1, 2, \ldots, H$:

   - Use lasso with top h markers, main effects from step 1, and interactions between top h markers and treatment.
   - Estimate λ_1 based on CV with a focus on μ_{A*}^h obtained from h markers: $A^*(\mathbf{X}_l^h)$.

4. Choose h that maximizes μ_{A*}^h. Done.

Step 1 of this algorithm is suggested in order to stabilize estimates of the mean function $\mathcal{E}[Y_j | \mathbf{X}_j, S_j]$ used to estimate U_l and T_l. It may not be needed for genotype markers. This model selection targets out-of-sample estimation of the optimal population outcome. The algorithm is limited to a small number of candidate models. There may be other search procedures but Gunter et al. [6] used simulations to compare their algorithm to standard lasso and found it performs slightly better.

The work of Gunter et al. [6] offers a focus on model development with the goal of defining a treatment selection function. These authors target an optimal result at the population level.

7 Resemblance Between Relatives

Some individuals in a clinical trial may be related to each other, whether or not this is by design. Here "related" means members of the same family. There is also a low-level evolutionary relatedness that results in a low level of inbreeding within a study population. Because relatedness depends on previous generations it is necessary to work with the coefficients F and θ, and extensions of these, rather than the within-population coefficient f.

To extend the earlier treatment, it may now be supposed there is an arbitrary number of alleles at a trait/response locus, and the genetic value for genotype $T_r T_s$ is written as

$$G_{rs} = \mu_0 + \alpha_r + \alpha_s + \delta_{rs}$$

where

$$\mu_0 = \sum_r \sum_s p_r p_s G_{rs} = G_{..}$$

$$\alpha_r = \sum_s p_s G_{rs} - \mu = G_{r.} - G_{..}$$

$$\delta_{rs} = G_{rs} - \mu - \alpha_r - \alpha_s = G_{rs} - G_{r.} - G_{s.} + G_{..}$$

These imply that $\sum_r p_r \alpha_r = 0, \sum_r \delta_{rs} = 0$. The variance components are

$$\sigma_A^2 = 2 \sum_r p_r \alpha_r^2$$

$$\sigma_D^2 = \sum_r \sum_s p_r p_s \delta_{rs}^2$$

If several loci contribute to a trait, the effects of all alleles can be summed, and interactions (epistasis) introduced between loci. For an individual with alleles $T_{lr}, r = 1, 2$, at locus l:

$$Y = \mu + \sum_l \left[\sum_r \alpha_{lr} + \sum_r \sum_{r'} \delta_{lrr'} \right]$$

$$+ \sum_{l \neq l'} \left[\sum_r \sum_{r'} (\alpha\alpha)_{lr,l'r'} + \sum_r \sum_s \sum_{s'} (\alpha\delta)_{lr,l'ss'} + \sum_r \sum_{r'} \sum_s \sum_{s'} (\delta\delta)_{lrr',l'ss'} \right] + \cdots$$

The total genetic variance becomes

$$\mathrm{Var}(G) = \sigma_A^2 + \sigma_D^2 + \sigma_{AA}^2 + \sigma_{AD}^2 + \sigma_{DD}^2 + \cdots$$

where the variance components are

$$\sigma_A^2 = 2 \sum_l \sum_r p_{lr} \alpha_{lr}^2$$

$$\sigma_D^2 = \sum_l \sum_r \sum_{r'} p_{lr} p_{lr'} \delta_{lrr'}^2$$

$$\sigma_{AA}^2 = 2 \sum_{l \neq l'} \sum_r \sum_{r'} p_{lr} p_{l'r'} (\alpha\alpha)_{lr,l'r'}^2$$

$$\cdots$$

7.1   Trait Mean in Inbred Populations

Inbreeding, whether due to individuals having related parents or simply a consequence of populations being finite, affects the trait or response mean in a population. If random members of a population are inbred to an extent F relative to a reference or founder population, the genotype frequencies are

$$P_{rr} = p_r^2 + F p_r (1 - p_r)$$

$$P_{rs} = 2p_r p_s (1 - F), \quad r \neq s$$

The expected trait value is, therefore,

$$
\begin{aligned}
\mu_F &= \sum_r \sum_s P_{rs}(\mu_0 + \alpha_r + \alpha_s + \delta_{rs}) \\
&= \sum_r \left[F p_r + (1 - F) p_r^2 \right] (\mu_0 + 2\alpha_r + \delta_{rr}) \\
&\quad + \sum_{r \neq s} \left[p_r p_s (1 - F) \right] (\mu_0 + \alpha_r + \alpha_s + \delta_{rs}) \\
&= F \sum_r p_r (\mu_0 + 2\alpha_r + \delta_{rr}) + (1 - F) \sum_r \sum_s p_r p_s (\mu_0 + \alpha_r + \alpha_s + \delta_{rs}) \\
&= F \left(\mu_0 + \sum_r p_r \delta_{rr} \right) + (1 - F)(\mu_0) \\
&= \mu_0 + FH
\end{aligned}
$$

This result uses the notation $H = \sum_r p_r \delta_{rr}$ where the δ's terms are as defined in the non-inbreeding case. The mean in an inbred population changes with the degree of inbreeding and the degree of dominance.

For a trait affected by multiple loci, the mean is also affected by the two-locus inbreeding coefficient and the degree of dominance by dominance epistasis.

7.2   Genetic Variance in Inbred Populations

For the trait variance, it is necessary to find the expected value of the square of the linear model for trait values. Using a similar approach as that for the mean:

$$
\begin{aligned}
\mathcal{E}(G_{rs}^2) &= F \sum_r p_r (\mu_0^2 + 4\alpha_r^2 + \delta_{rr}^2 + 4\mu_0 \alpha_i + 2\mu_0 \delta_{rr} + 4\alpha_r \delta_{rr}) \\
&\quad + (1 - F) \sum_{r,s} p_r p_s (\mu_0^2 + \alpha_r^2 + \alpha_s^2 + 2\alpha_r \alpha_s + 2\mu_0 \alpha_r + 2\mu_0 \alpha_s \\
&\qquad + 2\mu_0 \delta_{rs} + 2\alpha_r \delta_{rs} + 2\alpha_r \delta_{rs} + \delta_{rs}^2) \\
&= F \left[\mu_0^2 + 4 \sum_r p_r \alpha_r^2 + \sum_r p_r \delta_{rr}^2 + 2\mu_0 \sum_r p_r \delta_{rr} + 4 \sum_r p_r \alpha_r \delta_{rr} \right] \\
&\quad + (1 - F) \left(\mu_0^2 + 2 \sum_r p_r \alpha_r^2 + \sum_{r,s} p_r p_s \delta_{rs}^2 \right)
\end{aligned}
$$

The genetic variance becomes

$$\sigma_G^2 = 2(1+F)\sum_r p_r\alpha_r^2 + (1-F)\sum_{r,s} p_r p_s \delta_{rs}^2 + F\sum_r p_r \delta_{rr}^2$$

$$+ 4F\sum_r p_r\alpha_r\delta_{rr} - F^2\left(\sum_r p_r\delta_{rr}\right)^2$$

$$= (1+F)\sigma_A^2 + (1-F)\sigma_D^2 + 4FD_1 + FD_2 + F(1-F)H^2$$

to introduce $D_1 = \sum_r p_r\alpha_r\delta_{rr}$ and $D_2 = \sum_r p_r\delta_{rr}^2$. This expression for variance allows for inbreeding but not for linkage disequilibrium among the trait loci. For two equally frequent alleles, $D_1 = 0, D_2 = 0$. For additive traits, $H = D_1 = D_2 = 0$.

For a trait affected by multiple loci, the variance in an inbred population involves the two-locus inbreeding coefficient F_{11} as well as the usual one locus coefficient:

$$\sigma_G^2 = (1+F)\sigma_A^2 + (1-F)\sigma_D^2 + (1+2F+F_{11})\sigma_{AA}^2$$

$$+ (1-F_{11})\sigma_{AD}^2 + (1-2F+F_{11})\sigma_{DD}^2 + \dots$$

It is not always the case that $F_{11} = F^2$. This expression for variance allows for inbreeding but not for linkage disequilibrium among the trait loci.

7.3   Genetic Covariance for Two Individuals

If J, J', with genotypes $T_r T_s$ and $T_{r'} T_{s'}$, are two members of a population, the covariance of trait values for the two individuals rests on the covariance of their genetic values which, in turn, rests on their joint genotypic frequencies:

$$\text{Cov}(G_J, G_{J'}) = \mathcal{E}(G_J G_{J'}) - \mathcal{E}(G_J)\mathcal{E}(G_{J'})$$

$$\mathcal{E}(G_J G_{J'}) = \sum_{r,s,r',s'} P_{rs,r's'} G_{rs} G_{r's'}$$

For one individual P_{rs} can be written in terms of allele frequencies and the inbreeding coefficient F. For two individuals $P_{rs,r's'}$ needs an expanded set of probabilities that alleles are identical by descent (ibd).

A complete description of the ibd status among four alleles a, b, c, d carried by two individuals J, J' with alleles ab and cd requires 15 measures, as opposed to the two, F and $1-F$, for one individual. If there is no need to distinguish between the identity status for maternal and paternal alleles, the 15 ibd states can be collapsed into the nine states shown in Fig. 4. Solid lines in that figure join alleles that are identical by descent. State S_3, shown as identity among alleles a, b, c also represents identity among alleles a, b, d. Note here that a, b, c, d are labels to distinguish one allele from another: they do not indicate allelic type.

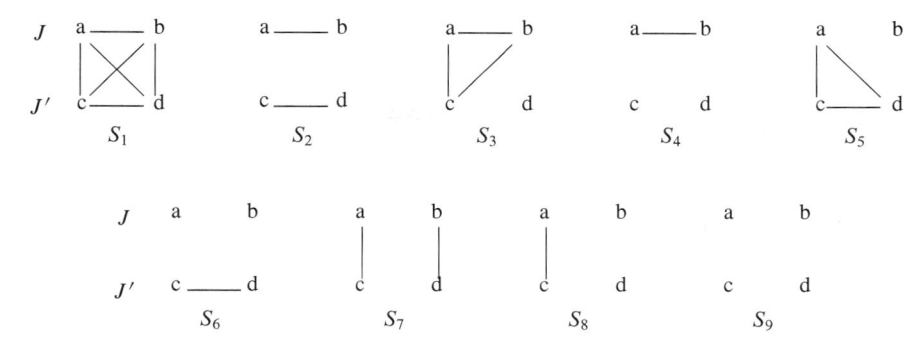

Fig. 4 Reduced identity states S for two individuals $J(a, b)$ and $J'(c, d)$

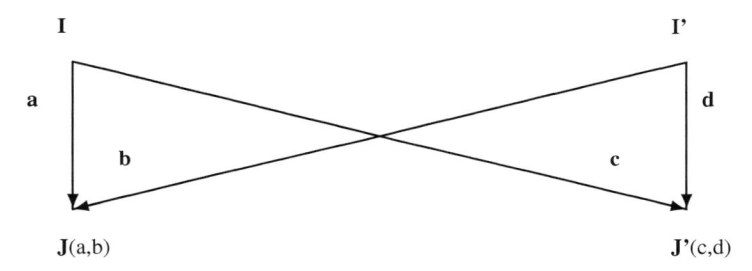

Fig. 5 IBD coefficients for Sibs J, J' from unrelated parents I, I'

The coancestry coefficient $\theta_{JJ'}$ referred to earlier is the probability that a random allele from $J(ab)$ is ibd ($\equiv$) to a random allele from $J'(cd)$:

$$\theta_{JJ'} = \frac{1}{4} [\Pr(a \equiv c) + \Pr(a \equiv d) + \Pr(b \equiv c) + \Pr(b \equiv d)]$$

$$= \Delta_1 + \frac{1}{2}(\Delta_3 + \Delta_5 + \Delta_7) + \frac{1}{4}\Delta_8$$

For non-inbred relatives

$$\theta = \frac{1}{2}\Delta_7 + \frac{1}{4}\Delta_8$$

As an example, the pedigree for two non-inbred sibs J, J' with parents I, I' is shown in Fig. 5.

Non-inbred Relatives When neither individual is inbred, neither a, b nor c, d are ibd. There are only three states and the three probabilities are often written as $k_2 = \Delta_7, k_1 = \Delta_8$ or $k_0 = \Delta_9$ to indicate the number of pairs of ibs alleles carried by the two individuals. Values of these three probabilities for some common relationships are shown in Table 8.

Table 8 Identity coefficients for common non-inbred relatives

Relationship	k_2	k_1	k_0	$\theta = \frac{1}{2}k_2 + \frac{1}{4}k_1$
Identical twins	1	0	0	$\frac{1}{2}$
Full sibs	$\frac{1}{4}$	$\frac{1}{2}$	$\frac{1}{4}$	$\frac{1}{4}$
Parent child	0	1	0	$\frac{1}{4}$
Double first cousins	$\frac{1}{16}$	$\frac{3}{8}$	$\frac{9}{16}$	$\frac{1}{8}$
Half sibs[a]	0	$\frac{1}{2}$	$\frac{1}{2}$	$\frac{1}{8}$
First cousins	0	$\frac{1}{4}$	$\frac{3}{4}$	$\frac{1}{16}$
Unrelated	0	0	1	0

[a]Also grandparent grandchild and avuncular (e.g., uncle niece)

Table 9 SNP genotype probabilities for pairs of relatives

Genotypes	General	Non-inbred
AA, AA	$\Delta_1 p_A + (\Delta_2 + \Delta_3 + \Delta_5 + \Delta_7)p_A^2$ $+(\Delta_4 + \Delta_6 + \Delta_8)p_A^3 + \Delta_9 p_A^4$	$k_0 p_A^4 + k_1 p_A^3 + k_2 p_A^2$
aa, aa	$\Delta_1 p_a + (\Delta_2 + \Delta_3 + \Delta_5 + \Delta_7)p_a^2$ $+(\Delta_4 + \Delta_6 + \Delta_8)p_a^3 + \Delta_9 p_a^4$	$k_0 p_a^4 + k_1 p_a^3 + k_2 p_a^2$
Aa, Aa	$2\Delta_7 p_A p_a + \Delta_8 p_A p_a + 4\Delta_9 p_A^2 p_a^2$	$4k_0 p_A^2 p_a^2 + k_1 p_A p_a + 2k_2 p_A p_a$
AA, Aa	$\Delta_3 p_A p_a + (2\Delta_4 + \Delta_8)p_A^2 p_a + 2\Delta_9 p_A^3 p_a$	$2k_0 p_A^3 p_a + k_1 p_A^2 p_a$
Aa, AA	$\Delta_5 p_A p_a + (2\Delta_6 + \Delta_8)p_A^2 p_a + 2\Delta_9 p_A^3 p_a$	$2k_0 p_A^3 p_a + k_1 p_A^2 p_a$
aa, Aa	$\Delta_3 p_A p_a + (2\Delta_4 + \Delta_8)p_A p_a^2 + 2\Delta_9 p_A p_a^3$	$2k_0 p_A p_a^3 + k_1 p_A p_a^2$
Aa, aa	$\Delta_5 p_A p_a + (2\Delta_6 + \Delta_8)p_A p_a^2 + 2\Delta_9 p_A p_a^3$	$2k_0 p_A p_a^3 + k_1 p_A p_a^2$
AA, aa	$\Delta_2 p_A p_a + \Delta_4 p_A p_a^2 + \Delta_6 p_A^2 p_a + \Delta_9 p_A^2 p_a^2$	$k_0 p_A^2 p_a^2$
aa, AA	$\Delta_2 p_A p_a + \Delta_6 p_A p_a^2 + \Delta_4 p_A^2 p_a + \Delta_9 p_A^2 p_a^2$	$k_0 p_A^2 p_a^2$

7.4 Joint Genotypic Probabilities for Relatives

The set of identity measures $\Delta_i = \Pr(S_i)$ for identity states S_i allow the joint genotypic probabilities to be written as in Table 9 for SNPs. These in turn allow for the covariance in trait values to be found for any pair of relatives.

7.5 Genetic Covariance for Non-inbred Relatives

The general expression for covariance can be shown to be

$$\mathcal{C}_{JJ'} = 2\theta_{JJ'}\sigma_A^2 + \Delta_7 \sigma_D^2 + (4\Delta_1 + \Delta_3 + \Delta_5)D_1$$
$$+ \Delta_1 D_2 + (\Delta_1 + \Delta_2 - F_J F_{J'})H^2$$

Table 10 Genetic covariances of common non-inbred relatives

Relationship	Genetic covariance
Identical twins	$\sigma_A^2 + \sigma_D^2$
Full sibs	$\frac{1}{2}\sigma_A^2 + \frac{1}{4}\sigma_D^2$
Parent-child	$\frac{1}{2}\sigma_A^2$
Double first cousins	$\frac{1}{4}\sigma_A^2 + \frac{1}{16}\sigma_D^2$
Half sibs[a]	$\frac{1}{4}\sigma_A^2$
First cousins	$\frac{1}{8}\sigma_A^2$
Unrelated	0

[a] Also grandparent–grandchild and avuncular (e.g., uncle–niece)

When J and J' are the same individual, $\theta_{JJ'} = (1 + F)/2$, $\Delta_1 = F$ and $\Delta_7 = (1 - F)$. The other seven Δ's are zero, so

$$\mathcal{C}_{JJ} = V_I = (1 + F)\sigma_A^2 + (1 - F)\sigma_D^2 + 4FD_1 + FD_2 + F(1 - F)H^2$$

as expected.

For non-inbred relatives

$$\mathcal{C}_{JJ'} = \left(k_2 + \frac{1}{2}k_1\right)\sigma_A^2 + k_2\sigma_D^2$$

and values for common relationships are shown in Table 10.

7.6 Heritability

Trait and response values have both genetic and environmental components. The simplest model of $Y = G + E$ leads to the variance of trait values among individuals J in a non-inbred population of unrelated individuals:

$$\text{Var}_J = \sigma_A^2 + \sigma_D^2 + \sigma_E^2$$

This is also referred to as the phenotypic variance σ_P^2.

For an additive trait and for individuals that have no shared environment, the variance–covariance matrix for a sample of related pairs I, I' and inbred individuals I has elements

$$\text{Var}_J = (1 + F_I)\sigma_A^2 + \sigma_E^2$$

$$\text{Cov}_{JJ'} = 2\theta_{JJ'}\sigma_A^2$$

The narrow-sense heritability h^2 is defined as $h^2 = \sigma_A^2/\sigma_P^2$. The correlation of additive trait values for pairs of non-inbred individuals related to an extent $\theta_{JJ'}$ is, therefore,

$$\rho_{JJ'} = 2\theta_{JJ'}h^2$$

Traditional methods for estimating heritability have used trait values measured for sets of individuals whose relationship is known from their family membership. It is common, for example, to take measurements on monozygotic (MZ) and dizygotic (DZ) twins and make use of the relationships

$$\text{Var}_J = \sigma_A^2 + \sigma_D^2 + \sigma_E^2$$
$$\text{Cov}_{MZ} = \sigma_A^2 + \sigma_D^2$$
$$\text{Cov}_{DZ} = \frac{1}{2}\sigma_A^2 + \frac{1}{4}\sigma_D^2$$

where any environmental correlations have been ignored. It is a simple matter to estimate the three variance components, and hence heritability, by the method of moments from these three equations although maximum likelihood methods are used in practice.

The SNP profiles of individuals in a study can be used to estimate the *actual* inbreeding and coancestry coefficients. These, in turn, lead to estimates of the additive genetic variance and hence the heritability of a complex trait. Although heritability is a statistical construct, depending on allele frequencies in the study population, rather than a biological quantity, it is of interest. The heritability explained by markers found to be associated with a trait or response variable can be compared to prior values based on family pedigrees in order to check on the completeness of the genetic study. There has been discussion of "missing heritability" when the genetic estimates are less than prior values ([20] and references therein). This chapter will conclude with a discussion of estimating inbreeding and relatedness.

7.7 Estimation of Actual Inbreeding

Individual-specific inbreeding coefficients F can be estimated under the assumption that all loci have the same coefficient, interpreted as the probability of identity by descent (ibd). Many loci are needed. At locus l, write p_l for the frequency of A_l and code the genotypes $A_l A_l, A_l a_l, a_l a_l$ as $X_l = 2, 1, 0$. These coding variables have the properties $\mathcal{E}(X_l) = 2p_l$, $\text{Var}(X_l) = 2p_l(1 - p_l)(1 + F)$.

Then one moment estimator is formed by summing over loci $l, l = 1, 2, \ldots L$:

$$\hat{F}_1 = \frac{1}{L}\sum_{l=1}^{L}\frac{(X_l - 2p_l)^2}{2p_l(1 - p_l)} - 1$$

Another one is

$$\hat{F}_2 = \frac{1}{L}\sum_{l=1}^{L}\frac{X_l^2 - (1 + 2p_l)X_l + 2p_l^2}{2p_l(1 - p_l)}$$

If the p_l are known, both these are unbiased. The second one has a smaller variance.

The variances can be reduced by an alternative weighting over loci:

$$\hat{F}_1^a = \frac{\sum_{l=1}^{L}(X_l - 2p_l)^2}{\sum_{l=1}^{L} 2p_l(1 - p_l)} - 1$$

$$\hat{F}_2^a = \frac{\sum_{l=1}^{L}[X_l^2 - (1 + 2p_l)X_l + 2p_l^2]}{\sum_{l=1}^{L} 2p_l(1 - p_l)}$$

To avoid having to choose among different moment estimates, and to reduce variance, it may be preferable to use maximum likelihood estimation. An iterative method makes use of Bayes' theorem. If F represents the probability the individual in question has two ibd alleles at a locus, i.e. is inbred at that locus,

$$\Pr(A_l A_l |\text{inbred}) = p_l, \Pr(A_l A_l |\text{Not inbred}) = p_l^2$$

$$\Pr(A_l a_l |\text{inbred}) = 0, \Pr(A_l a_l |\text{Not inbred}) = 2p_l(1 - p_l)$$

$$\Pr(a_l a_l |\text{inbred}) = 1 - p_l, \Pr(a_l a_l |\text{Not inbred}) = (1 - p_l)^2$$

From Bayes' theorem then

$$\Pr(\text{inbred}|A_l A_l) = \frac{\Pr(A_l A_l |\text{inbred}) \Pr(\text{inbred})}{\Pr(A_l A_l)} = \frac{F}{F + p_l(1 - F)}$$

$$\Pr(\text{inbred}|A_l a_l) = 0$$

$$\Pr(\text{inbred}|a_l a_l) = \frac{F}{F + (1 - p_l)(1 - F)}$$

This suggests an iterative scheme: assign an initial value to F, and then average the updated values over loci. If G_l is the genotype at locus l, the updated value F' is

$$F' = \frac{1}{L} \sum_{l=1}^{L} \Pr(\text{inbred}|G_l)$$

This value is then substituted into the right-hand side and the process continues until convergence.

7.8 Estimation of Actual Relatedness

A moment estimate makes use of observed identity in state (ibs), as shown in Table 11. If N_0, N_1, N_2 are the number of loci in ibs state $i; i = 0, 1, 2$ then

$$\Pr(\text{ibs} = 0) = \Pr(\text{ibs} = 0|\text{ibd} = 0) \Pr(\text{ibd} = 0)$$

Table 11 Identity in state categories for two individuals

ibs state	Genotypes	Probability[a]
2	$(AA, AA), (aa, aa), (Aa, Aa)$	$(p^2 + q^2)^2 k_0 + k_1(p^3 + pq + q^3) + k_2$
1	$(AA, Aa), (Aa, AA), (aa, Aa), (Aa, aa)$	$4pq(p^2 + q^2)k_0 + 2pqk_1$
0	$(AA, aa), (aa, AA)$	$2p^2q^2k_0$

[a] $q = 1 - p$

summed over loci to provide

$$N_0 = \Pr(\text{ibd} = 0) \sum_l 2p_l^2(1 - p_l)^2$$

leads to a moment estimate

$$\Pr(\text{ibd} = 0) = \frac{N_0}{\sum_l 2p_l^2(1 - p_l)^2}$$

From

$$\Pr(\text{ibd} = 1) = \Pr(\text{ibs}=1|\text{ibd} = 0)\Pr(\text{ibd} = 0)$$
$$+ \Pr(\text{ibs}=1|\text{ibd} = 1)\Pr(\text{ibd} = 1)$$

summed over loci to provide

$$N_1 = \Pr(\text{ibd} = 0) \sum_l 4p_l(1 - p_l)[p_l^2 + (1 - p_l)^2] + \Pr(\text{ibd} = 1) \sum_l 2p_l(1 - p_l)$$

a moment estimate of k_1 is obtained. Use is made of the previously estimated k_0:

$$\Pr(\text{ibd} = 1) = \frac{N_1 - \sum_l 4p_l(1 - p_l)[p_l^2 + (1 - p_l)^2]\Pr(\text{ibd} = 0)}{\sum_l 2p_l(1 - p_l)}$$

The remaining coefficient k_2 is found from the result $k_0 + k_1 + k_2 = 1$. In practice, this method is not robust to small allele frequencies and it can return invalid estimates.

A moment estimator for the coancestry $\theta_{jj'}$ between individuals j and j', rather than the three k's is:

$$\hat{\theta}_{jj'} = \frac{1}{L} \sum_{l=1}^{L} \frac{(X_{lj} - 2p_l)(X_{lk} - 2p_l)}{2p_l(1 - p_l)}$$

where $X_{lj}, X_{lj'}$ are $2, 1, 0$ if j, j' are (AA, Aa, aa), respectively, at locus l. An alternative way of combining over loci is

$$\hat{\theta}_{jj'a} = \frac{\sum_{l=1}^{L}[(X_{lj} - 2p_l)(X_{lj'} - 2p_l)]}{\sum_{l=1}^{L}[2p_l(1 - p_l)]}$$

These are both unbiased but they have different variances.

An iterative procedure for maximum likelihood estimation of relatedness is analogous to that for the inbreeding coefficient, and it uses all six distinct pairs of genotypes shown in Table 9 (combining pairs of rows with the same probabilities) with probabilities depending on allele frequencies for that SNP and on a set of three k parameters that are assumed to be the same for all SNPs.

If S is the observed pair of genotypes, Table 9 provides the conditional probabilities $\Pr(S|D_i)$ where the D_i represent the identity states (the relationship). The probability of ibd state D_i is k_i. An iterative algorithm for estimating the k's from observed genotypes S_l at SNP l is based on Bayes' theorem for the probability of descent state $D_i, i = 0, 1, 2$:

$$\Pr(D_i|S_l) = \frac{\Pr(S_l|D_i)\Pr(D_i)}{\Pr(S_l)}$$

The procedure begins with initial estimates of the $k_i = \Pr(D_i)$. The denominator is calculated from the law of total probability by adding over the three descent states:

$$\Pr(S_l) = \sum_i \Pr(S_l|D_i)\Pr(D_i) = \sum_i \Pr(S_l|D_i)k_i$$

The updated estimates are obtained by averaging over L loci:

$$k_i' = \frac{1}{L}\sum_{l=1}^{L}\left(\frac{\Pr(S_l|D_i)k_i}{\sum_j \Pr(S_l|D_j)k_j}\right), \quad i = 0, 1, 2$$

These updated values are then substituted into the right-hand side and the process continued until the likelihood no longer changes (or changes by less than some specified small amount) where

$$\text{Likelihood} = \prod_{l=1}^{L}\left[\sum_i \Pr(S_l|D_i)k_i\right]$$

It will be better to monitor changes in the log-likelihood.

8 Discussion

The current availability of dense sets of marker SNPs for the human genome is having a large impact on genetic studies and offers new possibilities for clinical trials. This chapter offers a unified basis for the analysis of marker and response data, emphasizing the central importance of linkage disequilibrium between marker locus and the genes that affect response. It is convenient to phrase the development of association mapping in the language of quantitative genetics, using additive and nonadditive components of variance.

A novel feature of dense SNP data is that good estimates can be made of actual inbreeding and relatedness. These estimates are more relevant than values predicted from family pedigree, and all that are available in the absence of family data.

In biomedical research genetic markers can be used both to infer causes of disease and to identify treatments that are tailored to the individual. However, the dimensionality of genomic markers has challenged us to develop new methods that are appropriate for a large number of statistical comparisons and to develop computational methods that allow high-dimensional regression. In the broader context, the use of biological annotation is also essential for both viewing the relevance of empirical associations and to structure analysis in order to focus on those markers with the highest expectation for association with the outcomes under study.

The continued expansion of molecular technologies will challenge the biostatistical community to develop appropriate methodology so that reliable conclusions can be obtained from new measurements. Ultimately, meaningful collaboration between quantitative scientists and biomedical investigators will lead to the understanding of the mechanisms leading to disease onset, progression, and response to treatment.

Acknowledgements This work was supported in part by NIH grants GM 075091, HG 004464, HG 005157, HL 072966 and TR 000423.

References

1. Bansal V, Libiger O, Torkamani A, Schork NJ (2010) Statistical analysis strategies for association studies involving rare variants. Nature Reviews Genetics 11:773–785
2. Burton PR, Clayton DG, Cardon LR, Craddock N, Deloukas P et al (2007) Genome-wide association stidy of 14,000 cases of seven common diseases and 3,000 shared controls. Natire 447:661–676.
3. Cornelis MC, Agrawal A, Cole JW, Hansel NN, Barnes KC, Beaty TH, Bennett SN, Bierut LJ, Boerwinkle E, Doheny KF, Feenstra B, Feingold E, Fornage M, Haiman CA, Harris EL, Hayes MG, Heit JA, Hu FB, Kang JH, Laurie CC, Ling H, Manolio TA, Marazita ML, Mathias RA, Mirel DB, Paschall J, Pasquale LR, Pugh EW, Rice JP, Udren J, van Dam RM, Wang X, Wiggs JL, Williams K, Yu K (2010) The gene, environment association studies consortium (GENEVA): maximizing the knowledge obtained from GWAS by collaboration across studies of multiple conditions. Genet Epidemiol 34:364–372
4. Dahlman I, Eaves IA, Kosoy R et al (2002) Parameters for reliable results in genetic association studies in common disease. Nat Genet 30:149–150
5. Daly AK (2010) Genome-wide association studies in pharmacogenomics. Nat Rev Genet 11:241–246
6. Gunter L, Zhu J, Murphy S (2007) Variable selection for optimal decision making. Artif Intell Med 4594:149–154
7. Hastie T, Tibshirani R (1993) Varying coefficient models. J R Stat Soc Series B 55:757–796
8. Hill WG, Goddard ME, Visscher PM (2008) Data and theory point to mainly additive genetic variance for complex traits. PLoS Genet 4:e1000008
9. Hoerl AE (1962) Application of ridge analysis to regression problems. Chem Eng Prog 58: 54–59
10. Jarvik JG et al (2009). Surgery versus non-surgical therapy for carpal tunnel syndrome: a randomized parallel group trial. Lancet 374:1074–1081

11. Kallmes DF, Comstock B, Heagerty PJ et al (2009) A randomized clinical trial for vertoblasty for osteoporotic compression fractures. N Engl J Med 361:569–579

12. Laurie CC, Doheny KF, Mirel DB, Pugh EW, Bierut LJ, Bhangale T, Boehm F, Caporaso NE, Cornelis MC, Edenberg HJ, Gabriel SB, Harris EL, Hu FB, Jacobs K, Kraft P, Landi MT, Lumley T, Manolio TA, McHugh C, Painter I, Paschall J, Rice JP, Rice KM, Zheng X, Weir BS for the GENEVA Investigators (2010) Quality control and quality assurance in genotypic data for genome-wide association studies. Genet Epidemiol 34:591–602

13. Nyholt DR (2004) A simple correction for multiple testing for single-nucleotide polymorphisms in linkage disequilibrium with each other. Am J Hum Genet 74:765–769

14. Pritchard JK, Donnelly P (2001) Case? control studies of association in structured or admixed populations. Theor Popul Biol 60:227–237

15. Sitlani C, Heagerty PJ, Longitudinal structural mixed models as tools for characterizing the accuracy of markers used to select treatment (submitted)

16. Tibshirani R (1996) Regression shrinkage and selection via the lasso. J R Stat Soc Series B 58:267–288

17. Wakefield JC (2009) Bayes factors for genome-wide association studies: comparison with P-values. Genet Epidemiol 33:79–86

18. Wu TT, Chen YF, Hastie T, Sobel E, Lange K (2009) Genome-wide association analysis by lasso penalized logistic regression. Bioinformatics 25:714–721

19. Zou H, Hastie T (2005) Regularization and variable selection via the elastic net. J Roy Stat Soc Series B 67:301–320.

20. Zuk O, Hechter E, Sunyaev SR, Lander ES (2012) The mystery of missing heritability: genetic interactions create phantom heritability. Proc Natl Acad Sci USA, vol 109, pp 1193–1198

Addresses for Contact Authors (in the same order as the papers)

David L. DeMets
Department of Biostatistics & Medical Informatics
University of Wisconsin-Madison
610 Walnut Street
Madison, WI 53726, USA
email:demets@biostat.wisc.edu

Ross L. Prentice
Public Health Sciences
Fred Hutchinson Cancer Resarch Center
1100 Fairview Ave. N., Seattle, WA 98109, USA
email:rprentic@WHI.org

Steven G. Self
Public Health Sciences, Vaccine and Infectious Disease
Fred Hutchinson Cancer Research Center
1100 Fairview Ave. N., Seattle, WA 98109, USA
email:sself@fhcrc.org

Robert T. O'Neill
Office of Biostatistics
FDA Center for Drug Evaluation and Research
10903 New Hampshire Avenue
Silver Spring, MD 20993-0002, USA
email:Robert.ONeill@fda.hhs.gov

Richard Simon
Biometric Research Branch
National Cancer Institute
9000 Rockville, MD 20892-7434, USA
email:rsimon@nih.gov

T.R. Fleming and B.S. Weir (eds.), *Proceedings of the Fourth Seattle Symposium
in Biostatistics: Clinical Trials*, Lecture Notes in Statistics 1205,
DOI 10.1007/978-1-4614-5245-4, © Springer Science+Business Media New York 2013

Bruce S. Weir
Department of Biostatistics
University of Washington
Seattle, WA 98195-7232, USA
bsweir@uw.edu

Janet Wittes
Statistics Collaborative, Inc
1625 Massachusetts Ave., NW; Suite 600
Washington, DC 20036, USA
email: janet@statcollab.com

Christy Chuang-Stein
Statistical Research and Consulting Center
Pfizer Inc.
5857 Stoney Brook, Kalamazoo, MI 49009, USA
email:christy.j.chuang-stein@pfizer.com

Thomas R. Fleming
Department of Biostatistics
University of Washington
Seattle, WA 98195-7232, USA
email:tfleming@uw.edu

Robert Temple
FDA Center for Drug Evaluation and Research
10903 New Hampshire Avenue
Silver Spring, MD 20993-0002, USA
email:Robert.Temple@fda.hhs.gov

Scott S. Emerson
Department of Biostatistics
University of Washington
Seattle, WA 98195-7232, USA
email:semerson@uw.edu

Referees
(in alphabetical order)

Garnet Anderson, Fred Hutchinson Cancer Research Center, Seattle, WA, USA
Christy Chuang-Stein, Pfizer, Inc., Kalamazoo, MI, USA
Yates Coley, University of Washington, Seattle, WA, USA
Andrea Cook, Group Health Research Institute, Seattle, WA, USA
James Dai, Fred Hutchinson Cancer Research Center, Seattle, WA, USA

David DeMets, University of Wisconsin-Madison, Madison, WI, USA
Ruth Etzioni, Fred Hutchinson Cancer Research Center, Seattle, WA, USA
Daniel Gillen, University of California, Irvine, CA, USA
Ziding Feng, Fred Hutchinson Cancer Research Center, Seattle, WA, USA
Thomas Fleming, University of Washington, Seattle, WA, USA
Erin Gabriel, University of Washington, Seattle, WA, USA
Ted Gooley, Fred Hutchinson Cancer Research Center, Seattle, WA, USA
Navneet Hakhu, University of Washington, Seattle, WA, USA
Antje Hoering, Cancer Research and Biostatistics, Seattle, WA, USA
John Kittelson, University of Colorado at Denver, Denver, CO, USA
Brian Leroux, University of Washington, Seattle, WA, USA
Gregory Levin, University of Washington, Seattle, WA, USA
Caitlin McHugh, University of Washington, Seattle, WA, USA
Jennifer Nelson, Group Health Research Institute, Seattle, WA, USA
Robert O'Neill, Food and Drug Administration, Silver Spring, MD, USA
Megan Othus, Fred Hutchinson Cancer Research Institute, Seattle, WA, USA
David Prince, University of Washington, Seattle, WA, USA
Giancarlo Sal y Rosas, University of Washington, Seattle, WA, USA
Steve Self, Fred Hutchinson Cancer Research Center, Seattle, WA, USA
Richard Simon, National Cancer Institute, Rockville, MD, USA
Kelly Stratton, University of Washington, Seattle, WA, USA
Ching-Yun Wang, Fred Hutchinson Cancer Research Center, Seattle, WA, USA
Bruce Weir, University of Washington, Seattle, WA, USA
Janet Wittes, Statistics Collaborative, Inc., WA, USA
Leila Zelnick, University of Washington, Seattle, WA, USA

Printed by Publishers' Graphics LLC
BT20130315.19.21.39